Current Topics in Neonatology Number 3

Current Topics in Neonatology Number 3

edited by

Thomas N. Hansen
Chairman, Department of Pediatrics,
The Ohio State University,
Chief Executive Officer, Children's Hospital,
Columbus, Ohio, USA

and

Neil McIntosh
Chairman and Professor of Child Life and Health
Department of Child Life and Health,
The University of Edinburgh,
Edinburgh, UK

W.B. SAUNDERS
London • Edinburgh • New York • Philadelphia • Sydney • Toronto

W.B. SAUNDERS
A Division of Harcourt Brace and Company Limited

ISBN 0–7020–2348–5

British Library Cataloguing in Publication Data
A catalogue record for this book is available from the British Library

Library of Congress Cataloging in Publication Data
A catalog record for this book is available from the Library of Congress

Commissioning Editor: Maria Khan
Project Manager: Louise Cook
Project Supervisor: Mark Sanderson
Printed in Hong Kong

Contents

Contributors *vii*
Contents of *Current Topics in Neonatology* Number One *ix*
Contents of *Current Topics in Neonatology* Number Two *xi*
Preface *xiii*

1. Renal Function and Failure in the Newborn 1
Andrea Turner and George B. Haycock

2. Rational Antibiotic Approach in a Neonatal Unit 24
Jennifer A. Royle and David Isaacs

3. Human Milk and the Preterm Infant 43
Anthony F. Williams

4. What is an Adequate Blood Pressure in the Preterm Newborn? 62
Steven Cunningham

5. Nutrition and the Brain 93
Forrester Cockburn

6. Development of the Gastrointestinal Tract 110
Tarja Ruuska and Peter Milla

7. Liquid Ventilation: Present and Immediate Future 140
Thomas H. Shaffer and Marla R. Wolfson

8. Bronchopulmonary Dysplasia: A Team Approach 157
Mary E. Wearden and James M. Adams

9. Using New Information in Retinopathy of Prematurity 174
Dale L. Phelps

10. Infections in Newborn Infants and the Potential for New Prevention and Treatment Strategies 200
Paola Papoff and Robert D. Christensen

11. Prenatal Diagnosis 232
Theresa L. Stewart and Diana W. Bianchi

12. What is New in the Management of Preterm Labor? 251
David S. McKenna and Jay D. Iams

Index 270

List of contributors

James M. Adams MD Medical Director, Social Care Nurseries, Associate Professor of Pediatrics, Section of Neonatology, Department of Pediatrics, Baylor College of Medicine, Houston, TX, USA.

Diana W. Bianchi MD Chief, Division of Genetics, Chief of Perinatal Genetics, and Associate Professor of Pediatrics, Obstetrics and Gynecology, New England Medical Center, Departments of Pediatrics, Obstetrics and Gynecology, Tufts University School of Medicine, Boston, MA, USA.

Robert D. Christensen MD Professor and Chief, Division of Neonatology, Department of Pediatrics, University of Florida College of Medicine, Gainesville, FL, USA.

Forrester Cockburn CBE, MD, FRCP, FRCPCH(Hons), DCH, MB ChB Emeritus Professor of Child Health, Department of Child Health, University of Glasgow, Royal Hospital for Sick Children, Glasgow, UK.

Steven Cunningham MB ChB, MRCP, PhD Lecturer, Department of Child Life and Health, University of Edinburgh, Edinburgh, UK.

George B. Haycock MB BChir, FRCP, DCH Ferdinand James de Rothschild Professor of Paediatrics, Department of Paediatrics, The Guy's, King's College and St Thomas' Hospitals Medical and Dental School, Guy's Hospital, London, UK.

Jay D. Iams MD Frederick P. Zuspan Professor of Obstetrics and Gynecology, Department of Obstetrics and Gynecology, Division of Maternal Fetal Medicine, Ohio State University, Columbus, OH, USA.

David Isaacs MB BChir, MD, MRCP, FRACP, FRCPH Clinical Professor, Department of Immunology and Infectious Diseases, The New Children's Hospital, Sydney, Australia.

David S. McKenna MD Assistant Professor, Department of Obstetrics and Gynecology, Division of Maternal and Fetal Medicine, Wright State University, OI, USA.

Peter J. Milla MSc, MBBS, FRCP, FRCPCH Professor of Paediatric Gastroenterology and Nutrition, Honorary Consultant Paediatric Gastroenterologist, Institute of Child Health and Great Ormond Street Hospital for Children NHS Trust, University College London Medical School, London, UK.

Paola Papoff MD Research Fellow Department of Pediatrics, Division of Neonatology, University 'La Sapienza', Rome, Italy.

Dale L. Phelps MD Professor of Pediatrics and Ophthalmology, Department of Pediatrics, University of Rochester, Rochester, NY, USA.

Jennifer A. Royle MB BS, FRACP Paediatrician and Fellow in Immunisation Research, Royal Children's Hospital, Melbourne, Victoria, Australia.

Tarja Ruuska MD, PhD Senior Lecturer in Paediatric Gastroenterology, Department of Paediatrics, Tampere University Hospital, Tampere, Finland.

Thomas H. Shaffer PhD Professor of Physiology and Pediatrics, Director, Respiratory Physiology Section, Temple University, Philadelphia, PA, USA.

Theresa L. Stewart MD Fellow, Maternal-Fetal Medicine and Genetics, Division of Genetics, New England Medical Center, Boston, MA, USA.

Andrea Turner MA, MB BChir, MRCP Specialist Registrar in Paediatrics, Department of Paediatrics, The Guy's, King's College and St Thomas' Hospitals Medical and Dental School, Guy's Hospital, London, UK.

Mary E. Wearden MD Assistant Professor of Paediatrics, Baylor College of Medicine, Texas Medical Center, Houston, TX, USA.

Anthony F. Williams DPhil, FRCP Senior Lecturer and Consultant in Neonatal Pediatrics, Regional Neonatal Unit, St George's Hospital, London, UK.

Marla R. Wolfson PhD Associate Professor of Physiology and Pediatrics, Department of Physiology, Temple University, Philadelphia, PA, USA.

Contents of Number One

1. Genital Mycoplasmas and Infection in the Neonate
   Andrew J. Lyon

2. Synchronous Intermittent mandatory Ventilation
   Anne Greenough

3. Near Infrared Spectroscopy
   John S. Wyatt

4. Fluid Management in the Extremely Preterm Infant
   Gunnar Sedin

5. Outcome of Infants Born at Less than 26 Weeks Gestation
   Victor Y.H. Yu, Elizabeth A. Carse and Margaret P. Charlton

6. Treating Pain in the Neonate
   Hans-Ulrich Bucher and Annemarie Bucher-Schmid

7. Antenatal Hormone Treatment to Prevent Lung Disease
   Roberta A. Ballard

8. Systematic Reviews of Randomized Trials in Neonatology
   John C. Sinclair

9. What Causes Neonatal Necrotizing Entercolitis and How Can It Be Prevented?
   David A. Clark and Mark J.S. Miller

10. Gene Therapy for the Lung
    Barbara Warner and Jonathan Wispe

11. Vertical Human Immunodeficiency Virus Infection
Mark W. Kline

12. Nitric Oxide Therapy in Infants with Persistent Pulmonary Hypertension
Michael R. Gomez

Contents of Number Two

1. Scoring Systems for Neonatal Illness
Andrew R. Wilkinson

2. Role of Sleeping Position in the Aetiology of the Sudden Infant Death Syndrome
Peter J. Fleming and Peter S. Blair

3. Management of the Asphyxiated Infant
Mats Blennow and Hugo Lagercrantz

4. Management of the Infant with Inherited Metabolic Disease
Jean-Marie Saudubray, Philippe Jouvet and Hélène Ogier de Baulny

5. Neonatal Physiological Monitoring
Neil McIntosh

6. Erythropoietin Therapy in Preterm Infants
Michael Obalden and Rolf F. Meier

7. What Should We Do About Jaundice?
Daniel S. Seidman, Rena Gale and David K. Stevenson

8. Making Therapeutic Decisions for Newborns with Complex Congenital Heart Defects
David J. Fisher

9. Pharmacologic Prevention of Intraventricular Hemorrhage
Jan Goddard-Finegold

10. New Strategies for Mechanical Ventilation: What's New with the Oscillator
William E. Truog

11. Contemporary Understanding of the Pathophysiology and Management of Congenital Diaphragmatic Hernia
Robin H. Steinhorn, Philip L. Glick, Stuart O'Toole and Frederick C. Morin III

12. Role of Postnatal Steroids for Neonatal Chronic Lung Disease
Cynthia H. Cole and Ivan D. Frantz III

Preface

We have had many favourable comments following the first two volumes of *Current Topics in Neonatology* and we hope this third volume will be equally well received. The scientific basis of neonatology and the clinical areas of diagnosis and management are proceeding apace and as editors we believe we can bridge the natural gap with these volumes between cutting edge journal papers and the management provided by textbooks which is often out of date by the time of publication. We continue to strive for expertise using contributors from around the world as we recognise that sometimes local practice becomes a rather parochial 'gold standard'.

Thomas Hansen
Neil McIntosh

1999

1

Renal Function and Failure in the Newborn

Andrea Turner and George B Haycock

RENAL FUNCTION IN THE FETUS AND NEWBORN

Knowledge of renal function is a prerequisite for understanding renal dysfunction. The kidney of the newborn infant is different from that of the older child and adult, and that of the fetus is different again. This chapter describes the development of renal function in the human fetus and newborn, both premature and mature, and interprets the features of renal failure in infants by reference to the developmental process. Although much of the understanding of renal functional development is derived from studies of experimental animals, this review concentrates mainly on information obtained from humans, except where the invasive nature of the research has precluded human experimentation. The first part of the chapter emphasizes those aspects of development that are relevant to the pathophysiology of acute renal failure: several more general and comprehensive reviews of the subject are available.[1–5]

Morphological Development of the Kidney

The kidney develops from the most caudal segment of the nephrogenic ridge, *the metanephros*, a specialized population of mesodermal cells which condense around the tip of the ureteric bud from about 5 weeks' gestation. As the ureteric bud branches and rebranches, forming first the major calices, then the minor calices, and then the arborizing system of collecting ducts, nephron formation is induced in relation to the successive divisions of the duct system. Nephrogenesis proceeds centrifugally: nephrons that eventually lie deepest in the cortex (the *juxtamedullary* nephrons) are the first to be formed, and those in the most superficial (*subcapsular*) cortex are the last. The first few generations of nephrons atrophy without having functioned. The first permanent nephrons, and the production of urine, date from 8–10 weeks' gestation; the last nephrons are formed by 36 weeks. Although renal mass continues to increase rapidly after 36 weeks, this is due to enlargement of tubules, not the development of new nephrons. These processes are summarized in Figure 1.1.

Renal Function in the Human Fetus

Direct, invasive studies of renal function are ethically impossible in normal human fetuses. However, a good deal of information has been amassed by non-invasive techniques, as well as by more direct methods in fetuses who were being investigated for suspected renal abnormalities *in utero*, but who were found after birth to have normal renal function. The latter group of subjects are a reasonable surrogate for strictly normal fetuses as regards information on blood and urine composition. The Fetal Medicine Group at King's College Hospital, London, has published data in 3 separate papers that can be combined to calculate mean glomerular filtration rate (GFR), measured as creatinine clear-

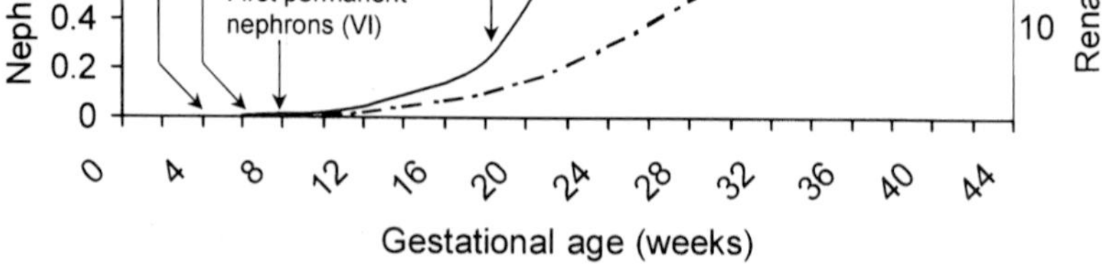

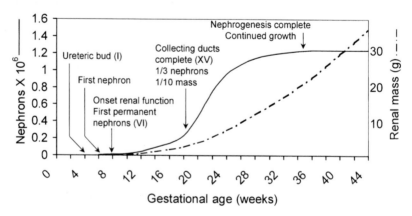

Figure 1.1 Development of the human kidney from conception to term. Roman numerals in parentheses indicate the number of generations of divisions from the ureteric bud. Redrawn from Ref. 1 with permission.

ance, in normal fetuses from 20 weeks' gestation to term. In the first of these,[6] blood samples were obtained from 344 singleton fetuses and biochemical analysis performed, including plasma creatinine and electrolyte concentrations. In the second,[7] fetal urine flow rate was estimated by extremely frequent ultrasonography of the fetal bladder in 85 healthy fetuses. Regression analysis of the slope of bladder filling against time was used to calculate urine flow rate (V). The third paper[8] measured urine biochemistry from fetuses with dilated urinary tracts; 27 of these fetuses survived with normal renal function or died of other causes but were not found to have normal kidneys at post-mortem examination. Although there is considerable scatter of values for all 3 variables (V, urine and plasma creatinine concentrations) mean values can be derived for each week of gestation, and using these creatinine clearance can be calculated from the formula:

$$C = \frac{U_{Cr} \cdot V}{P_{Cr}}$$

where C is clearance, V is urine flow rate and U_{Cr} and P_{Cr} are urine and plasma creatinine, respectively. These results for fetuses from 20 weeks' gestation to term are shown in Figures 1.2 and 1.3, and are compared with those for newborn babies of the same absolute gestational age but who had been born at least 3 days before the study.[9] It can be seen that, at all ages within the study period, creatinine clearance is substantially greater in the fetus than in the neonate.

The same data source can be used to calculate fractional sodium excretion (FE_{Na}), the proportion of filtered sodium excreted in the

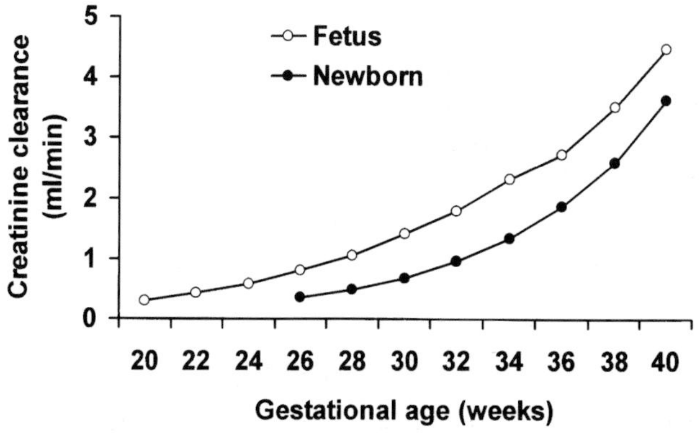

Figure 1.2 Creatinine clearance in the human fetus and newborn, not corrected for body size. Calculated from data published in references 4, 5, 6, 7.

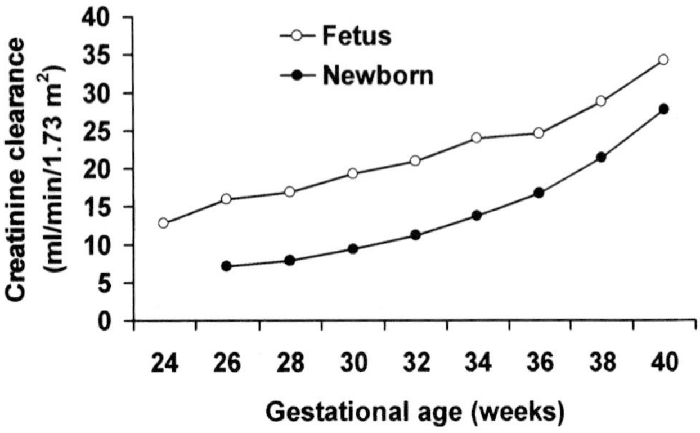

Figure 1.3 Creatinine clearance in the human fetus and newborn, corrected for body surface area. Calculated from data published in references 6, 7, 8 and 9.

urine. FE_{Na} is the excretion rate of sodium divided by its filtration rate, which reduces to:

$$FE_{Na} = \frac{\text{excretion Na}}{\text{filtration rate Na}} = \frac{U_{Na} \times P_{cr}}{U_{cr} \times P_{Na}}$$

In term infants, children and adults with normal renal function on a normal sodium intake, FE_{Na} is <1%. As shown in Figure 1.4, FE_{Na} is high in the fetus until term, and also in neonates before about 32 weeks' corrected gestation age, while in neonates from 33 weeks onward it is 'normal', i.e. <1%. As with creatinine clearance, FE_{Na} is much higher in the fetus than in the infant after birth. Although creatinine clearance has not been directly validated as a measure of GFR in human fetuses, the agreement with clearance of sodium iothalamate, a well documented marker for GFR, has been shown to be excellent in the sheep fetus.[10] These findings indicate that, compared with that of the newborn infant after birth, the fetal kidney is filtering and diuresing at a high rate. This is necessary to maintain the volume of the amniotic fluid which is constantly being swallowed and reabsorbed by the fetus. The consequences of failure of this replacement are well known (the Potter sequence).

Renal Function in the Newborn

Glomerular filtration and renal plasma flow

GFR is low in the newborn compared to the older individual. Average absolute values are about 0.5 ml/min at 28 weeks' gestation, increasing

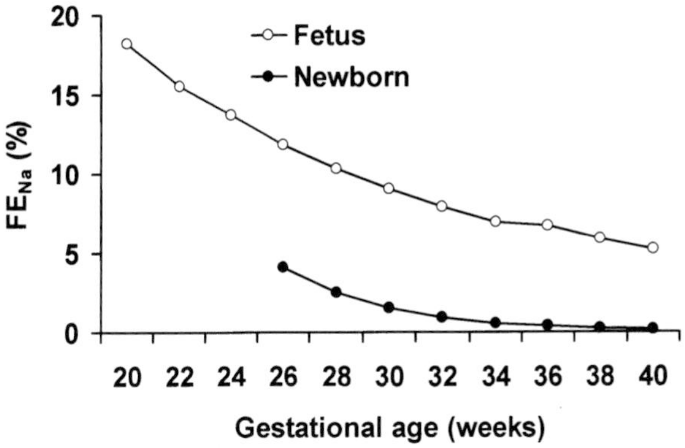

Figure 1.4 Fractional sodium excretion (FE_{Na}) in the human fetus and newborn. Calculated from data published in references 6, 7 and 8.

to about 4 ml/min at term, i.e. about 8-fold (Figure 1.2). When corrected for body surface area, GFR increases only by a factor of 3 over the same time interval, from 10 ml/min/1.73 m^2 at 28 weeks' gestation to 30 ml/min/1.73 m^2 at term (Figure 1.3). These data were obtained by measuring creatinine clearance: many other studies using other methods, including inulin clearance, give essentially identical values. The rationale for correcting GFR for surface area in the newborn has been challenged. However, even if it is corrected for total body water[12] or weight,[13] there is still a substantial increase from 28 weeks' gestation until term. This increase continues after birth, the mean value rising to about 50 ml/min/1.73 m^2 at 1 month, 80 ml/min/1.73 m^2 at 6 months, 100 ml/min/1.73 m^2 at 1 year and reaching the adult value of 125 ml/min/1.73 m^2 at 18 months.[13]

As previously mentioned, the large rise in GFR observed during the first weeks of life is not due to new nephron formation. It has been shown in animals that the main determinant of changes in GFR in young animals is change in renal plasma flow (RPF), and that the observed rise in RPF is due to a fall in renal vascular resistance.[14, 15] Evidence from the newborn of several species shows that RPF and GFR are low because the arterioles of the middle and outer layers of the renal cortex are tightly vasoconstricted, to the extent that the glomeruli contained in them are filtering little or not at all. This is logical in that the deepest (juxtamedullary) nephrons are the first to be formed and would therefore be expected to be functionally the most mature in the neonatal period. Sequential vasodilatation, proceeding in a centrifugal pattern, leads to the progressive recruitment of successive layers of glomeruli to the filtration process, until the whole complement is functioning after several days (in rodents) or weeks (in dogs).[16–19]

RPF and GFR are driven by the arterial pressure and regulated by constriction and dilatation of the afferent and efferent glomerular arterioles. The balance between constriction and dilatation is largely modulated by the balance between angiotensin II (AII, vasoconstrictor) and prostaglandins (PGs, vasodilator). AII constricts the efferent arteriole more than the afferent, thus maintaining filtration pressure. PGs dilate both. Inhibition of synthesis of AII with angiotensin converting enzyme inhibitors causes unopposed vasodilatation and a sharp fall in GFR; this can lead to acute renal failure in the fetal and neonatal kidney.[20, 21] Conversely, inhibition of prostaglandin synthesis with non-steroidal anti-inflammatory drugs in the newborn can also lead to acute renal failure, in this case due to unopposed vasoconstriction.[22–24] Vasodilators such as tolazoline can also lead to acute renal failure in newborn infants.[25]

Autoregulation of renal blood flow in the newborn

Like other vital organs such as the brain and heart, the kidney has the ability to regulate its own blood flow across a wide range of perfusion pressure. This is due to reflex changes in the tone of the resistance vessels and occurs in the isolated perfused kidney, indicating its independence of humoral and nervous control. This phenomenon is known as *autoregulation* of blood flow. It is present in the newborn and very young animal,[26] although the range of blood pressures across which it is effective increases with age, reflecting the physiological rise in blood pressure that takes place over time (Figure 1.5). This explains why RPF and GFR remain fairly constant during changes in blood pressure secondary to external influences such as exercise and changes in hydration. The capacity for autoregulation is not unlimited, however, and below a minimum necessary perfusion pressure, RPF, and therefore GFR, decline as a function of falling pressure. In these circumstances, even if the kidney has suffered no intrinsic damage, renal function may be inadequate for the needs of the organism, a condition known as *pre-renal failure*.

Proximal tubular function

The most important function of the proximal tubule is reabsorption of most of the salt and water contained in the glomerular ultrafiltrate, and almost all of the nutritionally and physiologically important solutes (glucose, amino acids, phosphate and bicarbonate). In the adult, about two-thirds of filtered salt and water are reabsorbed in this segment. In newborn infants, studied by clearance techniques,[27] a much smaller pro-

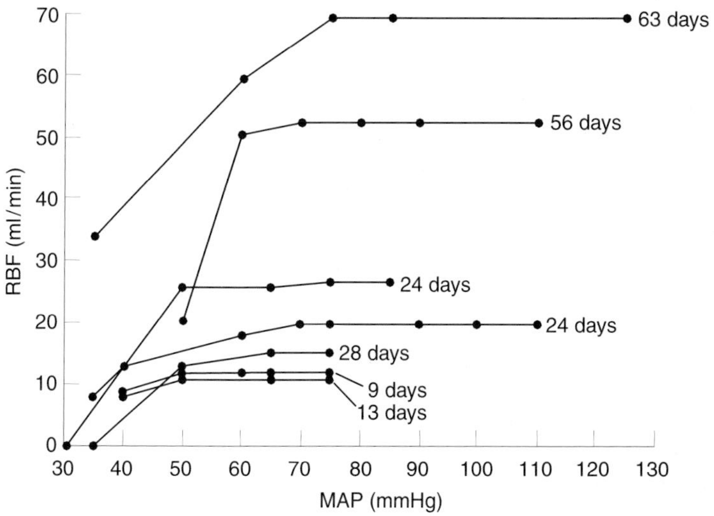

Figure 1.5 Autoregulation of blood flow in the canine kidney. Each line represents a single animal whose age in days is shown. The range of mean arterial pressure (MAP) across which autoregulation occurs increases with the age of the animal. RBF = renal blood flow. Below the autoregulatory range, RBF (and glomerular filtration rate) decline with further reductions in MAP, a condition of pre-renal failure. Reproduced from Ref. 2 with permission.

portion of filtered volume is reabsorbed in the proximal tubule in infants born at or near term and this proportion is even lower in preterm infants born at a mean gestational age of about 30 weeks. Similar findings have been obtained in newborn dogs[28] and rats.[29] Despite this, term infants conserve salt and water extremely efficiently. This can only be explained by a compensatory increase in the proportion of the filtered load reabsorbed distally. The fact that very preterm infants are renal salt losers in the first few days of life suggests that the distal nephron has not matured sufficiently to compensate for the low proximal reabsorption rates. In summary, the proportion of filtered salt and water reabsorbed in the proximal tubule in the early postnatal period is very low in very preterm infants, and increases progressively with maturity. From about 32 weeks' gestation, frank urinary sodium loss is prevented by high rates of reabsorption in the distal tubule, but in very low birth weight infants the distal tubule is unable to compensate and urinary sodium losses are high, leading to negative sodium balance and hyponatraemia unless corrective measures are taken.[9, 30] This tendency to urinary salt loss is exaggerated in some forms of neonatal acute renal failure.[31]

Proximal tubular reabsorption of organic nutrient solutes is less complete in premature infants than in older individuals. This has been shown for amino acids;[32] the data for glucose are somewhat contradictory but the evidence suggests a small rise in the renal glucose threshold with time when preterm and term infants are compared.[33] The proximal tubular bicarbonate threshold, likewise, is very low at birth in preterm infants (18.6 mmol/l, 95% confidence limits 17.5–19.3), rising to 20.3 mmol/l (19.3–21.2) at 21 days.[34] The mean value for term infants in early infancy is about 22 mmol/l.[35] Another proximal tubular reabsorptive function that undergoes significant maturation between 32 weeks' gestation and term is that for the low molecular weight protein β-2 microglobulin;[36] moreover, fractional excretion of this and other low molecular weight proteins is depressed to a greater degree in preterm than in term infants by aminoglycoside toxicity[37] and asphyxia.[36, 38] These and other data indicate that, in general, the proximal tubule is functionally immature in newborn and especially very preterm infants, and is more vulnerable to ischaemic and toxic insults than that of the older individual.

Loop of Henle and distal tubule

Sodium, potassium and chloride are reabsorbed without water in the thick ascending limb (TAL) of the loop of Henle, and in the absence of antidiuretic hormone (ADH) this continues in the distal convoluted tubule and collecting duct, leading to production of urine more dilute than plasma. Clearance studies performed under maximal water diuresis[27] show that the capacity to dilute the urine is greater in term infants (minimum urine osmolality 52.9 + 9.4 mOsmol/kg H_2O) than in those born at about 32 weeks' gestation (67.5 + 23.2 mOsmol/kg H_2O). The difference, though statistically significant ($p < 0.0025$), is small and indicates that even quite premature infants reabsorb sodium well in distal nephron segments. The same process of active electrolyte reabsorption in the TAL is the first step in the generation of medullary interstitial hypertonicity, which when amplified by the medullary countercurrent system of multipliers (descending and ascending limbs of the loop of Henle) and exchangers (vasa recta) provides the tubule-to-interstitium osmotic gradient for water reabsorption when the collecting ducts are made permeable to water by ADH. Children and adults can concentrate urine to about 1200 mOsmol/kg H_2O, about 4 times the concentration of plasma. Healthy newborn infants can only achieve a value of about 600 mOsmol/kg H_2O on a physiological diet, but when dietary protein is increased leading to a higher than normal plasma urea concentration urine can be concentrated to 900–1000 mOsmol/kg H_2O.[39] In extremely premature babies (<32 weeks' gestation), the upper limit is about 550 mOsmol/kg H_2O, even though ADH secretion appears to respond appropriately to both osmolar and non-osmolar stimuli.[40, 41]

Another important function of the distal tubule is excretion of non-volatile acid (NVA) generated by metabolism (mainly sulphuric, phosphoric and organic acids). Since, at physiological pH, the sodium concentration of the extracellular fluid exceeds that of hydrogen ion (H^+) by a huge margin (>10^6), the conjugate base (e.g. sulphate or lactate) is filtered as the sodium salt and the associated H^+ is secreted into the distal tubular fluid, mainly in the collecting duct. The capacity to excrete enough H^+ depends on the ability of the tubule to transport H^+ against a concentration gradient (i.e. to lower urinary pH below that of plasma) and the presence of sufficient buffer in the urine. The two most important urinary buffers are inorganic phosphate (P_i) and ammonium (NH_4^+), the latter being synthesized from glutamine by tubule cells. Newborn infants, including those born preterm, can lower urine pH adequately (<5.4).[42] The capacity to excrete an acid load, however, is less than that of more mature individuals.[43] This is probably due to 3 factors:

- low GFR;
- low urinary P_i excretion; and
- limited ability of the infant tubule to synthesize NH_4^+.

The normal physiological state of a newborn infant is one of marked anabolism, and on a physiological diet (human milk) production of NVA is minimal since virtually all the protein in the diet is incorporated into new tissue. Preterm infants given an unphysiologically high protein intake generate NVA from the excess protein. This can overwhelm the kidney's ability to excrete the resulting H^+, leading to the syndrome of late metabolic acidosis (LMA) of prematurity.[44] The combination of catabolism and reduced renal function, e.g. in the sick newborn with incipient or actual acute renal failure, can also lead to severe and rapidly progressive acidosis. LMA should not be confused with the mild acidosis seen in normal preterm infants, which is due to a low proximal tubular bicarbonate threshold.[34]

NEONATAL ACUTE RENAL FAILURE

Definition

Acute renal failure (ARF) is the clinical syndrome resulting from an abrupt reduction in the GFR, such that normal extracellular fluid volume and composition can no longer be maintained. There is no consensus of opinion as to what change in GFR is required to make a diagnosis of ARF in the neonate. Chevalier *et al*[31] used a plasma creatinine (P_{Cr}) >1.5 mg/dl (132.6 μmol/l), a definition which has since been adopted by other groups.[45, 46] Many groups, however, have defined ARF clinically in terms of oliguria and a raised blood urea nitrogen (BUN). BUN is influenced by many extrarenal factors, e.g. dehydration and protein catabolism, and is a less reliable indicator of reduced GFR than the P_{Cr}. While the presence of oliguria has frequently been taken as a prerequisite for the diagnosis of neonatal ARF, non-oliguric ARF can also occur.[31, 47]

Incidence

The reported incidence of ARF varies and depends on the definition used, with non-oliguric ARF probably being under recognized. Norman and Asadi[48] found the incidence of ARF, defined in terms of elevated BUN and oliguria, to be 6% of consecutive admissions to the neonatal intensive care unit (NICU). Stapleton *et al*[45] carried out a prospective study of all babies admited to their NICU over a 4-month period and found an 8% incidence of ARF.

Aetiology

Neonatal ARF may be classified into 4 categories:

- *Pre-renal failure* – hypoperfusion, secondary to either hypovolaemia or hypotension, in an otherwise normal kidney. Prolonged, untreated pre-renal failure can progress to intrinsic renal failure.
- *Intrinsic renal failure* – acute damage to the renal parenchyma. In the neonate, primary renal diseases, such as glomerulonephritis, are extremely rare and this category consists largely of ATN, interstitial nephritis and vascular causes.
- *Post-renal failure* – obstruction to the flow of urine through the urinary tract.
- *Congenital chronic renal failure* – since the excretory needs of the fetus are met by the placenta, congenital abnormalities of the renal tract present in the newborn with a clinical picture similar to infants with true ARF.

The commonest causes of ARF are given in Table 1.1.

Table 1.1 Causes of renal failure in the newborn.

PRE-RENAL FAILURE	INTRINSIC RENAL FAILURE
Hypovolaemia	Acute tubular necrosis
Haemorrhage	Prolonged hypoperfusion and/or hypoxia
Twin–twin transfusion	— birth asphyxia
Placental abruption	Nephrotoxins
Intracranial haemorrhage	— aminoglycosides
Dehydration	— NSAIDs
Third space loss	Tubular lumen obstruction
Normovolaemic hypotension	— haemoglobinurea
Reduced cardiac output	— myoglobinuria
— congenital heart disease	
— post-bypass	Infection/inflammation
— post-asphyxial	Acute pyelonephritis
Vasodilation	Interstitial nephritis
— sepsis	
— vasodilator drugs	Vascular
	Renal artery thrombosis
Hypoxia	Renal vein thrombosis
Respiratory distress syndrome	DIC
Other cardiorespiratory disease	
POSTRENAL FAILURE	CONGENITAL RENAL FAILURE
Urinary tract obstruction	
Posterior urethral valves	Reduced nephron number
Neuropathic bladder	Bilateral renal agenesis
Bilateral pelviureteric junction obstruction	Bilateral renal dysplasia
	— multicystic
	— refluxing
	Recessive polycystic disease

Diagnosis

Neonatal ARF most often presents with typical abnormal biochemical findings discovered during investigation of the sick neonate (Table 1.2). There is commonly oliguria (urine output <1 ml/kg/24 h) or anuria with signs of fluid overload, e.g. peripheral oedema, hypertension and occasionally pulmonary oedema, as a consequence of continuation of normal fluid intake in the presence of unrecognized oliguria.

Evidence of reduced GFR is essential to the diagnosis of ARF. Although a raised BUN has frequently been used as a marker for

Table 1.2 Typical biochemical changes in acute renal failure.

Increased	Decreased
Creatinine	Sodium*
Urea	Bicarbonate
Uric acid	Calcium
Hydrogen ion	
Potassium	

*Sodium concentration is usually, although not invariably, reduced due to ongoing hypotonic fluid administration before renal failure is recognized.

neonatal ARF, it is influenced by many extrarenal factors and the P_{Cr} is therefore a more reliable guide. The normal P_{Cr} varies with the gestation, birth weight and age of the baby but a reasonable value for diagnosis of ARF is $>$132.6 μmol/l or 1.5 mg/dl.

The other biochemical changes reflect accumulation of products of metabolism, e.g. urate, leakage of intracellular constituents into the plasma, e.g. potassium, inorganic phosphate, and failure of tubular reabsorption of plasma constituents, e.g. sodium, bicarbonate and calcium (Table 1.2).

Imaging

Pre-renal failure and ATN are diagnosed primarily on history, clinical and biochemical signs. However, ultrasonography of the kidneys and urinary tract should be performed in all cases to exclude congenital causes and post-renal failure. Renal vein thrombosis will also be confirmed or excluded by this investigation.

Urinary indices

Analysis of the urine composition helps differentiate pre-renal failure and ATN (Table 1.3). Pre-renal failure, the physiological response of the kidney to hypoperfusion, results in avid sodium and water retention, producing 'good quality' urine with a high osmolality, low sodium and high urea and creatinine concentrations. In contrast, ATN results in urine of poor quality, with a composition similar to that of glomerular filtrate, since the damaged tubules are unable to modify it appropriately.

The fractional excretion of sodium (FE_{Na}) and the renal failure index (RFI) are the indices that best discriminate between these 2 conditions.[49, 50] FE_{Na} is calculated as described above and RFI by the formula;

Table 1.3 Urinary indices in pre-renal failure and acute tubular necrosis.

Test	Pre-renal failure	Acute tubular necrosis
Urine urea	High	Low
U:P	High (>10)	Low
Urine creatinine	High	Low
U:P creatinine	High (>40)	Low
Urine osmolality	High (>500 mOsmol/kg)	Low (~300 mOsmol/kg)
U:P osmolality	High (>2)	Low (~1)
Urine specific gravity	High (>1025)	Low (~1010)
Urine sodium	Low (<10 mmol/l)	High (>20 mmol/l)
FE_{Na}	Low (<1%)	High (>2.5%)
RFI	Low (<1)	High (>2.5)

U = urine; P = plasma; FE_{Na} = fractional excretion of sodium; RFI = renal failure index.

$$RFI = \frac{U_{Na} \times P_{cr}}{U_{cr}}$$

where U and P refer to urine and plasma concentrations, and the subscripts Na to sodium and Cr to creatinine. An FE_{Na} of >2.5% and an RFI of >3.0 are consistent with intrinsic ARF, although some infants with prerenal failure may also have a high FE_{Na}.[50] As premature infants have very high sodium excretion rates,[9] these indices are unreliable in this population, although in infants of 29–31 weeks' gestational age an RFI of 8 or an FE_{Na} of >6% is diagnostic of intrinsic ARF.[51]

The ultimate proof of the diagnosis of pre-renal failure is an improvement in urine output and renal function following a fluid challenge of 10 ml/kg of isotonic saline or colloid administered over 1 hour. This should be given only to babies with no evidence of circulatory overload.

Conservative Management

Fluid balance

Meticulous attention to fluid balance is essential. Hypovolaemia should be urgently corrected with isotonic fluid or colloid according to clinical assessment of the circulating volume. Fluid losses, e.g. urine output and gastrointestinal losses, must be accurately measured and, providing the clinical condition allows it, the infant should be regularly weighed. Maintenance fluid is then calculated as insensible loss plus urine output and adjusted according to clinical assessment of the patient. In the newborn, insensible loss is approximately 1150 ml/m^2 body surface area daily (60–80 ml/kg/day).[52] This is increased in low birth weight and premature infants and in those nurtured under radiant warmers, and is reduced by around 30% in mechanically ventilated infants where respiratory water loss is negligible.

Nutrition

Nutrition is an important consideration in ARF and may be severely limited by the imposed fluid restriction. Provision of adequate energy is necessary in order to promote anabolism and prevent catabolism which potentiates hyperkalaemia and acidosis. Enteral nutrition is preferred if the patient's condition allows, but parenteral nutrition may be necessary. If adequate nutrition is impossible because of the limited fluid volume available, dialysis is indicated.

Hyperphosphataemia

Hyperphosphataemia is managed by the addition of oral calcium carbonate to feeds. This binds phosphate, rendering it insoluble, thereby reducing intestinal absorption. The use of aluminium hydroxide as a phosphate binder should be avoided in neonates because of the risk of neurotoxicity.

Hyperkalaemia

Acute hyperkalaemia is a medical emergency since it may cause potentially lethal cardiac arrhythmias. Hypocalcaemia and hypomagnesaemia, both of which frequently occur in ARF, potentiate the toxic effect of hyperkalaemia on the heart. It is therefore important to maintain normocalcaemia using 10% calcium gluconate (0.1–0.2 ml/kg) as necessary.

Temporary interventions can be taken to shift potassium from the extracellular fluid into cells including:

- IV salbutamol (4 μg/kg over 5 min) – this has been shown to be a safe and highly effective treatment in hyperkalaemic infants and children.[53] Nebulized salbutamol is also effective in children[54] and, although not formally evaluated in neonates, the authors' experience suggests that this route is effective in this age group.
- IV glucose and insulin infusion (12 units soluble insulin in 100 ml 25% glucose – 5 ml/kg given over 30 min) – this is highly effective and has an additive effect with salbutamol. The blood glucose concentration must be closely monitored during and after treatment since fluctuations commonly occur.
- IV sodium bicarbonate (1 mmol/kg).

These measures shift potassium from the extracellular to the intracellular compartment but do not eliminate it from the body. They are, therefore, only temporarily effective, allowing time to prepare for dialysis. Oral/rectal cation exchange, e.g. calcium polystyrene sulphate, are effective in permanent removal of potassium from the body but may be complicated by bowel obstruction and perforation, and are best avoided in sick newborns who are already at risk of necrotizing enterocolitis.

Acidosis
Metabolic acidosis should be treated with sodium bicarbonate in a dose sufficient to normalize the plasma pH and bicarbonate. If correction cannot be achieved within the infant's fluid allowance, dialysis should be considered.

Management by Dialysis

Dialysis is now regarded as a routine therapy for ARF in the neonate. Both peritoneal and haemodialysis are possible in infants weighing <1 kg. The main indications for dialysis are given in Table 1.4.

The term dialysis refers to the removal of small solutes across a semipermeable membrane by diffusion down their concentration gradient. The membrane may be the peritoneum, separating blood in the splanchnic vessels from dialysis fluid within the peritoneal cavity, or may be synthetic, as in haemodialysis, with blood and dialysis fluid pumped on opposite sides of the membrane. This process differs from filtration, in which there is convective removal of plasma water and small solutes as a result of a pressure gradient across a highly permeable membrane. Treatments can result in pure dialysis, pure filtration, or, more often, both.

Peritoneal dialysis
Peritoneal dialysis (PD) is the modality of choice in most neonates, the advantage being relative ease of access and technical simplicity in comparison with haemodialysis. PD can be carried out via either a temporary catheter, inserted using the Seldinger technique at the cotside, or via a surgically placed catheter. Insertion of a semi-rigid temporary catheter may be complicated by perforation of bowel or major blood vessels, so use of a soft sialistic Tenckhoff catheter is preferred. To avoid overdilation of the entry site, which may result in leakage around the site of insertion, a 13 FG catheter can be inserted then replaced through the same hole with a larger 16 FG catheter.[55] In very low birth weight infants, in whom

Table 1.4 Indications for dialysis in acute renal failure.

Fluid removal
Volume overload
To 'make space' for drug administration and nutrition
Correction of biochemical imbalance
Hyperkalaemia
Severe metabolic acidosis
Hyperphosphataemia/hypocalcaemia

insertion of this size of catheter is not feasible, PD can be carried out via an angiography catheter,[56] intravenous cannula or thoracic drain.[57] Infants as small as 380 g have been successfully dialysed using such techniques. A relative contraindication to PD is major abdominal surgery, although there have been reports of success in some cases.[58, 59]

The fill volume is calculated from the patient's weight. An initial fill volume of 10–20 ml/kg is usually used, increasing up to 30 ml/kg as tolerated. Larger fill volumes may splint the diaphragm and cause respiratory embarrassment. The dialysate is run into the abdomen by gravity. An automatic cycler, e.g. the 'Pac-X' machine, will perform this function, and with paediatric lines has a minimum cycle volume of 50 ml. Therefore, in low birth weight infants, where a smaller cycle volume is required, dialysis must be performed manually.

It may be more difficult to achieve adequate ultrafiltration in neonates than in older children because their relatively larger functional peritoneal surface area, more permeable peritoneal membrane, and higher energy requirement all cause rapid absorption of glucose from the peritoneal cavity into the blood. This leads to loss of the osmotic gradient required to drive the convective transport of water from blood to the peritoneal cavity.[60] Shorter dwell times, relatively larger volumes and higher dialysate glucose concentrations, help to overcome this problem.

The commonest complications of PD are given in Table 1.5.

Haemofiltration and haemodialysis

There are occasions when PD fails or is contraindicated necessitating the use of haemofiltration and/or haemodialysis. While it is preferable to perform these techniques continuously in order to avoid swings in intravascular volume and biochemistry, intermittent haemodialysis has been used successfully in neonates.[60, 61]

Continuous arteriovenous haemofiltration. The simplest technique is continuous arteriovenous haemofiltration (CAV_H) in which an artery and a vein are cannulated and blood is driven across a suitable filter, e.g.

Table 1.5 Complications of peritoneal dialysis.

Hyperglycaemia
Catheter-related problems
Viscus perforation during insertion*
Fluid leakage
Catheter blockage
Exit-site infection
Peritonitis
Haemodynamic/ventilatory instability

* This serious complication is rare with good technique, especially if the catheter is inserted over a guide wire.

'Amicon minifilter') by the patient's own systemic blood pressure (Figure 1.6A). The technique was first described in a neonate in 1985[62] and has since been widely used.

Arterial access can be obtained via the umbilical or femoral vessels and venous access via the umbilical, femoral or jugular veins. A systemic blood pressure of at least 40 mmHg is required to maintain adequate flow across the filter and if necessary a volumetric infusion pump can be inserted into the circuit to improve this.[63] The ultrafiltration pressure can be increased by increasing the vertical height between the filter and the collection vessel and further adjusted by applying gentle suction with a pump across the filter (Figure 1.6A). The pump also prevents excessive ultrafiltration. Using this system ultrafiltration rates of up to 5 ml/kg/h have been achieved.[64] Replacement fluid can be infused into the venous port of the circuit if desired.

Most infants will tolerate a maximum extracorporeal volume of 10% of their blood volume. The smallest extracorporeal volume that can currently be achieved with CAV_H is 12 ml (using an Amicon minifilter and neonatal lines). Low birth weight infants will therefore require blood priming of the circuit prior to initiation of treatment. Various combinations of whole blood, packed cells, plasma and albumin have been used for priming filtration and dialysis circuits in neonates.[61, 62, 65, 66] Banked blood may have a potassium concentration of up to 20 mmol/l;[67] therefore fresh whole blood is preferable. The citrate anticoagulant may cause sudden hypocalcaemia leading to the recommendation, by Coulthard and Vernon, of using fresh whole blood anticoagulated with heparin.[55]

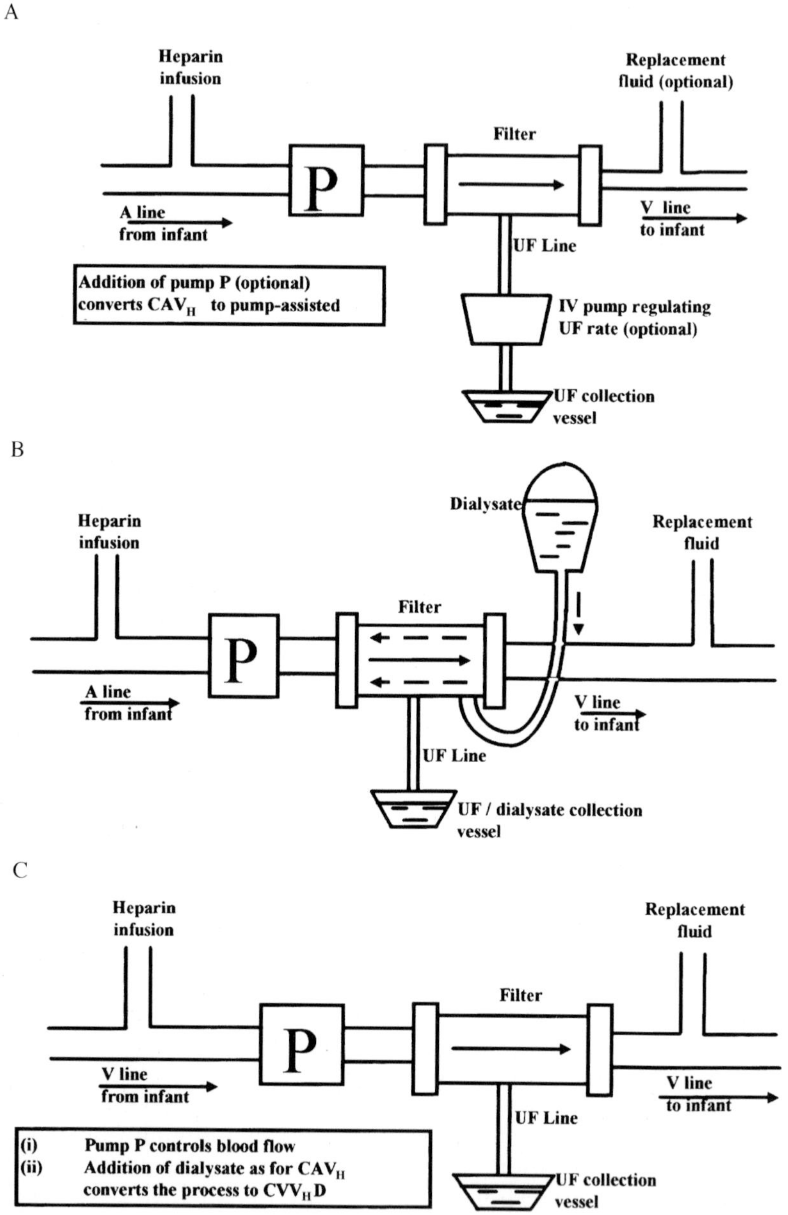

Figure 1.6 Schematic diagrams of (A) continuous arteriovenous haemofiltration; (B) continuous arteriovenous haemodiafiltration; and (C) continuous venovenous haemofiltration circuits. A = arterial; V = venous; UF = ultrafiltrate. Solid arrows: direction of blood flow. Dashed arrows: direction of dialysate flow. Other abbreviations and explanation are given in the text.

Heparin infusion is required to prevent clotting of the circuit. This is infused into the arterial port at a rate of 5–15 IU/kg/h following an initial bolus of 25–100 IU/kg. The infusion rate is adjusted, ideally according to the activated clotting time measured at the cotside, although laboratory measured activated partial thromboplastin times can be used. In many neonates, the haematocrit is relatively high and the mean arterial pressure relatively low, resulting in sluggish flow across the filter and a requirement for increased heparinization in order to prevent clotting. Where systemic heparinization is contra-indicated, heparin can be infused into the arterial port and protamine into the venous port.

Haemofiltration provides solute removal by convection but not diffusion. Occasionally this solute removal is inadequate. If so, diffusive clearance can be added by running dialysis fluid through the ultrafiltrate compartment of the filter in the opposite direction to blood flow, thereby converting the process to haemodiafiltration (Figure 1.6B).[68, 69]

A major disadvantage of CAV_H in the neonate is the requirement for arterial access which can be difficult to obtain, and in the case of brachial and femoral lines carries a risk of limb ischaemia and later reduced limb growth. CAV_H may not be possible in patients who are hypotensive or have poor cardiac function.

Continuous venovenous haemofiltration. An alternative technique is continuous venovenous haemofiltration (CVV_H), in which access is obtained either via 2 venous lines or a single double-lumen venous line, and a pump is used to control blood flow through the circuit (Figure 1.6C). Unfortunately, systems specifically designed for CVV_H in the neonate are not currently available.

Yorgin *et al*[66] first described CVV_H in a neonate in 1990, using a standard dialysis unit to control blood flow. Bunchman *et al*[70] have successfully adapted a 'Gambro AK-10' haemodialysis machine for CVV_H and, using an 'Amicon minifilter' and neonatal lines, have reduced the extracorporeal circuit volume to 38 ml. Blood priming is therefore required in infants weighing <4.5 kg. Alternatively, a volumetric infusion pump can be used to regulate blood flow.[71] This allows a lower blood flow and requires less technical support than does use of a standard dialysis machine. However, there is an increased risk of air embolus, since the circuit does not contain a bubble trap and air detector.

More recently, a manual syringe-driven technique has been described which allows venovenous ultrafiltration and haemodialysis to be performed in infants weighing <1000 g, the smallest to whom the technique has been applied being 630 g.[72] The technique is very labour intensive although automation may be possible in the future. As for

CAV_H, dialysis can be added to CVV_H by running dialysate through the filter in the opposite direction to blood flow.

In virtually all cases dialysis is possible in the neonate with ARF. Peritoneal dialysis remains the technique of first choice, although advances continue to be made in CAV_H and CVV_H. Ultimately, the choice of dialysis modality depends upon the individual patient and the technical support available within the unit.

REFERENCES

1. Spitzer A. Renal physiology and functional development. In: Edelmann CM Jr (ed) *Pediatric Renal Disease*. Boston: Little, Brown, 1978, pp 25–128.
2. Guignard J-P and John EG. Renal function in the tiny, premature infant. *Clin Perinatol* 1986;**13**: 377–401.
3. Arant BS Jr. Postnatal development of renal function during the first year of life. *Pediatr Nephrol* 1987;**1**: 308–313.
4. Robillard JE, Porter CC and Jose PA. Structure and function of the developing kidney. In: Holliday MA *et al* (eds) *Pediatric Nephrology*. Baltimore: Williams & Wilkins, 1994, pp 21–39.
5. Chevalier RL. Developmental renal physiology of the low birth weight preterm newborn. *J Urol* 1996;**156**: 714–719.
6. Moniz CF *et al*. Normal reference ranges for biochemical substances relating to renal, hepatic and bone function in fetal and maternal plasma during pregnancy. *J Clin Pathol* 1985;**38**: 468–472.
7. Rabinowitz R *et al*. Measurement of fetal urine production in normal pregnancy by real-time ultrasonography. *Am J Obstet Gynecol* 1989;**161**: 1264–1266.
8. Nicolaides KH *et al*. Fetal urine biochemistry in the assessment of obstructive uropathy. *Am J Obstet Gynecol* 1992;**166**: 932–937.
9. Al-Dahhan J *et al*. Sodium homeostasis in term and preterm neonates. I. Renal aspects. *Arch Dis Child* 1983;**58**: 335–342.
10. Adzick NS *et al*. Development of a fetal renal function test using endogenous creatinine clearance. *J Pediatr Surg* 1985;**20**: 602–607.
11. McCance RA and Widdowson EM. The correct physiological basis on which to compare infant and adult renal function. *Lancet* 1952;**ii**: 860–862.
12. Coulthard MG and Hey EN. Weight as the best standard for glomerular filtration in the newborn. *Arch Dis Child* 1984;**59**: 373–375.
13. Goldsmith DI. Clinical and laboratory evaluation of renal function. In: Edelmann CMJ (ed) *Pediatric Kidney Disease*. Boston: Little, Brown & Co, pp 213–224.
14. Gruskin AB, Edelmann CM Jr and Yuan S. Maturational changes in renal blood flow in piglets. *Pediatr Res* 1970;**4**: 7–13.

15. Aperia A and Herin P. Development of glomerular perfusion rate and nephron filtration rate in rats 17–60 days old. *Am J Physiol* 1975;**228**: 1319–1325.
16. Jose PA *et al.* Intrarenal blood flow distribution in canine puppies. *Pediatr Res* 1971;**5**: 335–344.
17. Spitzer A and Brandis M. Functional and morphologic maturation of the superficial nephrons. *J Clin Invest* 1974;**53**: 279–287.
18. Aschinberg LC *et al.* Neonatal changes in renal blood flow distribution in puppies. *Am J Physiol* 1975;**228**: 1453–1461.
19. John E, Goldsmith DI and Spitzer A. Quantitative changes in the canine glomerular vasculature during development: physiologic implications. *Kidney Int* 1981;**20**: 223–229.
20. Martin RA *et al.* Effect of ACE inhibition on the fetal kidney: decreased renal blood flow. *Teratology* 1992;**46**: 317–321.
21. O'Dea RF *et al.* Treatment of neonatal hypertension with captopril. *J Pediatr* 1988;**113**: 403–406.
22. Buderas S *et al.* Renal failure in two preterm infants: toxic effect of prenatal maternal indomethacin treatment? *Br J Obstet Gynaecol* 1993;**100**: 97–98.
23. Kaplan BS *et al.* Renal failure in the neonate associated with *in utero* exposure to non-steroidal anti-inflammatory agents. *Pediatr Nephrol* 1994;**8**: 700–704.
24. Reyes JL and Melendez E. Effects of eicosanoids on the water and sodium balance of the neonate. *Pediatr Nephrol* 1990;**4**: 630–634.
25. Trompeter RS, Chantler C and Haycock GB. Tolazoline and acute renal failure in the newborn [letter]. *Lancet* 1981;**i**: 1219.
26. Jose PA *et al.* Autoregulation of renal blood flow in the puppy. *Am J Physiol* 1975;**229**: 983–988.
27. Rodríguez-Soriano J *et al.* Renal handling of sodium in premature and full-term neonates: a study using clearance methods during water diuresis. *Pediatr Res* 1983;**17**: 1013–1016.
28. Kleinman LI. Renal sodium reabsorption during saline loading and distal blockade in newborn dogs. *Am J Physiol* 1975;**228**: 1403–1408.
29. Aperia A and Elinder G. Distal tubular sodium reabsorption in the developing rat kidney. *Am J Physiol* 1981;**240**: F487–491.
30. Al-Dahhan J *et al.* Sodium homeostasis in term and preterm neonates. III. The effect of salt supplementation. *Arch Dis Child* 1984;**59**: 945–950.
31. Chevalier RL, Campbell F and Brenbridge AN. Prognostic factors in neonatal acute renal failure. *Pediatrics* 1984;**74**: 265–272.
32. Brodehl J and Gellissen K. Endogenous renal transport of free amino acids in infancy and childhood. *Pediatrics* 1968;**42**: 395–404.
33. Arant BS Jr, Edelmann CM Jr and Nash MA. The renal reabsorption of glucose in the developing canine kidney: a study of glomerulotubular balance. *Pediatr Res* 1974;**8**: 638–646.
34. Schwarts GJ *et al.* Late metabolic acidosis: a reassessment of the definition. *J Pediatr* 1979;**95**: 102–107.
35. Albert MS and Winters RW. Acid-base equilibrium of blood in normal infants. *Pediatrics* 1966;**37**: 728–732.

36. Aperia A and Broberger U. Beta-2-microglobulin, an indicator of renal tubular maturation and dysfunction in the newborn. *Acta Paediatr Scand* 1979;**68**: 669–676.
37. Elinder G and Aperia A. Development of glomerular filtration rate and excretion of beta 2-microglobulin in neonates during gentamicin treatment. *Acta Paediatr Scand* 1983;**72**: 219–224.
38. Portman RJ, Kissane JM and Robson AM. Use of beta 2 microglobulin to diagnose tubulo-interstitial renal lesions in children. *Kidney Int* 1986;**30**: 91–98.
39. Edelmann CM Jr, Barnett HL and Stark H. Effect of urea on concentration of urinary nonurea solute in premature infants. *J Appl Physiol* 1966;**21**: 1021–1025.
40. Rees L *et al.* Hyponatraemia in the first week of life in preterm infants. Part I. Arginine vasopressin secretion. *Arch Dis Child* 1984;**59**: 414–422.
41. Marchini G and Stock S. Thirst and vasopressin secretion counteract dehydration in newborn infants. *J Pediatr* 1997;**130**: 736–739.
42. Manz F, Kalhoff H and Remer T. Renal acid excretion in early infancy. *Pediatr Nephrol* 1997;**11**: 231–243.
43. Hatemi N and McCance RA. Renal aspects of acid base control in the newly born. III. Response to acidifying drugs. *Acta Paediatr* 1961;**50**: 603–616.
44. Kildeberg P. Disturbances of hydrogen ion balance occurring in premature infants. II. Late metabolic acidosis. *Acta Paediatr* 1964;**53**: 517–526.
45. Stapleton FB, Jones D and Green R. Acute renal failure in neonates: incidence, etiology and outcome. *Pediatr Nephrol* 1987;**1**: 314–320.
46. Karlowicz MG, Adelman RD. Nonoliguric and oliguric acute renal failure in asphyxiated term neonates. *Pediatr Nephrol* 1995;**9**: 718–722.
47. Grylak L *et al.* Nonoliguric acute renal failure in the newborn. *Am J Dis Child* 1982;**136**: 518–520.
48. Norman ME and Asadi FK. A prospective study of acute renal failure in the newborn infant. *Pediatrics* 1979;**63**: 475–479.
49. Mathew OP *et al.* Neonatal renal failure: usefulness of diagnostic indices. *Pediatrics* 1980;**65**: 57–60.
50. Ellis EN and Arnold WC. Use of urinary indexes in renal failure in the newborn. *Am J Dis Child* 1982;**136**: 615–617.
51. Ishizaki Y *et al.* Evaluation of diagnostic criteria of acute renal failure in premature infants. *Acta Paediatr Jpn* 1993;**35**: 311–315.
52. Holliday MA and Segar WE. The maintenance need for water in parenteral fluid therapy. *Pediatrics* 1957;**19**: 823–832.
53. Murdoch IA, Dos Anjos R and Haycock GB. Treatment of hyperkalaemia with intravenous salbutamol. *Arch Dis Child* 1991;**66**: 527–528.
54. McClure RJ, Prasad VK and Brocklebank JT. Treatment of hyperkalaemia using intravenous and nebulized salbutamol. *Arch Dis Child* 1994;**70**: 126–128.
55. Coulthard MG and Vernon B. Managing acute renal failure in very low birthweight infants. *Arch Dis Child* 1995;**73**: F187–F192.
56. Steele BT *et al.* Acute peritoneal dialysis in infants weighing <1500 g. *J Pediatr* 1987;**110**: 126–129.

57. Sizun J *et al.* Peritoneal dialysis in the very low-birth-weight neonate (less than 1000 g). *Acta Paediatr* 1993;**82**: 488–489.
58. Mattoo TK and Ahmad GS. Peritoneal dialysis in neonates after major abdominal surgery. *Am J Nephrol* 1994;**14**: 6–8.
59. Alon U, Bar-Maor JA and Bar-Joseph G. Effective peritoneal dialysis in an infant with extensive resection of the small intestine. *Am J Nephrol* 1988;**8**: 65–67.
60. Bock GH *et al.* Hemodialysis in the premature infant. *Am J Dis Child* 1981;**135**: 178–180.
61. Sadowski RH, Harmon WE and Jabs K. Acute hemodialysis of infants weighing less than five kilograms. *Kidney Int* 1994;**45**: 903–906.
62. Lieberman KV, Nardi L and Bosch JP. Treatment of acute renal failure in an infant using continuous arteriovenous hemofiltration. *J Pediatr* 1985;**106**: 646–649.
63. Heney D, Brocklebank JT and Wilson N. Continuous arteriovenous haemofiltration in the newly born with acute renal failure and congenital heart disease. *Nephrol Dialysis Transplant* 1989;**4**: 870–876.
64. Bauer M and Stewart S. Renal failure following cardiac surgery in a 2.8 kg infant managed with continuous arteriovenous hemofiltration. *Ann Thorac Surg* 1988;**45**: 225–226.
65. Ronco C *et al.* Treatment of acute renal failure in newborns by continuous arterio-venous hemofiltration. *Kidney Int* 1986;**29**: 908–915.
66. Yorgin PD, Krensky AM and Tune BM. Continuous venovenous hemofiltration. *Pediatr Nephrol* 1990;**4**: 640–642.
67. Bunchman TE and Donckerwolcke RA. Continuous arterial-venous diahemofiltration and continuous veno-venous diahemofiltration in infants and children. *Pediatr Nephrol* 1994;**8**: 96–102.
68. Bishof NA *et al.* Continuous hemodiafiltration in children. *Pediatrics* 1990;**85**: 819–823.
69. Assadi FK. Treatment of acute renal failure in an infant by continuous arteriovenous hemodialysis. *Pediatr Nephrol* 1988;**2**: 320–322.
70. Bunchman TE *et al.* Continuous venovenous hemodiafiltration in infants and children. *Am J Kidney Dis* 1995;**25**: 17–21.
71. Ellis EN *et al.* Pump-assisted hemofiltration in infants with acute renal failure. *Pediatr Nephrol* 1993;**7**: 434–437.
72. Coulthard MG and Sharp J. Haemodialysis and ultrafiltration in babies weighing under 1000 g. *Arch Dis Child* 1995;**73**: F162–F165.

2

Rational Antibiotic Approach in a Neonatal Unit

Jennifer A. Royle and David Isaacs

Rational antibiotic use involves deciding which babies need antibiotics, which antibiotics, and for how long.

WHICH BABIES TO TREAT?

Early-Onset Sepsis

In this chapter, early-onset sepsis (EOS) is defined as sepsis occurring within 48 hours of delivery. Particular attention must be given to detecting (predicting) those babies at greater risk of sepsis.

Risk factors

Risk factors for EOS can be of assistance in predicting which babies may need antibiotics commenced immediately at birth, although about 25% of all babies with EOS have no maternal risk factors.[1] A septic looking baby with no risk factors for sepsis therefore needs immediate cultures and antibiotic treatment.

Table 2.1 lists the major risk factors for EOS. The single most reported risk factor is spontaneous preterm onset of labour, followed by prolonged rupture of membranes and maternal fever. These 3 risk factors are known to be associated with sepsis attributable to Group B streptococcus (GBS),[1] pneumococci[2] and enterococci.[3] Prolonged rupture of membranes has a continuum of increased risk: the greatest risk is after

Table 2.1 Risk factors for early-onset neonatal sepsis.

Spontaneous preterm onset of labour
Prolonged rupture of membranes
Maternal intrapartum fever
Signs of chorioamnionitis (e.g. smelly liquor)
Previous baby with group B streptococcal infection
Twin pregnancy

18 hours but the risk of sepsis increases when membranes are ruptured for > 12 hours.[1]

Signs of chorioamnionitis (e.g. smelly liquor) have been reported to be associated with an increased incidence of non-organism-specific sepsis.[1]

Preterm babies

When a term baby born to a woman with fever or prolonged rupture of membranes develops respiratory distress, sepsis is always first or second in the junior doctor's differential diagnosis. In contrast, a baby with respiratory distress following spontaneous preterm onset of labour is usually thought to have hyaline membrane disease (HMD) and sepsis is rarely considered.[5] However, the latter is the commonest risk factor for sepsis,[5] probably because bacteria can produce prostaglandin-like substances that induce labour. Effectively this means that almost all preterm babies with early-onset respiratory distress should start antibiotics, after taking cultures. Antibiotics can be safely withdrawn at 48–72 hours if cultures and other findings are not supportive of a diagnosis of sepsis. No laboratory tests, haematological or microbiological, have sufficient sensitivity to be used as the sole arbiter of which babies should receive antibiotics.

A preterm baby who develops early respiratory distress following an induced labour or caesarean section for maternal indications with no spontaneous onset of labour, does not necessarily need antibiotics if there are no risk factors for sepsis.

A normal chest X-ray (CXR) in a premature baby with respiratory distress should not deter one from commencing antibiotics when a sepsis risk factor is present. Classically, a fine generalized granularity is seen in HMD and patchy changes are seen in pneumonia, but variations occur in each condition and cases of early-onset pneumonia with GBS have been reported with a normal initial CXR.

Term baby with respiratory distress and no risk factors

HMD is rare in term babies, and respiratory distress at term should suggest the possibility of sepsis. Most term babies with respiratory distress will have a final diagnosis of transient tachypnoea of the newborn (TTN).

The initial CXR in TTN has a 'wet lung' appearance with increased vascular markings and often fluid in the horizontal fissure. An identical CXR appearance has been described in about 10% of cases of early-onset GBS pneumonia.[6] Most cases of early-onset pneumonia at term will have areas of focal consolidation or a generalized granularity mimicking HMD, so a normal or 'wet lung' CXR does not exclude pneumonia. Mifsud *et al* monitored tachypnoea routinely in all newborn babies and found this to be a useful indicator of EOS.[7] The earlier detection of the septic babies in this study prompted earlier antibiotic treatment and may have contributed to the decreased mortality.

Gram stains of gastric aspirates[8] and tracheal aspirates[9, 10] are only moderately reliable, with sensitivities of 77% and 74%, respectively, in predicting babies with early sepsis. These investigations can be used as an adjunct to aid diagnosis, but only bearing in mind that they will not identify all cases of early sepsis. Ingram *et al* reported that 3 of 16 (23%) babies with early-onset GBS pneumonia had negative gastric aspirates.[8]

Additional laboratory tests such as total neutrophil count, immature:total neutrophil (IT) ratio and serum C-reactive protein (CRP) level may help to decide whether to treat or observe term babies with respiratory distress, though one should be wary of taking false reassurance from negative results.[11]

Asymptomatic babies with risk factors

If a well baby has 2 or more risk factors for sepsis (e.g. spontaneous preterm onset of labour and prolonged rupture of membranes), a full septic screen should be performed and antibiotics commenced. When a single risk factor is present in an asymptomatic baby, there is no necessity to commence antibiotics, although the baby should be observed closely.

Maternal intrapartum antibiotics

Intrapartum maternal antibiotics are increasingly used and reduce the risk of neonatal colonization and sepsis due to GBS.[12] If the mother was given antibiotics intrapartum and the baby is subsequently born well, it can be difficult to decide whether or not to commence antibiotics.

The Centers for Disease Control and Prevention (CDC) recently published an algorithm outlining an approach to the management of a neonate born to a mother who received intrapartum antimicrobial prophylaxis (IAP) for prevention of early-onset GBS disease (Figure 2.1).[13] This algorithm is only a guideline: it is based on good sense rather than data, and is designed for GBS, rather than other causes of EOS.

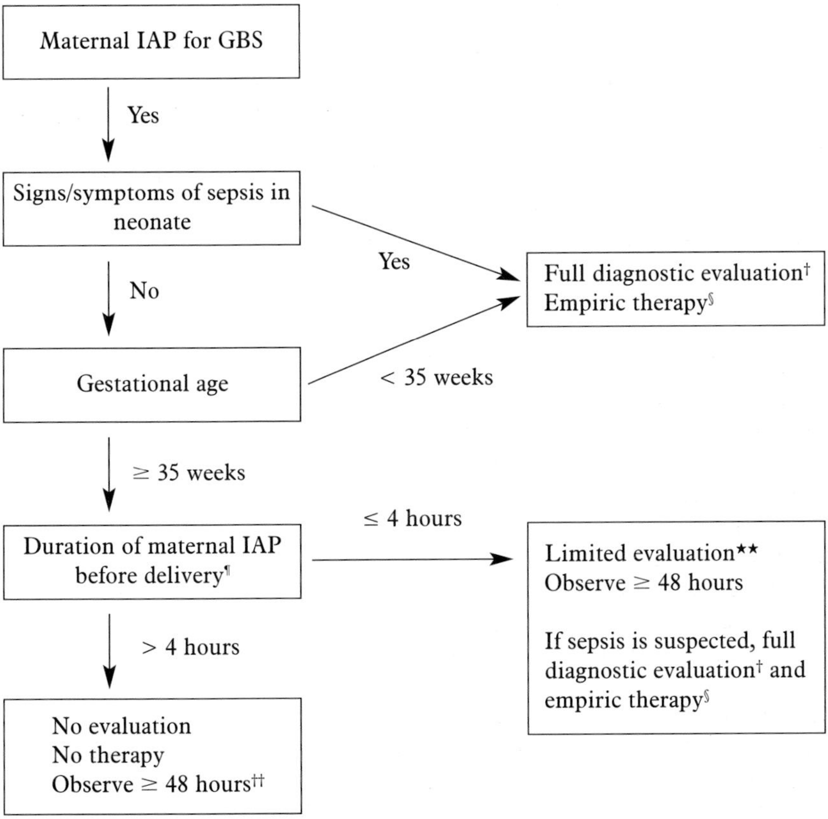

† Includes a complete and differential blood count, blood culture and chest X-ray if neonate has respiratory symptoms. Lumbar puncture is performed at the discretion of the physician.

§ Duration of therapy will vary depending on blood culture and cerebrospinal fluid (CSF) results and the clinical course of the infant. If these are unremarkable, duration of therapy may be as short as 48–72 hours.

¶ Duration of penicillin or ampicillin chemoprophylaxis.

** Complete and differential blood count and a blood culture.

†† Does not allow early discharge.

Figure 2.1 Centers for Disease Control 1996 algorithm for management of a neonate born to a mother who received intrapartum antimicrobial prophylaxis (IAP) for prevention of early-onset group B streptococcal (GBS) disease.

Positive urine GBS antigen test

Detection of streptococcal antigen can be used in an attempt to distinguish early-onset GBS pneumonia from HMD.[14–17] Ingram *et al* reported that latex particle agglutination (LPA) was more sensitive than countercurrent immunoelectrophoresis in detecting streptococcal antigen.[8] Concentrated urine has been shown to be the best body fluid to test (compared with serum and CSF). Bag urine samples are readily contaminated with skin bacteria, so although a negative bag urine LPA effectively excludes GBS infection, a positive LPA test on a bag specimen should be repeated on a sterile suprapubic aspirate (SPA) of urine. A positive LPA test (on an SPA from a symptomatic baby) is usually interpreted as meaning bacteraemia, and can be particularly useful when the mother has been treated with intrapartum antibiotics.

Some babies require empiric antibiotic treatment regardless of the LPA test, e.g. a term baby with respiratory distress and a risk factor (e.g. prolonged rupture of membranes). It is important to remember a negative antenatal maternal GBS vaginal culture does not exclude possible neonatal GBS infection, since 8% of women who are negative at the 28-week-gestation screening acquire GBS carriage by term.[1] In general, any symptomatic baby with a positive LPA test should be rapidly started on antibiotics after cultures are taken.

Management of asymptomatic babies with a positive LPA test is more difficult. In each case, an empirical decision will need to be made based on why the test was sent and the baby's gestation, etc. The more premature the baby, even if asymptomatic, the greater the justification for empiric antibiotic treatment.

Severe perinatal asphyxia

The decision to commence antibiotics acutely in the setting of severe perinatal asphyxia is made on an individual basis. Though most babies with perinatal asphyxia are not septic, up to 20% of babies with perinatal sepsis have respiratory depression requiring intubation.[18] Selecting these septic patients reliably is a difficult task. Both asphyxia and infection may cause pulmonary hypertension. The haematological picture is often abnormal in severe asphyxia; neutropenia may occur[19] and the CRP may be raised.[11]

Antibiotics should be commenced if a risk factor for sepsis (see Table 2.1) is present. There is no harm in starting a desperately sick newborn on antibiotics and reassessing their appropriateness after 2–3 days, once the initial situation has evolved and results of blood cultures, placental pathology and other investigations are available.

Meconium aspiration syndrome

Meconium aspiration may result from severe perinatal asphyxia. It has been argued that, although meconium is sterile, the plugging of airways resulting from meconium aspiration may predispose to secondary pneumonia. As is the case for severe perinatal asphyxia, it is not logical to prescribe antibiotics in case secondary pneumonia develops. Antibiotics are not routinely prescribed in meconium aspiration syndrome, but each baby should be assessed individually for the likelihood of sepsis. The presence of meconium during a preterm delivery is suggestive of infection, particularly Listeria infection.

Dirty procedures around delivery

In some babies, usually those with perinatal asphyxia or acute blood loss, intravenous catheters are inserted hurriedly, often in the delivery suite and under less than optimally sterile conditions. Antibiotics are often prescribed to cover such 'dirty' procedures. There is very little evidence that sepsis occurs as a result of dirty procedures or that it can be prevented by giving antibiotics. Nevertheless, the practice of giving antibiotics under these conditions is likely to continue, whatever is argued, and is probably relatively harmless if they are stopped early when cultures are negative.

Neutropenia

The commonest cause of transient neonatal neutropenia is maternal hypertensive disease of pregnancy.[20] Neutropenia is present at birth in about half of all babies whose mothers have pre-eclampsia.[21] Mouzinho *et al* reported a tendency for neutropenic neonates to be <30 weeks' gestation, weigh <1500 grams at birth, and born to mothers with more severe pregnancy-induced hypertension.[22] An increased risk of nosocomial infections has been reported in some studies,[21, 23] but not all.[22] As most reports suggest an increased risk of infection, a policy to culture and treat babies with early neutropenia empirically with antibiotics until the neutropenia resolves, even if they are symptom free, is rational.

Late-Onset Sepsis

This discussion refers to neonates >48 hours of age who are inpatients.

It is unusual for a previously well baby on the postnatal ward to develop sepsis, but if they do the initial signs are non-specific. These may include fever, tachypnoea, a cyanotic episode (apnoea, bradycardia or seizure) or perhaps a decrease in activity and poor feeding. Examination may reveal signs of respiratory distress (tachypnoea, nasal flare, grunt), tachycardia, fever, poor perfusion, rash, poor suck or a reduced conscious state. All of these signs alert the medical practitioner to send off investigations (blood, urine, CSF) and commence empiric antibiotics with the baby closely monitored in the special care or intensive care unit.

A ventilated baby with sepsis may present in an even more nonspecific way. Monitored infants may develop hypothermia or temperature instability rather than fever. Increased ventilatory or inotropic support, increased oxygen requirement, tachypnoea or tachycardia, a decrease in general activity, or poor colour (decreased perfusion) may indicate sepsis.

Critically ill neonates, in particular extremely premature ventilated babies on parenteral nutrition, are at greatest risk of developing late-onset sepsis (LOS). As for EOS, laboratory tests can be helpful in deciding which babies to treat, notably the serum CRP and the I:T ratio, but a clinical diagnosis of sepsis is an absolute indication for antibiotics. Lumbar puncture should be included routinely in the septic work-up for LOS because an abnormal result influences antibiotic choice.

Prophylactic Antibiotics

There are very few situations in which antibiotic prophylaxis has been shown to be effective in the neonatal period. Some neonatologists routinely prescribe antibiotics to babies requiring endotracheal intubation as prophylaxis against infection. In many situations intubated babies do require antibiotics, but this is to treat possible underlying sepsis, and a corollary of this is that the antibiotics can be ceased at 48–72 hours if cultures are negative.

There have been a number of recent papers on the use of prophylactic vancomycin to prevent coagulase-negative staphylococcal infections. The rationale is that this pathogen is the commonest cause of LOS affecting mainly the smallest, lowest gestation babies who were most ill on admission, causing prolongation of their hospital stay, significant morbidity and additional expenses.[24] Prophylactic vancomycin has been used in preterm neonates at a twice daily dose infused over 1 hour,[25] or as a continuous low-dose infusion given with parenteral nutrition.[26, 27] These studies report significant reductions in staphylococcal bacteraemia. Babies in the vancomycin arm of studies, however, may not grow staphylococcus as a contaminant (which is common in clinical practice) because the cultures are likely to be sterilized by the dose of vancomycin. Hence the visible benefit from vancomycin may appear exaggerated, with the control group having apparent episodes of bacteraemia as the cultures include more contaminants.[28]

Even if vancomycin does prevent coagulase-negative staphylococcal infections there are 2 dangers associated with its use:

- Preterm babies may be predestined by their degree of relative immunocompromise to develop septicaemia with any colonizing organism. Eradication of coagulase-negative staphylococci may merely allow more virulent organisms such as Gram-negative bacilli to colonize and invade.
- Vancomycin-resistant enterococci (VRE), which are normal bowel commensals and for which no antibiotics are available if sepsis occurs, may be selected.[29] VRE can be transmitted on the hands of personnel or by contaminated environmental surfaces and patient care equipment.[30–33] To prevent the emergence of VRE, vancomycin use should be severely restricted in neonatal units.[34, 35]

Prophylactic oral nystatin has been shown by Sims *et al*[36] to reduce fungal colonization and systemic fungaemia in very low birth weight babies being artificially ventilated.

WHAT ANTIBIOTIC TO USE?

The narrowest spectrum available of antibiotic should be used to cover the range of organisms causing sepsis in the neonatal unit. The antibiotics used should have been proven to be effective in treating cases of neonatal sepsis. There may be great variation in the organisms causing sepsis between regions, within regions and even locally within one hospital over time. Monitoring the episodes of sepsis in the nursery is vital. Recording the organisms causing systemic sepsis, assessing the outcome and closely following new trends in the emergence of resistant organisms is important. The empiric antibiotic policy of a unit is a dynamic policy which requires ongoing evaluation and possible changes depending on what is happening in the unit.

Early-Onset Sepsis

Penicillin or ampicillin are generally used together with an aminoglycoside (usually gentamicin) as empiric treatment of EOS. In most industrialized countries, GBS is the organism responsible for the majority of EOS episodes and also the cause of high morbidity and mortality.[4, 37] An aminoglycoside is used with a penicillin because Gram-negative organisms, particularly *Escherichia coli*, are a common cause of EOS. *Listeria monocytogenes* is not uncommon in some countries, particularly France, and is effectively covered by penicillin/ampicillin and an aminoglycoside regimen. The third-generation cephalosporins, though safe in neonates,[38] are ineffective against Listeria and enterococci and therefore are inappropriate as monotherapy for EOS.[39]

Even with optimal treatment of suspected EOS the morbidity and mortality remains high. Prior to delivery, a large microbial load may have disseminated, often in a compromised fetus, without maternal antibodies. Strategies to improve the outcome of EOS should address prevention by identifying and treating with intrapartum antibiotics women at risk for delivering a septic baby.[1, 40, 41] In future, effective GBS vaccines for immunizing mothers will have a vast impact on the incidence of EOS.[42]

Late-Onset Sepsis

Three approaches to the choice of antibiotic policies for LOS are outlined below.

Treat the baby according to an empiric antibiotic policy

When LOS is suspected, a septic work-up should be performed and empiric treatment started immediately. Antibiotics should then be stopped early if cultures are negative and sepsis is unlikely. This is probably the best way of limiting the emergence of resistant organisms. If a large range of antibiotics is used simultaneously, multiple drug resistance is a danger. Use of a standard regimen will usually result only in selection of organisms resistant to a single antibiotic. Colonization with resistant organisms does not necessarily lead to sepsis with resistant organisms.[43, 44]

There is no 'ideal' antibiotic regimen for treating suspected LOS. At present, in most industrialized countries, LOS is most commonly caused by coagulase-negative staphylococci, Gram-negative enteric bacilli, enterococci (faecal streptococci) and *Staphylococcus aureus*. Recording and reviewing causes of sepsis within a single unit is vital to detect changes in the causative organisms. Meningitis will usually require an antibiotic selection different from the empiric choice, which stresses the importance of immediate lumbar punctures in the septic work-up.

The most commonly used regimens are a semi-synthetic penicillin or vancomycin together with an aminoglycoside or third-generation cephalosporin. The semi-synthetic penicillin used is a penicillinase-resistant penicillin such as cloxacillin or methicillin since effective staphylococcal cover is important. In units where methicillin-resistant *Staph. aureus* (MRSA) is a problem, vancomycin is preferred to the penicillin.

The disadvantage of using aminoglycosides is their potential to cause oto- and nephro-toxicity and the consequent need to monitor drug levels. The third-generation cephalosporins do not require monitoring of drug levels and penetrate CSF well. However, the antibiotic pressure exerted by the cephalosporins can lead to the emergence of resistant organisms,[45] although this is not always the case.[46] The main disadvantage of vancomycin use is the danger of selecting for vancomycin-resistant organisms, particularly enterococci. If there is no MRSA colonization, cloxacillin is preferred to vancomycin for initial empiric therapy, together with an aminoglycoside or third-generation cephalosporin. Although coagulase-negative staphylococci are a common cause of sepsis and are often methicillin resistant, they do not usually cause fulminant infection and there is time to await the results of cultures. If vancomycin is the empiric choice, it should be stopped as early as possible, e.g. after 48–72 hours, if cultures are negative.

Treat according to the organisms colonizing the baby
Many units perform routine surveillance cultures, but the value of this time-consuming and expensive surveillance has been questioned.[44, 47] The sensitivity of surface cultures predicting the organism causing sepsis is low.[44] Evans *et al* reported surface cultures to have a sensitivity of 56% when taken on the day of sepsis, 50% 1 day before sepsis, 32% 2 days before and <30% when taken earlier than this.[47] They also found a number of false positive or misleading surveillance cultures. Likewise, use of routine endotracheal cultures for the prediction of sepsis in ventilated babies is not reliable in predicting the pathogens that are isolated from the blood during episodes of sepsis.[48] Choosing antibiotics for LOS based on the result of an individual's latest surveillance culture has an unacceptable margin of error.

Treat according to the prevalent organisms colonizing babies in the neonatal unit
Making antibiotic choices based on the prevalent colonizing organisms in the unit is full of hazards. White *et al* reported fluctuations in colonization rates of ampicillin- and gentamicin-resistant organisms in faecal cultures, and no correlation between patterns of colonization and episodes of sepsis.[43]

When to Change the Unit's Empiric Antibiotic Policy

Colonization with resistant organisms alone is not sufficient to warrant changing the antibiotic policy of a unit. The first case of sepsis with a resistant organism should be a warning. A second case of resistant sepsis indicates that widespread colonization is likely and the unit's antibiotic policy should be changed to a regimen effective against the resistant organism. A decision has to be made whether to screen other babies for colonization of the respiratory or gastrointestinal tract. This may not be appropriate immediately. Surveillance is most valuable to assess if a resistant organism no longer exists in a unit, or only exists in a few babies who can be isolated. The outbreak antibiotic policy should be continued for a few weeks after no further case of sepsis with the resistant organism has occurred. The pre-epidemic policy can then be reinstated for all babies in the general unit and those in isolation should continue with the amended policy.

DURATION OF ANTIBIOTICS

The promotion of rapid initiation of antibiotics when sepsis is suspected contrasts with the insistence that antibiotics should be ceased at 48–72 hours if blood cultures are negative. Pichichero and Todd studied the duration of culture incubation required to determine bacteraemia in the newborn infant: 96% of positive blood cultures had grown at 48 hours and 98% at 72 hours.[49] Stopping antibiotics at 48–72 hours when cultures are negative appears to be safe and practical.[50]

Long courses of antibiotics are known to select for antibiotic-resistant organisms.[51] Neonates often become colonized with an abnormal (more virulent) selection of Gram-negative enteric organisms, such as Citrobacter, Enterobacter and Klebsiella species, once a course of antibiotics exceeds 72 hours.[52] The risk of systemic candidiasis, particularly to premature babies, is increased with a longer duration of antibiotics.[53] Antibiotic toxicity, especially from aminoglycoside, is reduced by stopping unnecessary courses early. Significant cost reduction is made if antibiotics are stopped at 48 hours in terms both of drugs and of measuring serum aminoglycoside levels.

Not all clinical situations are straightforward when the 48-hour culture result becomes available. Various common situations are outlined below.

Negative Blood Cultures: But the Baby Looked Septic

How often no growth from blood cultures in the presence of bacteraemia (i.e. false negatives) occurs in the neonatal period is not known. Situations arise where it is felt the baby looks and acts septic and the blood cultures are negative. Squire *et al* reported that 7 of 39 babies (18%) who died from infection had positive pre-mortem blood cultures.[54] Webber *et al* reported negative blood cultures in 9 of 20 cases with clinical GBS pneumonia.[5] These 9 babies were heavily colonized with GBS and had clinical pneumonia. It is well recognized that a significant minority of patients with meningitis have negative (presumably false negative) blood cultures,[55, 56] once again highlighting the need to include a lumbar puncture in the initial septic work-up.

EOS occurs secondary to ascending or transplacental infection and heavy colonization is an almost invariable concomitant with the septicaemia. If a baby strongly suspected to have EOS is heavily colonized and has negative cultures (blood, CSF, urine), it seems reasonable to complete a full course of antibiotics. In this situation, heavy colonization with probable pathogens such as GBS or *Listeria monocytogenes* should increase the suspicion of sepsis. If systemic and surface cultures are negative, EOS is unlikely and antibiotics can be stopped at 48–72 hours.[50]

In suspected LOS, colonization is a poor indicator of clinical sepsis; many well babies are colonized with potential pathogens.[47]

Diligent attention to withdrawal of antibiotics when sepsis is unlikely is very important.

Negative Blood Culture: Mother had Intrapartum Antibiotics

Intrapartum antibiotics prevent GBS septicaemia and also reduce the proportion of babies colonized from 50% to 10%.[12] The concern is that the maternal antibiotics may increase the number of false negative blood cultures.[57] Once a newborn has had antibiotics started following maternal intrapartum antibiotics, the decision to stop antibiotics in the neonate is difficult (see Figure 2.1). It would be reasonable to stop neonatal antibiotics at 48–72 hours if superficial and systemic cultures (ear, blood) are sterile, and GBS antigenuria is not detected. A 7–10 day course should be completed if GBS antigenuria is present and probably also if the superficial cultures show heavy colonization with a clinical picture suggestive of sepsis.

Positive Blood Culture: ? A Contaminant

Contaminants of blood cultures can occur at the time of sampling the blood or subsequently in the laboratory. The fiddly technique required to take blood from a neonate causes more contaminants in neonatal cultures than in older age groups. Neonates are extremely susceptible to infection though, and may become infected with organisms of low virulence. If it is decided that a blood culture isolate is a contaminant, antibiotics should be stopped. Cultures which take 3 or more days to grow and those containing more than one organism are particularly likely to be contaminants (see p. 37). In the rare cases in which antibiotics were not commenced at the time of blood sampling, repeat blood cultures are necessary. Cases have been described of asymptomatic but persistent bacteraemia.[58] Factors to take into consideration in deciding whether or not a growth from a blood culture is a contaminant are described below.

The organism

The commonest contaminants are not surprisingly those that colonize the skin. Table 2.2 charts blood culture isolates which are almost invariably significant, often significant and those which are almost always a contaminant.[59] Gram-negative organisms, for example, should never be considered a contaminant. In disseminated candidiasis it is not uncommon to find that an earlier growth of candida from a blood culture was dismissed as a probable contaminant.[53] Coagulase-negative staphylococci are the commonest organisms causing LOS and also in many centres the commonest blood culture contaminant. Deciding whether a blood culture growing coagulase-negative staphylococcus reflects a true episode of LOS can be difficult. Rapid growth of the organism in pure culture in all bottles inoculated and associated abnormal laboratory findings (e.g. rising CRP, decreasing platelets) support true sepsis.

How the sample was taken

Recording whether a blood culture sample was taken with ease and considered by the doctor taking it to be a good (sterile) sample can assist interpretation of the result. It should be recorded in the patient's notes at the time of the blood test from which site and what technique was used to take the sample. In addition, recording in the notes the clinical and laboratory indications for performing the test will help to decide in 2 days' time whether the antibiotic course should be completed in view of the possible contaminant result. Inoculating blood into the culture bottles prior to filling other tubes, blood gas machine sites, etc., also reduces the chance of a contaminant. Water-loving organisms such as Pseudomonas or Acinetobacter grow around many environmental sites and can mimic an outbreak if repeated contaminants (pseudobacteraemias) occur.

Discussion of the possible contaminant result with the microbiology laboratory

Septicaemia is generally associated with large numbers of bacteria on culture and contamination of blood cultures with small numbers. Hence rapid growth of an organism is more likely to indicate true sep-

Table 2.2 Significance of blood culture isolates.

Significance	Organisms
Almost always significant	Group B streptococcus *Streptococcus pneumoniae* *Listeria monocytogenes* *Haemophilus influenzae* Group A streptococcus Group C/G streptococci *Neisseria meningitidis* *Neisseria gonorrhoeae* Gram-negative bacilli Candida and other fungi
Sometimes significant (about 50%)	*Staphylococcus aureus* Coagulase-negative staphylococci (*Staph. epidermidis,* etc) Enterococci (*Streptococcus faecalis, Strep. faecium, Strep. bovis,* etc.)* *Streptococcus viridans* group (including *Strep. mitis, Strep. mitior, Strep. milleri, Strep. sanguis,* etc.) Clostridium species Multiple isolates (polymicrobial)
Almost always contaminants	Diphtheroids Propionibacterium Bacillus species

* In early-onset sepsis, may be significant, late-onset usually contaminants.

ticaemia whereas delayed growth is more likely to be due to contamination. Some laboratories perform quantitative or semi-quantitative blood cultures, which can help distinguish contamination from sepsis. Multiple organisms in blood cultures are usually, but not always, contaminants.

Septicaemia

A clinically septic baby with a positive blood culture or urine GBS antigen test should be prescribed a 'full course' of intravenous antibiotics. What constitutes a full course for septicaemia or pneumonia is currently believed to be 7–10 days. As further research evolves, the duration may be based on firm data. Individual variation will exist: if a baby remains clinically ill, the duration of intravenous treatment should be extended. *Listeria monocytogenes* septicaemia is treated for 14 days because it is an intracellular pathogen.

Meningitis requires longer treatment. Most meningitis pathogens, e.g. GBS, require 2–3 weeks of intravenous treatment and Gram-negative meningitis requires at least 21 days, often more, because of ventriculitis. A lumbar puncture must be performed as part of the septic work-up. If the CSF has not been sampled initially for fear of causing respiratory compromise, it should be performed as soon as is clinically safe. The later a lumbar puncture is performed, the more difficult the results are to interpret and a partially treated meningitis may be missed.[55, 56]

SUMMARY

- Start antibiotics early, stop them early.
- Babies with early-onset respiratory distress should receive antibiotics if they have one or more maternal risk factors: spontaneous onset of preterm labour (<37 weeks' gestation), maternal fever (>37.5°C), prolonged rupture of membranes (>18 hours), signs of chorioamnionitis (smelly liquor).
- Spontaneous preterm labour is the commonest risk factor for sepsis, and the one most often forgotten by junior doctors.
- Babies with 2 or more risk factors for sepsis should be started on antibiotics even if they are asymptomatic.
- Prophylactic antibiotics are virtually never indicated.
- Antibiotic use should be as narrow spectrum as possible to cover likely organisms, not broad spectrum.
- Penicillin or ampicillin and an aminoglycoside are preferred for early-onset sepsis.
- Cloxacillin or methicillin and an aminoglycoside are preferred for late-onset sepsis, unless there is widespread colonization with MRSA (in which case, use vancomycin and an aminoglycoside) or with other resistant organisms, or unless other local organisms dictate a different antibiotic policy.
- Antibiotics should be stopped after 2–3 days if blood cultures are negative even if the baby 'looked septic': exceptions to this rule are pneumonia, clinical sepsis plus heavy colonization with a likely pathogen (GBS, Listeria) or clinical sepsis plus GBS antigenuria.
- Antibiotics should be continued for 7–10 days for proven septicaemia with most organisms (blood culture positive or GBS

antigenuria), 14 days for Listeria septicaemia, 2–3 weeks for GBS meningitis and at least 21 days for Gram-negative meningitis.

REFERENCES

1. Boyer KM, Cadzala CA, Burd LI *et al.* Selective intrapartum chemoprophylaxis of neonatal group B streptococcal early-onset disease. I. Epidemiologic rationale. *J Infect Dis* 1983;**148**: 795–801.
2. Bortolussi R, Thompson TR and Ferrieri P. Early-onset pneumococcal sepsis in newborn infants. *Pediatrics* 1977;**60**: 352–355.
3. Dobson SRM and Baker CJ. Enterococcal sepsis in neonates: Features by age at onset and occurrence of focal infection. *Pediatrics* 1990;**85**: 165–171.
4. Bradley JS. Neonatal infections. *Pediatr Infect Dis* 1985;**4**: 315–320.
5. Webber S, Wilkinson AR, Lindsell D *et al.* Neonatal pneumonia. *Arch Dis Child* 1990;**65**: 207–211.
6. Baker CJ and Edwards MS. Group B streptococcal infections. In: Remington JS and Klein JO (eds) *Infectious Diseases of the Fetus and Newborn Infant,* 3rd edn. Philadelphia: WB Saunders, pp 742–881.
7. Mifsud A, Seal D, Wall R and Valman B. Reduced neonatal mortality from infection after introduction of respiratory monitoring. *Br Med J* 1988;**296**: 17–18.
8. Ingram DL, Pendergrass EL, Bromberger PI *et al.* Group B streptococcal disease. *Am J Dis Child* 1980;**134**: 754–758.
9. Sherman MP, Goetzman BW, Ahlfors CE and Wennberg RP. Tracheal aspiration and its clinical correlates in the diagnosis of congenital pneumonia. *Pediatrics* 1980;**65**: 258–263.
10. Sherman MP, Chance KH and Goetzman BW. Gram's stains of tracheal secretions predict neonatal bacteraemia. *Am J Dis Child* 1984;**138**: 848–850.
11. Da Silva O, Ohlsson A and Kenyon C. Accuracy of leukocyte indices and C-reactive protein for diagnosis of neonatal sepsis: a critical review. *Pediatr Infect Dis J* 1995;**14**: 362–366.
12. Boyer KM and Gotoff SP. Early-onset neonatal group B streptococcal disease with selective intrapartum chemoprophylaxis. *N Engl J Med* 1986;**314**: 1665–1669.
13. Centers for Disease Control. Prevention of perinatal group B streptococcal disease: a public health perspective. *MMWR* 1996;**45**: 1–23.
14. Boyle RJ, Chandler BD, Stonestreet BS and Oh W. Early identification of sepsis in infants with respiratory distress. *Pediatrics* 1978;**62**: 744–750.
15. Siegel JD and McCracken GH. Detection of group B streptococcal antigens in body fluids of neonates. *J Pediatr* 1978;**93**: 491–492.
16. Edwards MS and Baker CJ. Prospective diagnosis of early-onset group B streptococcal infection by countercurrent immunoelectrophoresis. *J Pediatr* 1979;**94**: 286–288.

17. Edwards MS, Kasper DL and Baker CJ. Rapid diagnosis of type III group B streptococcal meningitis by latex particle agglutination. *J Pediatr* 1979;**95**: 202–205.
18. Gluck L, Wood HF and Fousek MD. Septicaemia of the newborn. *Pediatr Clin North Am* 1966;**13**: 1131–1148.
19. Manroe BL, Weinberg AG, Rosenfeld CR and Browne R. The neonatal blood count in health and disease. I. Reference values for neutrophilic cells. *J Pediatr* 1979;**95**: 89–98.
20. Rodwell RL, Taylor KMCD, Tudehope DI and Gray PH. Hematologic scoring system in early diagnosis of sepsis in neutropenic newborns. *Pediatr Infect Dis J* 1993;**12**: 372–376.
21. Koenig JM and Christensen RD. Incidence, neutrophil kinetics, and natural history of neutropenia associated with maternal hypertension. *N Engl J Med* 1989;**321**: 557–562.
22. Mouzinho A, Rosemfeld CR, Sanchez PJ and Risser R. Effect of maternal hypertension on neonatal neutropenia and risk of nosocomial infection. *Pediatrics* 1992;**90**: 430–435.
23. Cadnapaphornchai M and Faix RG. Increased nosocomial infection in neutropenic low birth weight (2000 grams or less) infants of hypertensive mothers. *J Pediatr* 1992;**121**: 956–961.
24. Gray JE, Richardson DK, McCormick and Goldmann DA. Coagulase-negative staphylococcal bacteremia among very low birth weight infants: relation to admission illness severity, resource use, and outcome. *Pediatrics* 1995;**95**: 225–230.
25. Moller JC, Nachtrodt G, Tegtmeyer FK *et al.* Prophylactic low-dose vancomycin treatment in very-low-birth-weight infants. *Dev Pharmacol Ther* 1992;**19**: 178–182.
26. Kacica MA, Horgan MJ, Ochoa L *et al.* Prevention of gram-positive sepsis in neonates weighing less than 1500 grams. *J Pediatr* 1994;**125**: 253–258.
27. Spafford PS, Sinkin RA, Cox C *et al.* Prevention of central venous catheter-related coagulase-negative staphylococcal sepsis in neonates. *J Pediatr* 1994;**125**: 259–263.
28. Horgan MJ, Kacica MA and Venezia RA. Prophylactic vancomycin for very-low-birthweight infants (letter; comment). *Lancet* 1992;**340**: 1046–1047.
29. Gin AS and Zhanel GG. Vancomycin-resistant enterococci. *Ann Pharmacother* 1996;**30**: 615–624.
30. Rhinehart E, Smith N, Wennersten C *et al.* Rapid dissemination of beta-lactamase producing aminoglycoside-resistant *Enterococcus faecalis* among patients and staff on an infant and toddler surgical ward. *N Engl J Med* 1990;**323**: 1814–1818.
31. Karanfil LV, Murphy M, Josephson A *et al.* A cluster of vancomycin-resistant *Enterococcus faecium* in an intensive care unit. *Infect Control Hosp Epidemiol* 1992;**13**: 195–200
32. Livornese LL, Dias S, Samel C *et al.* Hospital-acquired infection with vancomycin-resistant *Enterococcus faecium* transmitted by electronic thermometers. *Ann Intern Med* 1992;**117**: 112–116.

33. Boyce JM, Opal SM, Chow JW *et al.* Outbreak of multidrug-resistant *Enterococcus faecium* with transferable *vanB* class vancomycin resistance. *J Clin Microbiol* 1994;**32**: 1148–1153.
34. Centers for Disease Control. Recommendations for preventing the spread of vancomycin resistance. *MMWR* 1994;**44**: 1–13.
35. Edmiston CE. Vancomycin resistance: when failure becomes an opportunity for leadership. *Ann Pharmacother* 1996;**30**: 680–682.
36. Sims ME, Yoo Y, You H *et al.* Prophylactic oral nystatin and fungal infections in very-low-birthweight infants. *Am J Perinatol* 1988;5: 33–39.
37. Australasian Study Group For Neonatal Infections. Early-onset group B streptococcal infections in Aboriginal and non-Aboriginal infants. *Med J Aust* 1995;**163**: 302–306.
38. Mulhall A, de Louvois J, James J. Pharmacokinetics and safety of ceftriaxone in the neonate. *Eur J Pediatr* 1985;**144**: 379–382.
39. Isaacs D and Wilkinson AR. Antibiotic use in the neonatal unit. *Arch Dis Child* 1987;**62**: 204–208.
40. Jeffery HE, McIntosh EDG. Antenatal screening and non-selective intrapartum chemoprophylaxis for group B streptococcus. *Aust NZ J Obstet Gynaecol* 1994;**34**: 14–19.
41. Gilbert GL, Isaacs D, Burgess MA *et al.* Prevention of neonatal group B streptococcal sepsis: Is routine antenatal screening appropriate? *Aust NZ J Obstet Gynaecol* 1995;**35**: 120–126.
42. Baker CJ, Rench MA, Edwards MS *et al.* Immunisation of pregnant women with a polysaccharide vaccine of group B streptococcus. *N Engl J Med* 1988;**319**: 1180–1185.
43. White RD, Townsend TR, Stephens MA and Moxon ER. Are surveillance of resistant enteric bacilli and antimicrobial usage among neonates in a newborn intensive care unit useful? *Pediatrics* 1981;**68**: 1–4.
44. Isaacs D, Wilkinson AR and Moxon ER. Surveillance of colonisation and late-onset septicaemia in neonates. *J Hosp Infect* 1987;**10**: 114–119.
45. Modi N, Damjanovic V and Cooke RWI. Outbreak of cephalosporin resistant *Enterobacter cloacae* infection in a neonatal intensive care unit. *Arch Dis Child* 1987;**62**: 148–151.
46. Spritzer R, Kamp HJVD, Dzoljic G and Sauer PJJ. Five years of cefotaxime use in a neonatal intensive care unit. *Pediatr Infect Dis J* 1990;**9**: 92–96.
47. Evans ME, Schaffer W, Federspiel CF *et al.* Sensitivity, specificity and predictive value of body surface cultures in a neonatal intensive care unit. *JAMA* 1988;**259**: 248–252.
48. Slagle TA, Bifano EM, Wolf JW and Gross SJ. Routine endotracheal cultures for the prediction of sepsis in ventilated babies. *Arch Dis Child* 1989;**64**: 34–38.
49. Pichichero ME and Todd JK. Detection of neonatal bacteraemia. *J Pediatr* 1979;**94**: 958–960.
50. Isaacs D, Wilkinson AR and Moxon ER. Duration of antibiotic courses for neonates. *Arch Dis Child* 1987;**62**: 727–744.
51. Lacey RW. Evolution of microorganisms and antibiotic resistance. *Lancet* 1984;**ii**: 1022–1025.

52. Goldman DA, Leclair J and Macone A. Bacterial colonisation of neonates admitted to an intensive care environment. *J Pediatr* 1978;**93**: 288–293.
53. Weese-Mayer DE, Fondriest DW, Brouilette RT and Shulman ST. Risk factors associated with candidemia in the neonatal intensive care unit: a case-control study. *Pediatr Infect Dis J* 1987;**6**: 190–196.
54. Squire E, Favara B and Todd J. Diagnosis of neonatal bacterial infection: hematologic and pathologic findings in fatal and nonfatal cases. *Pediatrics* 1979;**64**: 60–64.
55. McIntyre P and Isaacs D. Lumbar puncture in suspected neonatal sepsis (annotation). *J Paediatr Child Health* 1995;**31**: 1–2.
56. Visser VE and Hall RT. Lumbar puncture in the evaluation of suspected neonatal sepsis. *J Pediatr* 1980;**96**: 1063–1067.
57. Adamkin DH, Marshall E and Weiner LB. The placental transfer of ampicillin. *Am J Perinatol* 1984;**1**: 310–311.
58. Albers WH, Tyler CW and Boxerbaum B. Asymptomatic bacteremia in the newborn infant. *J Pediatr* 1966;**69**: 193–197.
59. Isaacs D and Moxon ER. *Neonatal Infections*. Oxford: Butterworth Heinemann, 1991, pp 49–50.

3

Human Milk and the Preterm Infant

Anthony F. Williams

> *'The food for infants is human milk; it is, with certain exceptions, the only one which ought to be given to weaklings and newly born children.'*
> (P Budin, 1902)

Despite Budin's early enthusiasm,[1] controversy persists about the suitability of human milk for preterm infants. Over 60 years ago it was observed that premature infants fed on half-skimmed cow's milk showed faster rates of growth and nitrogen retention.[2] The more recent appearance of special formulas for preterm infants led some to conclude 'breast is not necessarily best'.[3] Yet 'feeding' and 'nutrition' are not synonymous where the newborn infant is concerned. Outcome may be measured in dimensions other than growth.[4]

'NON-NUTRITIONAL' OUTCOMES OF FEEDING

Human milk is a tissue, consisting of living cells in a matrix of immune, trophic and other factors as well as nutrients. *In vitro* evidence suggests that such factors play a part in extrauterine adaptation and protection of the newborn but sceptics could argue that they merely function to protect the breast. Animal studies have limited value as species differ in functional maturity at birth and mechanisms of immunity. Although the provision of passive mucosal immunity by breastfeeding is now well understood, questions remain about the clinical relevance of many other milk components. For example, human milk lactoferrin (molecular weight 78 kDa) is absorbed by breastfed babies and appears in their urine about 24 hours later.[5] Could other trophic factors be absorbed and what might be their role?

Much epidemiological evidence on the benefits of breastfeeding term babies is beset by problems of confounding as socioeconomic and educational factors strongly influence infant feeding practice.[6] For preterm infants, however, limited evidence is available from randomized controlled studies that human milk modifies outcome.

Infection

In a Delhi study, hospitalized low birth weight infants were allocated to receive human milk only, formula only, formula mixed with fresh milk or formula with colostrum.[7] Human milk feeding significantly reduced risk of superficial, systemic and enteric infection: the more human milk babies received, the lower the risk. Further randomized studies showed that Holder-pasteurized (63°C for 30 min) milk was as effective as fresh unless mixed with any formula.[8] The possibility of formula contamination was excluded by culture, suggesting that human milk had a protective effect.

Feed Tolerance and Necrotizing Enterocolitis

Human milk is better tolerated than formula. Infants weighing <1850 g randomly allocated to donor breast milk tolerated enteral feeding significantly earlier than those receiving preterm formula.[9] This could reflect more rapid gastric emptying,[10] accelerated gastrointestinal adaptation[11] or differences in the endocrine response to feeding.[12]

Although several feeding variables have been associated with necrotizing enterocolitis (NEC), most studies are flawed by small size or their selection of controls.[13] Pathogenesis probably requires ischaemic mucosa, substrate in the gut lumen and colonization by pathogenic bacteria.[14] A 6–10 fold increase in NEC was found among formula-fed infants in a retrospective study of almost 1000 infants weighing <1850 g,[15] the majority of whom had been randomly allocated to receive donor human milk, term or preterm formula alone or in combination with the mother's own breast milk. The effect was most marked among more mature babies. Three further observations were relevant to clinical practice: mixing human milk with formula was protective; pasteurized milk was effective (see Milk Banks below); and, whereas postponing enteral feeding with formula reduced the risk of NEC, postponing human milk feeding did not.

Diet, Growth and Neurological Development

Two randomized trials[16, 17] have shown that very low birth weight (VLBW) infants fed on *donor* human milk grow more slowly than those fed preterm formula. Although a randomized study of feeding mother's own milk would be unethical, a third study[18] included a group fed pasteurized human milk from donors who delivered prematurely ('preterm milk'). Their growth rates were similar to those of babies fed preterm formula and significantly faster than those of a term donor milk group. Diet allocation was sequential rather than randomized but this small study (n = 20/group) is the only unbiased comparison of feeding 'term' or 'preterm' human milk.

The long-term importance of early growth, particularly weight gain, remains debatable. Much interest now focuses on neurodevelopmental outcome. An early study[19] compared Bayley scale measurements at 9 months of babies <1850 g at birth randomly allocated to receive solely banked human milk or preterm formula in the neonatal period. The difference was not statistically significant despite large differences in early growth rate.[16] In contrast, the same group noted large differences in developmental outcome at 18 months between babies fed a preterm or term formula.[20] Pooled analysis of these parallel randomized studies (which used the same preterm formula) confirmed that donor human milk was associated with better neurological outcome than term formula,[21] a surprising finding as pasteurized 'drip' donor milk of very low energy content was used (mean [SD]: 460 [70] kcal/l).[16]

Although no randomized studies are available, provision of mother's own milk for preterm babies has been associated with an intelligence quotient advantage of 8.3 points at 7 years of age, after adjustment for identifiable confounding factors.[22] However, the possibility that maternal intention to breastfeed was a proxy for other aspects of parenting cannot be excluded.

If, as these and other findings[6] suggest, human milk promotes neurological development, the mechanism remains unclear. There is very limited evidence to support speculation that the n–3: n–6 long chain polyunsaturated fatty acid (LCPUFA) of human milk[23] is responsible. The functional implications of differences in brain lipid composition[24] attributed to early diet have not been characterized in sufficiently large studies and the potential role of many other human milk constituents (e.g. growth factors, sialic acid)[25] on brain development is unexplored.

NUTRITIONAL ASPECTS AND SUPPLEMENTATION

Term and Preterm Milk

There are many qualitative differences between milk produced by mothers delivering at term ('term milk') or before term ('preterm milk'),[26] but whether they reflect mammary epithelial 'leakiness' associated with early parturition or the effect of expressing lower volumes of milk is still unclear.[27] Sodium and protein content are inversely proportional to the volume expressed, and the composition of 'preterm milk' is similar to that produced at weaning. This may also explain the higher sodium content of hand-expressed milk.[28]

When breastfeeding the healthy infant, milk composition partly reflects appetite demand[29] but the demand–supply balance can be distorted by expression. In the case of a <1 kg baby, the mother is effectively feeding a pump with an inappropriately voracious appetite! Manipulating the expression regimen might theoretically adjust milk composition to the baby's requirements but there have been no formal studies, other than on separation of fore- and hind-milk.[30] Modification by maternal diet has been reported[31]: milk medium chain triglyceride content was increased but this offers no advantage for most preterm infants.

Although the variable composition of human milk is sometimes seen as a nuisance, it is important to remember that babies' nutritional requirements vary almost as widely. For example, there is a 2-fold difference between extremes of resting energy expenditure, and requirements for growth vary with the type of tissue made.[32] The reported weight velocity in a group of preterm babies varied from 8 to 24 g /kg/day,[16] even when formula of standard composition was fed. This emphasizes that many factors influence the growth of preterm babies and setting 'requirements' for such a heterogeneous group is an imprecise science. A means of individualizing intake by measuring nutritional response might be ideal. Can this be achieved when human milk is used?

Energy and Protein

At all protein intakes, nitrogen balance is affected by energy supply. Consequently these two aspects are considered together.

Energy

The average energy content of human milk is 700 kcal/l but it varies with fat content from <500 kcal/l (foremilk) to >900 kcal/l (hindmilk).

Fat absorption from human milk is very efficient, although it is reduced after heating to 63°C,[33] probably through inactivation of human milk bile-salt stimulated lipase. Fat may be lost by flotation and adherence to tubing during administration and peroxidation of polyunsaturated fatty acids can occur, although the latter is a greater problem with formula.[34] Milk energy content can be approximated simply using the 'creamatocrit' test,[35, 36] although it is unreliable for pasteurized or frozen milk. Other methods of measuring the macronutrient content for 'individualizing' supplements have been proposed.[37]

If a baby is not thriving on 200 ml/kg/day of human milk, consideration should be given to whether energy or protein intake needs to be supplemented. Assessment of protein:energy status can usefully complement measurement of fat intake. Blood urea concentration is a helpful pointer as it correlates with urinary nitrogen excretion.[38] This rises when energy supply is limiting or protein is provided to excess because it is oxidized rather than deposited in tissue. A blood urea >3 mmol/l in a baby *who is not thriving* commonly signifies energy deficiency or the presence of a catabolic state, such as that induced by steroid therapy.[39] Inappropriate use of protein supplements will further increase urea production and renal solute load. Increasing energy intake with hindmilk[30] or a fat/carbohydrate supplement (e.g. *Duocal*) is more appropriate. On the other hand, the baby with a low blood urea <1 mmol/l *who is not thriving* is likely to be protein deficient (Figure 3.1).[38, 40]

Protein

Human milk contains many more types of protein than formula. There are many ways of expressing protein content,[37] but the commonest is total nitrogen (measured by the Kjeldahl technique) multiplied by 6.38. About 25% of the nitrogen in human milk is 'non-protein' nitrogen,[41] a mixture of amino acids, urea, short peptides, nucleotides, amino-sugars, etc. Compared to formula, human milk protein digestibility is *low*[42] because about 20% consists of secretory immunoglobulin A and other immune proteins. These uncertainties about nitrogen bioavailability have led to suggestions that 5.18 would be a more suitable conversion factor than 6.38.[43] The efficiency with which *nutritional* protein is incorporated into tissue must be very high. Urea nitrogen, which accounts for up to 15% of nitrogen in milk,[44] may also be incorporated into protein though little is known about the effect of iatrogenic and other influences on the process in preterm babies.[45]

Several small studies, some uncontrolled, have shown faster mean rates of nitrogen retention and growth when human milk is supplemented with protein. Proteins from several sources have been used:

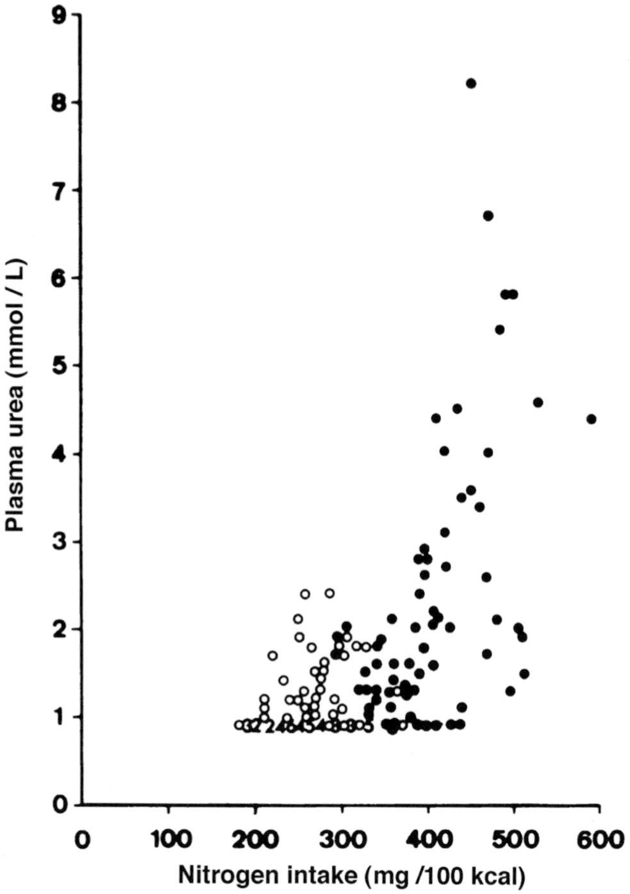

Figure 3.1 Influence of human milk nitrogen intake on plasma urea. Pooled weekly data from 28 babies weighing <1500 g at birth are shown. Nitrogen intake was varied by randomly allocating infants to high protein human formula (●) or low protein human formula (○). Numbers indicate replicate observations. Plasma urea shows a tendency to rise at intakes exceeding 400 mg/100 kcal indicating protein excess. At low protein intakes >50% of observations fall under 1 mmol/l and almost all at <2 mmol/l, indicating protein deficiency.[40]

human milk,[40, 46–50] human albumin,[51] 'meat'[48] and cow's milk.[50–52] The routine use of 'fortifiers' is now common, but is it really justified?

At an energy intake of 120–130 kcal/kg/day, provision of 3–3.5 g/kg/day human milk protein supports mean rates of growth and nitrogen retention comparable to those of the fetus during the last trimester of pregnancy.[40, 47] The human milk protein requirements of VLBW babies have been studied by converting donor milk into human 'formulae' of dissimilar protein content (high protein: 21 g protein/l; low protein: 12 g/l) but similar energy content (740 kcal/l).[40] 'Formula' composition approximated that of milk collected from mothers delivering at term ('low protein') or preterm ('high protein').[18] VLBW babies were randomly allocated to a human formula at birth and it was given alone or with any mother's own milk available to a maximum of 200 ml/kg/day. The 28 babies recruited therefore received a range of protein intakes between 2.0 and 4.2 g/kg/day. Babies in the 'high protein' group grew significantly more quickly. Balance studies undertaken every 3 weeks quantified the relationship between protein intake, nitrogen retention and growth. The composition of tissue deposited (18–21 mg nitrogen/g) was similar to that of fetal tissue (17–24 mg/g)[53] and the relationship between nitrogen intake (x) and retention (y) was given by (Figure 3.2):

$$y = -1477 + 290\ (\ln x \text{ mg/kg/day})$$

The validity of this relationship was confirmed by reference to other studies of the relationship between human milk nitrogen intake and retention (Figure 3.3). Solving the equation shows that fetal rates of nitrogen retention during the last trimester of pregnancy (340 mg/kg/day) could be achieved by feeding 3.4 g human milk protein/kg/day at the measured mean energy intake of 128 kcal/kg/day.

The mean protein content of milk produced by mothers of preterm babies during the first month of lactation[18, 53] is sufficient to meet these intakes if it is fed at 180–200 ml/kg/day. As at least 50% of mothers produce milk of adequate protein content, a selective, rather than routine, approach to protein supplementation seems more desirable. This can be based on the assessment of weight gain and blood urea concentration (see *Energy* above).

Wide variation in the protein content of preterm milk raises some questions about the safety of routine protein supplementation. In one study, it ranged from 12 to 25 g/l at 14 days postpartum.[53] Although adding a typical 0.7 g protein as 'fortifier' to each 100 ml of milk might be beneficial in the lower range, protein intake at the top could exceed 5.5 g/kg/day. Intakes exceeding 3.5 g/kg/day or a nitrogen:energy ratio >400 mg/100 kcal are most unlikely to help and are associated with rises in blood urea (Figure 3.1) and urinary nitrogen excretion.[38, 40]

The only published pragmatic study of routine human milk fortification was a large randomized controlled trial ($n \approx 140$/group) among infants weighing <1850 g. There was no overall benefit to short-term

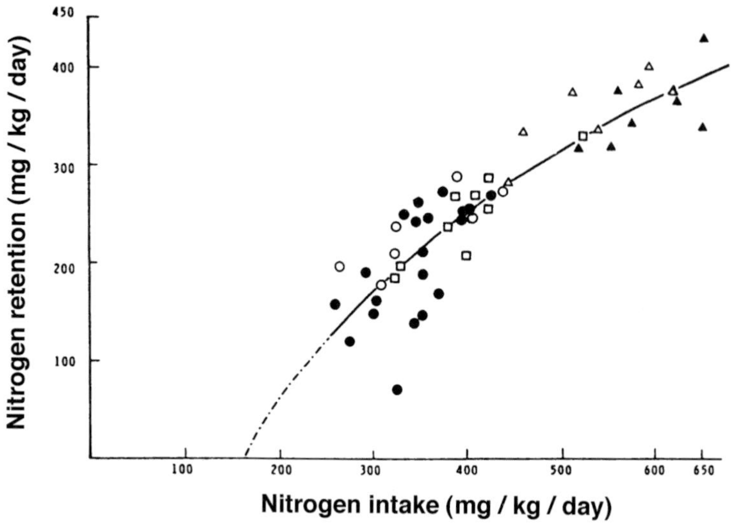

Figure 3.2 Relationship between human milk nitrogen intake and nitrogen retention. Results from fifty 3-day metabolic balances performed on 28 babies <1500 g at birth randomly allocated to diets (see text). Triangles indicate babies receiving 'high protein' human formula alone (▲) or mixed with mother's milk (△). Circles indicate babies receiving 'low protein' formula alone (●) or with mother's milk (○). Squares indicate babies receiving unmodified mother's milk only. Reproduced with permission from Ref 40.

growth or 18-month developmental outcome.[54] The 'fortified' group showed significantly higher mean plasma urea concentration ($p = 0.04$) which exceeded 5 mmol/l in 16% ($p = 0.02$). A further worrying aspect was the greater incidence of infection ($p = 0.04$) and NEC ($p = 0.12$) in 'fortified' babies. A small weight gain advantage associated with fortification (1.6 g/kg/day) was found in the subgroup given most human milk but seems unlikely to be of any short- or long-term benefit.

In summary, *routine* use of protein supplements ('fortifiers') does not seem to be justified by current evidence and has been associated with undesirable effects. Future research should concentrate on individualizing supplementation using measures of intake and indicators of protein:energy status.

Calcium, Phosphorus and Vitamin D

The fetus accrues 100–120 mg/kg/day of calcium and 60–75 mg/kg/day of phosphorus.[65] Human milk contains only about 35 mg of calcium/

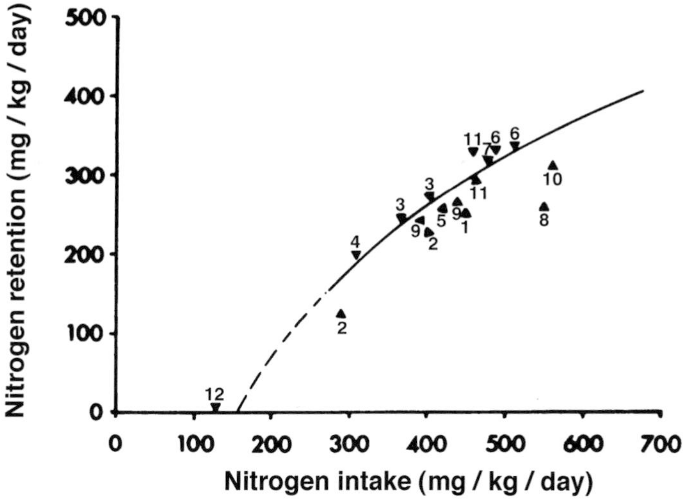

Figure 3.3 Relationship between human milk nitrogen intake and nitrogen retention. The curve was derived from experiments shown in Figure 3.2 (see text for equation). Numbered points indicate published data from other studies of human milk feeding: 1 = Ref. 53, 2 = 56, 3 = 57, 4 = 58, 5 = 59, 6 = 56, 7 = 64, 8 = 42, 9 = 60, 10 = 61, 11 = 62, 12 = 63.

100 ml and 15 mg of phosphorus/100 ml.[26] Phosphorus is needed both for lean tissue and bone and calcium almost entirely for bone. There they are deposited in a ratio given by the structure of hydroxyapatite ($Ca_5(PO_4)_3OH.F$). At low phosphorus intakes (e.g. from human milk), the lean tissue phosphorus requirement limits its availability for bone; at high phosphorus intake (e.g. from preterm formula), calcium may be limiting. The optimal Ca:P ratio therefore rises with intake from about 1.4:1 to 2:1. That of human milk (approximately 2:1) is thus inappropriately high for the small preterm infant with a low calcium intake.

Phosphorus

Phosphorus deficiency can occur when human milk is fed to a very preterm infant.[66] Hypercalciuria and sometimes hypercalcaemia are seen. Given the low calcium intake this seems paradoxical but emphasizes that calcium supplements alone have no value and can be harmful if given without phosphorus. Phosphorus deficiency is characterized biochemically by a plasma phosphorus concentration of <1.5 mmol/l or the absence of phosphaturia.[67] Ultimately, it results in metabolic bone disease of prematurity. A small randomized and blinded study in babies

<1250 g who were hypophosphataemic during the first 2 weeks of life showed that radiologically apparent metabolic bone disease was abolished by supplementation with 50 mg of phosphorus/day. Forty per cent of placebo-treated controls were affected.[67]

Vitamin D intake

Calcium absorption is greater with 1000 IU vitamin D/day than 400 IU, but is not further enhanced by doses >1000 IU/day;[68] 1000 IU/day is therefore sufficient and can be provided by, for example, 0.6 ml Abidec plus 600 IU calciferol.

Calcium

Calcium balance may be affected by many factors: drugs (e.g. diuretics, corticosteroids), nutrients (e.g. fatty acids, phosphates) and the molecular species used (e.g. phosphate, gluconate, glycerophosphate).[69] As the intake–response relationship can be unpredictable for calcium and phosphorus, an attempt has been made to adjust intake according to the calcium and phosphorus concentration of spot urine samples. If simultaneous calcium and phosphorus concentrations of >1.2 and >0.4 mmol/l, respectively, can be achieved, bone mineral content is greater.[70]

In the absence of monitoring, supplementation with calcium and phosphorus together can be haphazard; milk composition varies and supplements must be given at different times to avoid co-precipitation. Sixty milligrams of elemental calcium and 30 mg elemental phosphorus per 100 ml of milk have been recommended.[71] The uptake of calcium and phosphorus from 'fortifiers' also varies.[69, 72] Despite promoting a short-term advantage in bone mineral content (BMC), differences between 'fortified' and control infants in one study disappeared after 3 months.[74]

Long-term outcome

Although undermineralization is still detectable at 1 year in babies fed human milk,[75] catch-up occurs by 2 years.[76] Outcome in the longer term is not very clear. One study suggested ex-preterm infants still had reduced BMC in late childhood,[77] but a follow-up study of neonates <1850 g randomly allocated to donor human milk or preterm formula surprisingly showed that BMC at 5 years was *greater* among those fed donor milk and *inversely* correlated with early formula (hence calcium and phosphorus) intake.[78] More long-term data are clearly needed.

More also needs to be learned about the effect of early mineral intake on height: one study of factors influencing the length of ex-preterm infants at 18 months showed that both human milk feeding and elevated alkaline phosphatase concentration (>1200 IU/l) were independently associated with mean deficits of 0.9 cm and 1.6 cm, respectively.[79] The effect on later height is unknown.

HELPING MOTHERS BREASTFEED A PRETERM BABY

Demographic factors associated with low birth weight in the United Kingdom correlate with intention to bottle-feed. Moreover, birth may anticipate antenatal feeding education. Consequently, breastfeeding must be discussed with parents as early as possible. Health professionals sometimes fear this will increase parents' burden, though most mothers value this unique means of maintaining a physical link despite the separation as a result of early birth.

Mothers should be shown how to express as soon as possible and given written advice.* Milk yield is increased by frequent expression[80] (preferably every 3–4 hours) and 'double pumping' (i.e. simultaneous rather than sequential expression of both breasts) using an electric pump.[81] Milk should be collected in containers which can be easily cleaned and sterilized. Fat and leukocytes may be lost by adherence to glass, and immunoglobulin to stainless steel, polypropylene and polyethylene.[82, 83]

In 2 randomized studies, skin–skin contact ('kangaroo care') between a mother and her VLBW baby helped maintain lactation.[84, 85] This has other advantages too,[86] particularly where resources are limited. A randomized study in Ecuador demonstrated reductions in the cost of postneonatal care for VLBW infants and infectious morbidity.[87]

Babies can suck effectively from 32 weeks' postconceptional age onwards. Twelve of 17 VLBW babies consecutively admitted to a British neonatal unit started breastfeeding at a mean postnatal age of 11 days and 10 were fully breastfed at a mean age of 27 days.[88] Oxygen saturation is better maintained during breastfeeding than bottlefeeding in VLBW babies, including those with chronic lung disease.[89] If the mother cannot be present to breastfeed, gavage or cup feeding may be preferable to bottles: a descriptive study suggested that cup feeding from a postconceptional age of 30 weeks increased breastfeeding rate at discharge, though controlled studies are needed.[90]

If milk yield falls, advice on expression technique and frequency is probably more important than resort to drugs. An uncontrolled study

* For example *Expressing your breast milk*. Leaflet produced by the UK UNICEF Baby Friendly Initiative, 20 Guilford Street, London WC1N 1DZ.

of metaclopramide for prematurely delivered mothers demonstrated a rise in basal prolactin levels and a doubling of milk yield,[91] but evidence in mothers of term infants is inconsistent.[92] Metoclopramide is thus of uncertain value and is not licensed for this indication in the UK.

STORING AND ADMINISTERING HUMAN MILK

Human milk may contain pathogenic bacteria.[93] Some units routinely screen human milk before administration but this necessitates storage pending culture and so fresh milk is never given. A 14-month audit of bacteriologically screening human milk for 98 preterm infants <14 days old showed that all received coagulase-negative Staphylococci at least once, 41% *Staphylococcus aureus* and 64% Gram-negative bacilli. However, no adverse clinical events were ascribed to exposure[94] and coagulase-negative Staphylococci isolated from blood were of a different strain to those received in milk. As the available evidence suggests that fresh human milk reduces risk of infection,[7, 8] routine culture or pasteurization of milk to be fed to the mother's own baby seems to be unnecessary.

Hygienic expression technique and care to eliminate cross-infection risk from shared breast pumps are essential. Hand-expressed milk contains fewer bacteria.[95] Guidelines* on the collection and handling of a mother's own milk have recently been endorsed by the British Association for Perinatal Medicine amongst others. Expressed milk should be given to the baby as soon as possible or refrigerated. No significant growth occurs at 2–4°C for up to 48 hours[96] and bacterial content *falls* during refrigeration. Significant bacterial growth does not occur over 5[97] or 8 days[98] provided that milk is kept constantly at <4°C. Alternatively, it may be frozen at –20°C and thawed in a refrigerator for use. Once thawed, the milk is preferably used within 12 hours (24 hours at most)[4] because freezing impairs inhibitory activity to a greater degree than refrigeration,[98] possibly by killing cells.

Small bolus feeds are preferable to continuous infusion because significant bacterial growth may occur in both human milk and formula under such conditions.[99] Moreover, fat may be lost by adherence to tubes[100] and nutrients photodegraded, particularly riboflavin and vitamin A.[101] Peroxidation of lipid can also occur.[34] Feeds should be changed at 4-hour intervals[4] in the interests of bacteriological safety.

---

* *Guidelines for the collection, storage and handling of mother's breast milk to be fed to her own baby on a neonatal unit.* Available from the United Kingdom Association for Milk Banking, Milk Bank, Queen Charlotte's and Chelsea Hospital, Goldhawk Road, London W6 0XG.

Milk Banks

Milk banking is the collection, processing and storage of milk to feed babies other than the donor's own. Pooled human milk has been identified as a possible vector in only one reported case of HIV-1 infection,[102] but current United Kingdom Guidelines* require 3 independent safeguards against transmission of HIV and other viruses:

- selection of low-risk donors;
- serological screening; and
- heat-treatment of milk to a minimum of 56°C for 30 min (it is known that heating to 56°C[103] or 62.5°C[104] inactivates HIV inoculated into human milk).

Opinions on the place of banked human milk in neonatal care vary. In the UK, many new banks have opened but in Canada a statement discouraging the practice has been issued.[105]

SUMMARY

The complex composition of human milk clinically benefits preterm infants in ways formula cannot. It is better tolerated, reduces infective morbidity and probably stimulates neurological development in a way which is not understood. Although the composition of milk from term donors is suboptimal, that of own mother's milk is more appropriate though highly variable. Supplementation should take account of both this variability and the heterogeneous requirements of preterm infants as a group. The case for routinely supplementing a mother's milk with 'fortifiers' is weak and significant risks have been associated with this practice. Mothers should be encouraged to breastfeed however small their baby.

REFERENCES

1. Budin P. *The Nursling*. Translated by Maloney WJ. Caxton: London, 1907.
2. Gordon HH, Levine SZ, Wheatly MA and Marples E. Respiratory metabolism in infancy and childhood. The nitrogen metabolism in premature infants – comparative studies of human and cow's milk. *Am J Dis Child* 1937;**54**: 1030–1044.
3. Anonymous. Breast not necessarily best. *Lancet* 1988;**i**: 624–626.
4. Williams AF. Human milk and the preterm baby. *BMJ* 1993;**306**: 1628–1629.

* *Guidelines for the establishment and operation of human milk banks in the UK.* Royal College of Paediatrics and Child Health, London, 1994.

5. Hutchens TW, Henry JF, Yip T-T *et al.* Origin of intact lactoferrin and its DNA-binding fragments found in the urine of human milk fed preterm infants. Evaluation by stable isotopic enrichment. *Pediatr Res* 1991;**29**: 243–250.
6. British Paediatric Association, Standing Committee on Nutrition. Is breast-feeding beneficial in the UK? *Arch Dis Child* 1994;**71**: 376–380.
7. Naryanan I, Prakash K, Prabhakar AK and Gujral VV. A planned prospective evaluation of the anti-infective property of varying quantities of expressed human milk. *Acta Paediatr Scand* 1982;**71**: 441–445.
8. Naryanan I, Prakash K, Murthy NS and Gujral VV. Randomised controlled trial of effect of raw and Holder pasteurised human milk and of formula supplements on incidence of neonatal infection. *Lancet* 1984;**ii**: 1111–1112.
9. Lucas A. AIDS and human milk bank closures. *Lancet* 1987;**i**: 1092–1093.
10. Ewer AK, Durbin GM, Morgan MEI and Booth IW. Gastric emptying in preterm infants. *Arch Dis Child* 1994;**71**: F24–F27.
11. Heird WC, Schwartz SM and Hansen I. Colostrum induced enteric mucosal growth in beagle puppies. *Pediatr Res* 1984;**18**: 512–515.
12. Lucas A, Sarson DL, Blackburn AM, Adrian TE and Aynsley Green A. Breast *versus* bottle: endocrine responses are different with formula feeding. *Lancet* 1980;**i**: 1267–1269.
13. Williams AF. Role of feeding in the pathogenesis of necrotising enterocolitis. *Semin Neonatol* 1997; **2**: 263–271.
14. Koslowske AM. A unifying hypothesis for pathogenesis and prevention of necrotising enterocolitis. *J Pediatr* 1990;**117**: S68–S74.
15. Lucas A and Cole TJ. Breast milk and neonatal necrotising enterocolitis. *Lancet* 1990;**336**: 1519–1523.
16. Lucas A, Gore SM, Cole TJ *et al.* Multicentre trial on feeding low birthweight infants: effects of diet on early growth. *Arch Dis Child* 1984;**59**: 722–730
17. Tyson JE, Lasky RE, Mize CE *et al.* Growth, metabolic response and development in very low birth weight infants fed human milk or enriched formula. *J Pediatr* 1983;**103**: 95–104.
18. Gross SJ. Growth and biochemical response of preterm infants fed human milk or modified infant formula. *N Engl J Med* 1983;**308**: 237–241.
19. Lucas A, Morley R, Cole TJ *et al.* Early diet in preterm babies and developmental status in infancy. *Arch Dis Child* 1989;**64**: 1570–1578.
20. Lucas A, Morley R, Cole TJ *et al.* Early diet in preterm babies and developmental status at 18 months. *Lancet* 1990;**335**: 1477–1481.
21. Lucas A, Morley R, Cole TJ and Gore SM. A randomised multicentre study of human milk versus formula and later development in preterm infants. *Arch Dis Child* 1994;**70**: F141–F146.
22. Lucas A, Morley RM, Cole TJ, Lister G and Leeson-Payne C. Breast milk and subsequent intelligence quotient in children born preterm. *Lancet* 1992;**339**: 261–264.
23. Innis SM. Human milk and formula fatty acids. *J Pediatr* 1992; **120**: S56–61.
24. Farquharson J, Cockburn F, Patrick WA, Jamieson EC and Logan RW. Infant cerebral cortex phospholipid fatty acid composition and diet. *Lancet* 1992;**340**: 810–813.

25. Heine W, Wutzke KD and Radke M. Sialinsaure in muttermilch und sauglingsformelnahrungen. *Monatsschrift Kinderheilkunde* 1993;**141**: 946–950.
26. Williams AF. Lactation and infant feeding. In: McLaren DS, Burman D, Belton NR and Williams AF (eds) *Textbook of Paediatric Nutrition*, 4th edn. Edinburgh: Churchill Livingstone, 1991, pp 21–45.
27. Anderson GH. The effect of prematurity on milk composition and its physiological basis. *Fed Proc* 1984;**43**: 2438–2442.
28. Lang S, Lawrence CJ and Orme RL. Sodium in hand and pump expressed breast milk. *Early Hum Dev* 1994;**38**: 131–138.
29. Woolridge MW, Ingram JC and Baum JD. Do changes in pattern of breast usage alter the baby's nutrient intake? *Lancet* 1990;**336**: 395–397.
30. Valentine CJ, Hurst NM and Schanler RJ. Hindmilk improves weight gain in low birth weight infants fed human milk. *J Pediatr Gastroenterol Nutr* 1994;**18**: 474–477.
31. Silber GH, Hachey DL, Schanler RJ and Garza C. Manipulation of maternal diet to alter fatty acid composition of human milk intended for preterm infants. *Am J Clin Nutr* 1988;**47**: 810–814.
32. Brooke OG. Energy needs in infancy. In: Fomon SJ and Heird WC (eds). *Energy and Protein Needs in Infancy*. Orlando: Academic Press, 1986, pp 3–17.
33. Williamson S, Finucane E, Ellis E and Gamsu HR. Effect of heat treatment of human milk on absorption of nitrogen, fat, sodium, calcium and phosphorus by preterm infants. *Arch Dis Child* 1978;**53**: 555–563.
34. van Zoeren-Grobben D, Morson RMW, Ester WM and Berger HM. Lipid peroxidation in human milk and infant formula: effect of storage, tube feeding and exposure to phototherapy. *Acta Paediatr Scand* 1993;**82**: 545–549.
35. Lucas A, Gibbs JAH, Lyster RLJ and Baum JD. Creamatocrit: simple clinical technique for estimating fat concentration and energy value of human milk. *BMJ* 1978;**i**: 1018–1020.
36. Lemons JA, Schreiner RL and Gresham EL. Simple method for determining the caloric and fat content of human milk. *Pediatrics* 1980;**66**: 626–628.
37. Polberger S and Lonnerdal B. Simple and rapid macronutrient analysis of human milk for individualised fortification: basis for improved nutritional management of very low birth weight infants. *J Pediatr Gastroenterol Nutr* 1993;**17**: 283–290.
38. Polberger SKT, Axelsson IE and Raiha NCR. Urinary and serum urea as indicators of protein metabolism in very low birthweight infants fed varying human milk protein intakes. *Acta Paediatr Scand* 1990;**79**: 737–742.
39. Williams AF and Jones MG. Dexamethasone increases plasma amino acid concentrations in bronchopulmonary dysplasia. *Arch Dis Child* 1992;**67**: 5–9.
40. Williams AF. *Absorption, Tolerance and Utilisation of Human Milk Constituents by Very low Birth Weight Infants.* DPhil Thesis, University of Oxford, 1987.
41. Carlsson SE. Human milk non-protein nitrogen: occurrence and possible functions. *Adv Pediatr* 1985;**32**: 43–70.
42. Brooke OG, Wood C and Barley J. Energy balance, nitrogen balance and growth in preterm infants fed expressed breast milk, a premature infant formula and two low solute adapted formulae. *Arch Dis Child* 1982;**57**: 898–904.

43. Hambraeus L, Fransson G-B and Lonnerdal B. Nutritional availability of breast milk protein. *Lancet* 1984;**ii**: 167–168.
44. Harzer G, Franzke V and Bindels JG. Human milk non-protein nitrogen components: changing patterns of free amino acids and urea in the course of lactation. *Am J Clin Nutr* 1984;**40**: 303–309.
45. Jackson AA. Urea as a nutrient: bioavailability and role in nitrogen economy. *Arch Dis Child* 1994;**70**: 3–4.
46. Ronnholm KAR, Perheentupa J, Siimes MA. Supplementation with human milk protein improves growth of small premature infants fed human milk. *Pediatrics* 1986; **77**: 649–653.
47. Polberger SKT, Axelsson IA and Raiha NCR. Growth of very low birth weight infants on varying amounts of human milk protein. *Pediatr Res* 1989;**25**: 414–419.
48. Boehm G, Senger H, Friedrich M, Muller DM and Beyreiβ K. Protein supplementation of human milk for the nutrition of VLBW infants: Human milk protein *vs*. meat protein hydrolysate. *Klin Padiatr* 1990;**202**: 316–320.
49. Raschko PK, Hiller JL, Benda GI, Buist NRM, Wilcox K and Reynolds JW. Nutritional balance studies of VLBW infants fed their mothers' milk fortified with a liquid human milk fortifier. *J Pediatr Gastroenterol* 1989;**9**: 212–218.
50. Moro GE, Minoli I, Fulconis F, Clementi M and Raiha NCR. Growth and metabolic responses in low birth weight infants fed human milk fortified with a human milk protein or with a bovine milk protein preparation. *J Pediatr Gastroenterol Nutr* 1991;**13**: 150–154.
51. Boehm G, Muller M, Senger H and Rademacher C. Feeding premature babies with enriched human milk: EOPROTIN 60 compared with human albumin. *Kinderartzl Praxis* 1991;**59**: 293–298.
52. Kashyap S, Schulze KF, Forsyth M, Dell RB, Ramakrishnan R and Heird WC. Growth, nutrient retention and metabolic response of low birth weight infants fed supplemented and unsupplemented preterm human milk. *Am J Clin Nutr* 1990;**52**: 254–262.
53. Jackson AA, Shaw JCL, Barber A and Golden MHN. Nitrogen metabolism in the preterm infant: the possible essentiality of glycine. *Pediatr Res* 1981;**15**: 1454–1461.
54. Lucas A and Hudson G. Preterm milk as a source of protein for low birth weight infants. *Arch Dis Child* 1984;**59**: 831–836.
55. Lucas A, Fewtrell MS, Morley R *et al.* Randomised outcome trial of human milk fortification and developmental outcome in preterm infants. *Am J Clin Nutr* 1996;**64**: 142–151.
56. Atkinson SA, Bryan MH and Anderson GH. Human milk feeding in premature neonates: Protein, fat and carbohydrate balances in the first two weeks of life. *J Pediatr* 1981;**99**: 617–624.
57. Putet G, Senterre J, Rigo J and Salle B. Nutrient balance, energy utilisation and composition of weight gain in very low birth weight infants fed pooled human milk or a preterm formula. *J Pediatr* 1984;**105**: 79–85.

58. Roberts SB and Lucas A. The effect of two extremes of dietary intake on protein accretion in preterm infants. *Early Hum Dev* 1985;**12**: 301–307.
59. Senterre J. Nitrogen balances and protein requirements of preterm infants. In: Visser HKA (ed) *Nutrition and Metabolism of the Fetus and Infant*. The Hague: Martinus Nijhoff, 1979, pp 193–212.
60. Whyte RK, Haslam RC, Vlainic C *et al.* Energy balance and nitrogen balance in growing low birth weight infants fed human milk or formula. *Pediatr Res* 1983;**17**: 891–898.
61. Voyer M, Senterre J, Rigo J, Charlas P and Satge P. Human milk lacto-engineering. Growth, nitrogen metabolism and energy balance in preterm infants. *Acta Paediatr Scand* 1984;**73**: 302–306.
62. Schanler RJ, Garza C and Nichols BL. Fortified mothers' milk for very low birth weight infants: Results of growth and nutrient balance studies. *J Pediatr* 1985;**107**: 437–445.
63. Pencharz PB, Steffee WP, Cochran W, Scrimshaw NS, Rand WM and Young VR. Protein metabolism in human neonates: nitrogen balance studies, estimated obligatory losses of nitrogen and whole-body turnover of nitrogen. *Clin Sci Mol Med* 1977;**52**: 485–498.
64. Chessex P, Reichman BL, Verellen GJE *et al.* Quality of growth in premature infants fed their own mother's milk. *J Pediatr* 1983;**102**: 107–112.
65. Ziegler EE, O'Donnell AM, Nelson SE and Fomon SJ. Body composition of the reference fetus. *Growth* 1976;**40**: 329–341.
66. Carey DE, Goetz CA, Horak E and Rowe JC. Phosphorus wasting during phosphorus supplementation of human milk feedings in preterm infants. *J Pediatr* 1985;**107**: 790–794.
67. Holland PC. Wilkinson AR, Diez J and Lindsell DRM. Prenatal deficiency of phosphate, phosphate supplementation and rickets in very low birth weight infants. *Lancet* 1990;**335**: 697–701.
68. Senterre J and Salle B. Calcium and phosphorus economy of the preterm infant and its interaction with vitamin D and its metabolites. *Acta Paediatr Scand* 1982;**296 (Suppl)**: 85–92.
69. Schanler RJ and Abrams SA. Postnatal attainment of intrauterine macromineral accretion rates in low birth weight infants fed human milk. *J Pediatr* 1995;**126**: 441–447.
70. Pohlandt F. Prevention of postnatal bone demineralisation in very low birth weight infants by individually monitored supplementation with calcium and phosphorus. *Pediatr Res* 1994;**35**: 125–129.
71. Greer FR, Steichen JJ and Tsang RC. Calcium and phosphate supplements in breast milk-related rickets. *Am J Dis Child* 1982;**136**: 581–583.
72. Schanler RJ, Abrams SA and Garza C. Bioavailability of calcium and phosphorus in human milk fortifiers and formula for very low birth weight infants. *J Pediatr* 1988;**113**: 95–100.
73. Greer F and McCormick A. Improved bone mineralisation and growth in premature infants fed fortified own mother's milk. *J Pediatr* 1988;**112**: 961–969.

74. Pettifor JM, Rajah R, Venter A *et al.* Bone mineralisation and mineral homeostasis in very low birth weight infants fed either human milk or fortified human milk. *J Pediatr Gastroenterol Nutr* 1989;**8**: 217–224.
75. Abrams SA, Schanler RJ, Tsang RC and Garza C. Bone mineralisation in former very low birth weight infants fed either human milk or commercial formula: One-year follow-up observation. *J Pediatr* 1989;**114**: 1041–1044.
76. Schanler RJ, Burns PA, Abrams SA and Garza C. Bone mineralisation outcomes in human milk-fed preterm infants. *Pediatr Res* 1992;**31**: 583–586.
77. Helm I, Landin LA and Nilsson BE. Bone mineral content in preterm infants at age 4 to 16. *Acta Paediatr Scand* 1985;**139**: 736–740.
78. Bishop NJ, Dahlenburg SL, Fewtrell MS, Morley R and Lucas A. Early diet of preterm infants and bone mineralisation at age five years. *Acta Paediatr* 1996;**85**: 230–236.
79. Lucas A, Brooke OG, Baker BA, Bishop N and Morley R. High alkaline phosphatase activity and growth in preterm neonates. *Arch Dis Child* 1989;**64**: 902–909.
80. deCarvalho M, Anderson DM, Giangregco A and Pittard WB. Frequency of milk expression and milk production by mothers of nonnursing premature neonates. *Am J Dis Child* 1985;**139**: 483–485.
81. Auerbach KG. Sequential and simultaneous breast pumping: a comparison. *Int J Nursing Studies* 1990;**27**: 257–265.
82. Goldblum RM, Garza C, Johnson CA, Harmist R, Nichols BL and Goldman AS. Human milk banking I. Effect of container upon immunological factors in human milk. *Nutr Res* 1981;**1**: 449–459.
83. Williamson MT and Murti PK. Effects of storage time, temperature and composition of containers on biologic components of human milk. *J Hum Lact* 1996;**12**: 31–36.
84. Whitelaw A, Heisterkamp G, Sleath K, Acolet D and Richards M. Skin to skin contact for very low birth weight infants and their mothers. *Arch Dis Child* 1988;**63**: 1377–1381.
85. Bier JA, Ferguson AE, Morales Y *et al.* Comparison of skin to skin contact with standard contact in low birth weight infants who are breastfed. *Arch Pediatr Adolescent Med* 1996;**150**: 1265–1269.
86. Anderson GC. Current knowledge about skin-to-skin (Kangaroo) care for preterm infants. *J Perinatol* 1991;**11**: 216–226.
87. Sloan L, Camacho LWL, Rojas EP and Stern C, Maternidad Isidro Ayora Study Team. Kangaroo mother method: randomised controlled trial of an alternative method of care for stabilised low birth weight infants. *Lancet* 1994;**344**: 782–786.
88. Pearce JL and Buchanan LF. Breastmilk and breastfeeding in very low birth weight infants. *Arch Dis Child* 1979;**54**: 897–899.
89. Bier JB, Ferguson A, Anderson L *et al.* Breastfeeding of very low birth weight infants. *J Pediatr* 1993;**123**: 773–778.
90. Lang S, Lawrence CJ and Orme RL. Cup feeding: an alternative method of infant feeding. *Arch Dis Child* 1994;**71**: 365–369.

91. Ehrenkranz RA and Ackerman BA. Metoclopramide effect on faltering milk production by mothers of premature infants. *Pediatrics* 1986;**78**: 614–620.
92. Renfrew MJ and RossMcGill H. *Enabling Women to Breastfeed. Interventions which Support or Inhibit Breastfeeding – A Structured Review of the Evidence.* London: The Stationery Office, 1998 (in press).
93. Carroll L, Osman M, Davies DP and McNeish AS. Bacteriological criteria for feeding raw breast milk to babies on neonatal units. *Lancet* 1979;**2**: 732–733.
94. Law BJ, Urias BA, Lertzman J, Robson D and Romance L. Is ingestion of milk-associated bacteria by premature infants fed raw human milk controlled by routine bacteriologic screening? *J Clin Microbiol* 1989;**27**: 1560–1566.
95. Liebhaber M, Lewiston NJ, Asquith MT and Sunshine P. Comparison of two methods of human milk collection. *J Pediatr* 1978;**92**: 236–237.
96. Larson E, Zuill R, Zier V and Berg B. Storage of human breast milk. *Infect Control* 1984;**5**: 127–130.
97. Sosa R and Barness L. Bacterial growth in refrigerated human milk. *Am J Dis Child* 1987;**141**: 111–112.
98. Pardou A, Serruys E, Mascart-Lemone F, Dramaix M and Vis HL. Human milk banking: influence of storage processes and of bacterial contamination on some milk constituents. *Biol Neonate* 1994;**65**: 302–309.
99. Botsford KB, Weinstein RA, Boyer KM, Nathan C, Carman M and Paton JB. Gram-negative bacilli in human milk feedings: Quantitation and clinical consequences for premature infants. *J Pediatr* 1986;**109**: 707–710.
100. Brooke OG and Barley J. Loss of energy during continuous infusion of breast milk. *Arch Dis Child* 1978;**53**: 344–345.
101. Bates CJ, Liu DS, Fuller NJ and Lucas A. Susceptibility of riboflavin and vitamin A in breast milk to photodegradation and its implications for the use of banked breast milk in infant feeding. *Acta Paediatr Scand* 1985;**74**: 40–44.
102. Nduati RW, John GC and Kreiss J. Postnatal transmission of HIV-1 through pooled breast milk. *Lancet* 1994;**344**: 1432.
103. Eglin RP and Wilkinson AR. HIV infection and pasteurisation of breast milk. *Lancet* 1987;**i**: 1093.
104. Orloff SL, Wallingford JC and McDougal JS. Inactivation of human immunodeficiency virus Type 1 in human milk; effects of intrinsic factors in human milk and of pasteurisation. *J Hum Lact* 1993;**9**: 13–17.
105. Canadian Paediatric Society. *Statement N95–03: Human Milk Banking and Storage*. Ottawa: Canadian Paediatric Society, 1995.

4

What is an Adequate Blood Pressure in the Preterm Newborn?

Steven Cunningham

Low placental resistance and a maternally regulated metabolism place few demands on the developing cardiovascular system of the fetus at 23–30 weeks' gestation. Within this environment, anatomical and physiological maturation of the cardiovascular control and feedback mechanisms can occur protected from undue stress. It is from this arena that the very low birth weight (VLBW) preterm infant is born; the immature cardiovascular system is immediately required to function independently in a metabolically demanding environment with a relatively high resistance circulation. Tissues which would normally be relatively inactive at these gestations are suddenly required to function and oxygen to enable them to do so. Unfortunately, it is not yet possible to accurately demand and repeatedly measure cellular metabolic requirements (especially cerebral) of the extreme preterm infant, and so to gauge under which circumstances the immature cardiovascular system can and cannot meet these requirements. Signs of poor perfusion are late markers of cellular dysfunction, and by the time they are recognized in the preterm infant significant cellular hypoxia may have occurred, leading to damage that may not be evident for many years.[1] Clinical management of blood pressure in the VLBW infant therefore requires a perspective of the fetal and preterm cardiovascular physiology and anatomy that will help decide when support should begin, what intervention should be given, and how best to judge the benefit (or not) of such treatment.

CARDIOVASCULAR FUNCTION AT 20–30 WEEKS' GESTATION AND ADAPTATIONS AT BIRTH

To understand how the cardiovascular system is able to respond to the acute exposure of immaturity that results from preterm birth, it is important to understand:

- the progression of cardiovascular development *in utero*; and
- how preterm birth influences the postnatal maturation of cardiovascular function and control

Cardiovascular function results from a complex interplay of ventricular size, contractility and compliance, peripheral vascular resistance and the neurohumoral control of the cardiovascular system in response to intrinsic and environmental demands. The VLBW newborn is born at a gestation when, *in utero*, the individual components of the system increasingly co-ordinate their functions. In animal models the study of the fetal cardiovascular system at gestations associated with preterm birth has been hindered by the inability of most species to survive preterm birth, and also because of species differences in cardiovascular maturation. The ability to study the human fetus *in utero* is increasing with current technology, but it still has a long way to go.

Myocardium of the Extreme Preterm Infant

By mid term the human fetal cardiovascular system is established in providing a blood supply to the low resistance fetal circulation with its minimal metabolic demands. At this stage of development the fetal heart has only 50% of the myocardial contractile mass of an adult heart (reducing force per unit area),[2] has a reduced ability for aerobic energy production (mitochondrial disorganization)[3] and also has a higher water content than the mature heart. The sarcomeres in the immature myocardium are reduced in number (but not size) and in their ability to utilize calcium.[2] The postnatal transition time from immature (low density sarcomere/high water content) to mature myocardium is poorly studied in the preterm infant, but this immaturity will undoubtedly compromise the compliance and contractility of the preterm myocardium through the early period of intensive care.

Relative Ventricular Size and Function

The relative size and compliance of the ventricles are important determinants of cardiovascular function. Ventricular mass changes throughout fetal development, with 24 weeks' gestation representing the point at which the mass of the right ventricle becomes greater than that of the left for the first time.[4] Ventricular dominance rapidly changes postnatally, with the left ventricle becoming dominant by 4 weeks of age in the term infant, the most rapid growth occurring in the first 10 days of life.[5, 6] The fetal myocardium has poor functional ability to cope with changes in afterload. If mean arterial blood pressure is artificially raised, the fetal heart will work against the rise in afterload by increasing heart rate rather than contractility;[7, 8] by term the ventricle can respond to increased afterload by greater utilization of preload.[7] Although ventricular compliance increases throughout gestation, the most significant changes occur in the first 3 postnatal weeks.[9–12] The physiological and morphological transition of the ventricles from a fetal to an 'adult' role does not occur in unison, so that the left ventricle achieves an adult pattern of function at a time when the right ventricle still behaves in a fetal mode.[2] Although these changes are well documented in the term infant, the relative changes in dominance and compliance are poorly documented in the preterm infant. The use of adult echocardiographic techniques may not give a true representation of function in the preterm infant, as they do not take into account the relative distortion of the preterm left ventricular wall and the effect this has on measures that are not adjusted for ventricular wall area.[1, 13]

Development of Vasculature and Resistance

Mean arterial blood pressure rises steadily from mid gestation (as shown in the sheep fetus), partly as a result of increased cardiac output, but also because after this point vascularity does not increase at the same rate as body size so that there is a relative increase in peripheral vascular resistance.[14, 15] Although relative peripheral vascular resistance increases (relative to body size), absolute values continue to fall throughout mid gestation with increasing peripheral vascularity. In late gestation, the deposition of elastin in large arteries is associated with an increase in peripheral vascular resistance and hence there is a rise in blood pressure (in sheep).[16] Blood volume (relative to body size) does not change from mid gestation onwards.[17]

Development of Cardiovascular Control

Changes in cardiovascular control occur throughout mid gestation. Parasympathetic control is present at 15 weeks and increases to term, progressively slowing the fetal heart rate. Sympathetic innervation occurs later and continues to develop after birth:[18] fetal heart rate is not slowed by β blockers (metoprolol) until 23–28 weeks gestation.[19] In the preterm lamb, catecholamine levels at preterm delivery are greater than those at term, but the physiological responses to them (blood pressure and heart rate) are not as great, indicating immature target tissue.[20] One of the great difficulties when studying the fetal autonomic system is determining when receptors which are histologically mature begin to function, and at what gestation they reach a full, mature level of function.[21] What influence preterm birth has on the rate of maturation is even more difficult to assess, and at present there is little data on this.[22] Baroreceptors have a functional ability to change blood pressure by 25 weeks' gestation,[23, 24] and chemoreceptors are sensitive to changes in arterial oxygen from 0.7 gestation (c28 weeks).[25] Baroreceptors can be reset during rises in blood pressure both *in utero* and at birth.[26, 27] Whereas such resetting occurs within 1 hour in the adult, the time taken in the preterm infant is unknown.

CLINICAL ASSESSMENT OF SUBOPTIMAL PERFUSION IN THE VERY LOW BIRTH WEIGHT INFANT

An adequate blood pressure is one that will provide all cells with sufficient glucose and oxygen for ATP production. Cells do not store oxygen and have limited supplies of glucose; they also have a poor ability to survive periods where supply does not meet demand and supply therefore has to be constant.[28] As it is not possible to measure cellular metabolic demand in a clinical setting, grosser indications of failed cellular metabolism must be relied upon; a falling blood pressure is an expression of extreme cardiovascular decompensation. By the time blood pressure begins to fall, serious and prolonged cellular hypoxia may have occurred unnoticed in 'watershed' areas. Earlier compensatory markers of impending hypotension may be less reliable in the VLBW infant, because of cardiovascular and autonomic immaturity, and it is often difficult to distinguish whether these markers indicate hypovolaemia or a myocardial problem. The weight given to each of the early signs of hypotension in assessing hypovolaemia (see below) varies between clinicians, and although echocardiography is helpful in assessing cardiac function, it is not usually available continually in the majority of neonatal units.

Signs of poor perfusion present in adults/older children may not be as clinically reliable in the preterm infant as:

- The preterm heart functions at a high resting rate and therefore has limited ability to increase its rate in response to impending hypotension.[29]
- Urine output may correlate poorly with renal perfusion in the first few days of life, particularly in sick infants.[30, 31]
- Good peripheral perfusion may be a sign of immaturity of α_2-adrenergic autonomic vasoconstrictor ability in the first few days of life.[25, 32–34]
- Acidosis may occur as a result of excess renal bicarbonate loss in the extreme preterm infant and so does not reflect poor peripheral perfusion.[35]
- Fluctuating central venous pressure may occur with respiratory instability[36] as well as with low preload.[37]
- The method of measurement may be important in accurately identifying low blood pressure.[38]

Intensive care support of the VLBW preterm infant should aim to provide a blood pressure which gives adequate oxygenation for the metabolic demands of all organs. This support should have enough reserve to cope with the fluctuations in stability that characterize preterm intensive care. If blood pressure is sufficient and pulmonary oxygen transfer is good, then small changes in either will probably be tolerated. In the unstable infant with pulmonary disease where blood oxygenation is poor and myocardial and pulmonary function are compromised by mechanical ventilation, it is important to optimize blood pressure to ensure tissue oxygenation is not compromised.

OBSERVED AND APPLIED MEASURES OF BLOOD PRESSURE IN THE PRETERM INFANT – DO THEY HELP WITH MANAGEMENT?

Observational Blood Pressure Studies

The precise mechanisms determining the level of arterial blood pressure after birth are unknown. Low arterial blood pressure can persist even after the ductus arteriosus has closed, and initial increases in left ventricular output appear to be independent of tissue oxygen demands.[39] The studies of blood pressure to date have mostly been concerned with providing a reference range from preterm infants, often with a lower limit (frequently the 10th centile) determined as being unacceptable. Such studies have varied in the numbers and birthweight of infants observed, the criteria for inclusion and exclusion of infants, the frequency and duration of observations and also the method of measurement of blood pressure used. Table 4.1 gives an overview of the studies which have established reference ranges for blood pressure from observation of preterm infants, demonstrating the differences in study format. Few studies have provided adequate long-term end points for their blood pressure observations other than a relation to intraventricular haemorrhage (IVH)/periventricular leukomalacia (PVL), which represent the crudest forms of cerebral injury in preterm infants. Distinct neurodevelopmental differences in relation to their peers in later childhood[40, 41] and the possibility of poor vascular programming determining later cardiovascular disease, may yet prove to be the repercussions of poor perfusion in the preterm newborn.[42]

The majority of studies (Table 4.1) show an increase in blood pressure with increasing gestational and postnatal age; some studies have demonstrated a temporary peak in pressures on day 3–4 of life, with a small reduction thereafter until day 7–8. No study has observed blood pressure in an unselected cohort of preterm infants given no cardiovascular support. Studies have often selected a group of what are considered to be 'normal' preterm infants and then excluded any other infants – usually those who have received blood pressure support. In such studies, the resulting reference ranges simply reflect the blood pressure policy of that unit during the study period; they are not able to demonstrate the natural variability of blood pressure within the preterm population or how that relates to tissue oxygenation and subsequent neurodevelopmental or respiratory outcome. What happens to the infants excluded from these studies is as interesting as what happens to those who were included, because they are the ones that are problematical and for whom some reference to outcome is needed.

Of the studies included in Table 4.1, those of Versmold *et al*,[43] Watkins *et al*[44] and Bada *et al*[45] are quoted most frequently. Versmold *et al*'s study was based on only a small number of infants of birth weight <1000 g. The studies by Watkins *et al* and Bada *et al* contained more infants, with the latter involving more frequent blood pressure observations (minute as opposed to hourly observations): blood pressure was related to IVH and PVL in both groups. Unfortunately, no information is given about infants receiving cardiovascular support in the Bada paper, and this may explain why the average mean blood pressure in infants <1000 g is frequently 5 mmHg less than the same group in

Table 4.1 Blood pressure studies in the preterm infant.

Study	Weight (g)	Measurement	Systolic (s) Diastolic (d) Mean (m)*	No. of infants	No. of days observed	No. of data points assessed	Exclusions (infants with/ receiving)	Criteria given for blood pressure intervention	Related to outcome
Kitterman *et al* (1969)[176]	1050–2000	Direct	s/d/m	14	0.5	672	'Unstable' infants	No	Survival of newborn period
Bucci *et al* (1972)[177]	<2500	Indirect	s	189	3	651	Severe respiratory disease, cardiovascular instability	No	Survival of newborn period
Versmold *et al* (1981)[43]	<1000	Direct	s/d/m	16	0.5	143	'Unstable' or receiving inotropes	No	No
Moscoso *et al* (1983)[178]	<1250	Direct	s/d/m	25	0.5	4500	Inotropes/colloid, IVH, infection, heart failure or poor trace	No	No
Adams *et al* (1983)[179]	<1500	Direct	m	15	2	36 000	Severe pulmonary disease or inotropes	No	No
Kollee *et al* (1986)[180]	<1250	Indirect	s/d/m	15	1	120	IVH, PDA, colloid, respiratory instability	No	No
Tan (1988)[181]	<1500	Indirect	s/d/m	45	70	765	Low agpars, respiratory distress, sepsis, PDA	No	No
Shortland *et al* (1988)[182]	<1500	Direct	s/d/m	32	6	4608	Inotropes or colloid	Poor urine output or increased toe/core temperature difference	No
Watkins *et* al (1989)[44]	<1500	Direct	m	131	4	5425	Dopamine, phenobarbitone, tolazoline, colloid	No	Cerebral ultrasound findings
Bada *et al* (1990)[45]	<1500	Direct	m	100	2	282 200	IVH (>grade 1) at <1 hour of age	No	Cerebral ultrasound findings
Spinnazola *et al* (1991)[183]	<750	Direct	s/d/m	12	7	829	Cardiovascular instability	Yes	No
Low *et al* (1991)[184]	<1500	Indirect	m	20	4	38 400	'Unstable' infants	No	Cerebral ultrasound findings

Powell *et* al (1992)[185]	<1500	Direct	m	27	7	272 160	Colloid, dopamine or dexamethasone	No	No
Greenough and Emery (1993)[186]	≤1500	Indirect	s	90	2	180	Colloid or inotropes, and non-ventilated infants	No	No
Hegyi *et al* (1994)[46]	<2000	Mixed	s/d (minimum/ maximum)	545	0.25	1090	Infants with any of 7 factors affecting blood pressure	No	No
Hegyi *et al* (1996)[47]	<2000	Mixed	s/d (minimum/ maximum)	545	7	15 260	Infants with any of 7 factors affecting blood pressure	No	No
Cunningham (1998)	<1500	Direct	m	232	7	2 338 560	Infants receiving inotropes or colloid >10 ml/kg; infants with grade 2–4 IVH	Yes	Cerebral ultrasound findings. Respiratory outcome. Developmental outcome at 2 years

* Average values unless stated.
IVH = intraventricular haemorrhage; PDA = patent ductus arteriosus.

Watkins' report. Clearly, at a mean blood pressure of 35 mmHg, 5 mmHg might be an important discrepancy. The 2 recent reports by Hegyi *et al* are a retrospective observation.[46, 47] Although these studies involve large numbers of infants and provide valuable baseline data, they do not help guide blood pressure management as they do not give any evidence to support the use of the references provided in terms of infant outcome. Other data[48] taken from a unit with a relatively high threshold for blood pressure support, provide a reference range from a large group of VLBW infants followed up intensively to discharge and then also at 2 years of age.

No group having developed reference blood pressure ranges has then reported a prospective evaluation of those ranges. Gill and Weindling studied blood pressure in the same unit that Watkins *et al* had earlier produced their reference blood pressure data and found that 35% of VLBW infants had a blood pressure below the 10th centile for gestation and postnatal age, as defined by Watkins *et al*, and would therefore be expected to need intervention.[44, 49] Bourchier and Weston used a definition for hypotension which made 38.6% of VLBW infants in their unit hypotensive in the first week of life.[50] Campbell used a definition of hypotension in infants ≤750 g, which qualified 52% of infants as needing epinephrine infusions.[51] Clearly, if cardiovascular support is be instigated in over one-third of preterm infants, a clearer idea is needed of the benefits of that support.

Blood Pressure 'Rules of Thumb'

Nearly all neonatologists agree that blood pressure below a certain limit has to be supported, but there is little agreement on what that limit should be.[52] Two rules of thumb appear to have been commonly adopted, probably because they are easy to remember. Neither has a significant scientific basis for its use.

A lower limit for mean blood pressure of 30 mmHg for all babies <31 weeks' gestation (or <1000 g) is one rule of thumb. This value was defined 'arbitrarily' by Barr *et al* in 1977,[53] because of a lack of other data, and has since been adopted and supported by others.[54] Szymonowicz *et al* prospectively applied this blood pressure limit and noted a reduction in the incidence of IVH, though their study used historical controls.[55] When Miall-Allen *et al* set a lower limit of 30 mmHg for mean blood pressure in 33 infants <31 weeks' gestation, they found infants with a blood pressure below this level for >1 hour had a significantly increased risk of ultrasonically detected cerebral injury;[56] this finding was repeated in an even smaller study.[57] Three studies have used this limit as a marker of success for interventions to raise blood pressure, though no study demonstrated an improvement in neurodevelopmental/respiratory outcome resulting from using this limit (as opposed to any other).[58–60] Cerebral blood flow appears to be independent of this value[61] and so Miall-Allen *et al*'s work needs updating.

The second, more liberal, rule of thumb commonly adopted is that mean blood pressure should not fall below an infant's gestational age (in completed weeks). This measure was supported by the British Association of Perinatal Medicine in 1992.[62] There is no evidence to support this rule. A study of 141 VLBW infants based in a unit using this policy demonstrated no association between the amount of time that an infant spent with a mean blood pressure below his gestational age (at which point support began) and an increased risk of IVH or death.[63] D'Souza *et al*, although they advocate treatment of hypotension, in a study of blood pressure in 34 preterm infants could not demonstrate any reduction in periventricular haemorrhage resulting from therapeutic intervention.[64] These findings contrast with other observational studies of blood pressure in the development of IVH (see below).

As the neonatal population has changed dramatically in the last 10–20 years,[65, 66] and as most studies in this time have shown an incremental increase in blood pressure with increasing weight, gestation (reflecting but greater than that *in utero*) and postnatal age, Barr *et al*'s arbitrary limit of 30 mmHg for all infants <31 weeks' gestation or the use of gestational age as a lower limit, may be too rigid and too simple to cover all situations. Clearly, prospective studies of the effects of blood pressure intervention are needed, but would need large multicentre composition.

SYSTEMIC EFFECTS OF CARDIOVASCULAR COMPROMISE IN THE VERY LOW BIRTHWEIGHT INFANT

Organs are either supply dependent (brain and heart) or independent (liver, spleen, gut, skin and kidney). Supply-dependent organs have less ability to increase blood flow and fractional extraction of oxygen, and therefore have a limited ability to cope with hypotension or hypoxia.[67] Whilst preterm infants have the ability to increase fractional extraction of oxygen in response to hypoxia,[68–70] their ability to autoregulate blood flow may be compromised by the immaturity of their feedback and control systems.[1, 19, 71]

Early hypotensive stress may also produce blood flow redistribution within an organ (with possible watershed hypoxia), even when total organ blood flow is maintained. The kidney, in response to falling blood pressure, redirects blood flow from the cortex to the medulla and within the cortex to the juxta-medullary nephrons.[72] The multifunctional liver creates a priority system of metabolic functions.[67] In the cerebral circulation too, there is preferential flow distribution during hypotensive stress.[73] A study has suggested that adult pigs can increase the microvascular distribution of blood during hypotension by capillary dilatation, but this capillary reserve is lacking in newborn piglets.[74] It is important to note these responses as most techniques available in a clinical setting only give estimates of total organ blood flow and cannot identify problems of intra-organ differential perfusion.

Cerebral Injury

The cerebral circulation in the preterm newborn is susceptible to loss of autoregulation, particularly during episodes of low blood pressure or hypoxia.[37, 71, 73, 75–77] Studies in animals[78–80] and humans[64, 81] have shown that hypotensive stress and not hypoxia is responsible for the greater degree of cerebral injury. Both studies in humans showed a significant association between hypotension (defined in each paper) and developmental delay at 1 and 2 years of age. Lou *et al* have also shown that low cerebral blood flow leads to later neurodevelopmental dysfunction.[82] The correlation, however, between cerebral blood flow measurements and later neurodevelopmental outcome is unclear.[83] Cerebral blood flow in the preterm infant averages 20 ml/100 g/min.[84] Mechanically ventilated preterm infants have a lower cerebral blood flow (10–12 ml/100 g/min) and therefore may be particularly susceptible to ischaemic brain injury.[85] Although Lou *et al* demonstrated brain atrophy in 6 of 10 infants who had cerebral blood flow <20 ml/100 g/min, normal outcome (at 6 months of age) has been demonstrated in preterm infants with flow rates as low as 5 ml/100 g/min.[86] Early reports using near infrared spectroscopy in preterm infants have suggested global cerebral blood flow may be poorly related to blood pressure:[61] this is not consistent with data from animal models.[73, 80] IVH has been most consistently associated with low[44, 55, 56, 87–90] and variable blood pressure[91–93] or a combination of both.[45] Variable blood pressure, if directly transmitted to the cerebral circulation in the absence of autoregulation, might produce haemorrhage.[37, 91, 94, 95] There have been no randomized trials to investigate the role of raising blood pressure in preventing IVH, though the stabilizing effects of pancuronium,[91, 96] phenobarbitone[65] and colloid[97, 98] have been investigated without finding consistent benefit. It is apparent therefore, that although low blood pressure is associated with a poorer neurodevelopmental outcome, blood pressure management can as yet be poorly adapted to minimize the risk of developmental delay.

Renal Effects

In adults, reduction in urine output is a good, if late, marker of poor renal perfusion.[67] In healthy preterm infants in the first few days of life, renal blood flow[99] and urine output[100] increase in association with (though in the first 24 hours apparently independent of) increases in mean blood pressure. Only 4–6% of cardiac output is distributed to kidneys in the first 12 hours after birth, increasing to approximately 10% thereafter:[101] animal studies have suggested that this increase is produced by a cell-mediated change in function independent of changing haemodynamics.[102] In the sick preterm infant, however, mechanical ventilation[103] and respiratory distress syndrome[104, 105] can reduce urine output independent of effects on blood pressure,[103] and it is therefore not always possible to use urine output as a sensitive marker of perfusion. The advent of surfactants and high frequency oscillation have somewhat obscured the distinct antidiuretic and diuretic phases of respiratory distress syndrome, and more work is needed to identify how well urine output can reflect adequacy of renal perfusion (blood pressure) in this new era.[106–108]

Myocardial Effects

Poor myocardial contractility is a common finding in infants with low blood pressure[109] but echocardiography would appear to be the only reliable method for its detection. Perfusion of the coronary arteries may be an important determinant of that dysfunction. Coronary artery perfusion occurs predominantly in diastole, and therefore factors which reduce diastolic pressure (peripheral vasodilatation, hypovolaemia or a large shunt through a patent ductus arteriosus) may reduce coronary artery perfusion and in doing so compromise cardiac contractility. It is unusual however to identify either early (raised ST segments/arrhthymias) or permanent coronary ischaemia in preterm infants, and so the contribution of poor coronary perfusion to low blood pressure (and vice versa) in the preterm infant is unclear. It has not yet been satisfactorily demonstrated whether or not coronary arteries have the ability to autoregulate in the preterm infant: dopamine receptors are present in the coronary arteries from an early gestation, though their ability to vasodilate has not been clearly demonstrated.[110–112] Coronary artery vasoconstriction can be mediated by acetylcholine in the preterm piglet.[113]

Gastrointestinal Effects

The hypothesis that ischaemia is a major aetiological factor in necrotizing enterocolitis has prompted much interest in the behaviour of gut blood flow in the preterm infant, particularly during episodes of cardiovascular compromise.[114] As a supply-independent organ, the adult gut responds to low blood pressure by vasodilatation and increased oxygen extraction. Oxygen extraction in the preterm can be extremely effective: perfusion pressure has to fall to ≤70% of its baseline value before cellular oxygen levels fall below 95% of their starting level.[68, 115, 116] Vasodilatation is less successful in immature animals and may be absent[117, 118] (despite the presence of vasodilatory adrenoreceptors).[119] Hypotension in preterm infants leads to a reduction in flow in the superior mesenteric artery (reversible by inotropes).[120] Unlike in term infants, stable preterm infants demonstrate a fall in blood pressure after a feed, though they are able to increase superior mesenteric artery blood flow velocity by increasing cardiac output.[34, 121] It is easy to postulate that the postprandial metabolic demands placed on the gut by an enteral feed might produce gut hypoxia if blood flow cannot meet these demands.

EFFECTS OF PATENT DUCTUS ARTERIOSUS ON BLOOD PRESSURE IN THE PRETERM

In the term infant, the ductus arteriosus closes at 10–15 hours of age in response to oxygen, though the biochemical basis for this remains poorly understood:[122] ductal closure can be induced by acetylcholine, indomethacin and glucocorticoids. Autonomic ganglia increase in number in the ductus with increasing gestation. These are absent in children with patent ductus arteriosus (PDA), indicating a role for the autonomic system in closure of the duct.[122] It is possible that relative autonomic immaturity may be responsible for failure of duct closure in the preterm term, as infusion of autonomic maturing glucocorticoids in preterm lambs and antenatal steroids in preterm infants, produce a significant reduction in patent ductus arteriosus.[123]

In a longitudinal study of 48 VLBW infants, Evans and Iyer found 3 distinct groups of behaviour of the ductus arteriosus after preterm birth: in 65% the ductus closed asymptomatically and spontaneously, the majority within 48 hours;[124] in 19% (representing those with the worst respiratory disease) closure was temporary, with a reopening of ductus at an average of 7 days of age; and in only 17% did the ductus progressively become symptomatic after only minimal constriction.

This finding is important as it shows that relatively few VLBW infants should have significant haemodynamic effects from their PDA in the first week of life, and it may also help to explain why in the preterm infant, the effects of PDA on systemic blood pressure are unclear. Clinical assessment of PDA is not reliable and echocardiography will remain a valuable tool in assessing haemodynamic significance.[125]

In animal studies, effective blood flow can be maintained in the presence of a patent ductus arteriosus by increased left ventricular contractility (Frank-Starling mechanism).[126] The reduction in afterload created by the PDA can improve left ventricular function in the face of moderate left to right shunts: it has even been postulated that the reduction in afterload created by a moderate shunt may give a physiological advantage to the immature and poorly compliant myocardium.

The effects of a PDA on blood pressure can be assessed by comparing infants with and without a PDA, or by comparing infant blood pressure before and after medical closure (with possible effects of surgery or medication on blood pressure allowed for). Evans and Iyer demonstrated that a haemodynamically significant PDA (determined echocardiographically) did not affect blood pressure in infants of birth weight 1000–1500 g, whereas blood pressure was lower than controls in infants <1000 g with a haemodynamically significant PDA in the first 5 days of life.[128] Mellander and Larsson found that blood pressure was only lower in infants with a haemodynamically significant PDA if they were ventilated[127] (presumably resulting from altered left ventricular function): ventilation, however, reduced blood pressure even in those infants without a PDA.[47] Medical treatment of a PDA with indomethacin has been associated with an increase in mean and systolic pressures following treatment.[128] The effects of PDA ligation on blood pressure are less clear with studies demonstrating either no change[129] or an increase[130, 131] in blood pressure post ligation.

INTERVENTIONS TO RAISE BLOOD PRESSURE

Plasma Expanders

The majority of clinicians initially treat poor perfusion with an aliquot of intravascular volume expander. Certainly, capillary leakage and large insensible fluid losses in the preterm predispose to hypovolaemia[132] and atrial filling may be compromised by mechanical ventilation if preload volumes are inadequate.[37, 133, 134] This is therefore a reasonable initial clinical response. However, blood volume and blood pressure correlate poorly in the preterm infant.[135, 136] It is possible that this lack of correlation in part reflects an individual maturity of peripheral vasoconstriction where infants who are able to vasoconstrict can maintain blood pressure in the face of falling blood volume, whereas those with poor peripheral autonomic control cannot.[32, 34, 137]

Infusion of plasma expanders offers a temporary increase in blood pressure in the majority of infants,[138, 139] the duration of effect increasing with increasing volume infused rather than increased concentration of plasma protein:[140] plasma proteins are rapidly lost in capillary leakage.[132] A delicate relationship, however, exists between cardiac contractility, preload, afterload and peripheral vascular resistance, which may be upset by acute large volume load (increased preload),[141, 142] and so volume should be given in small frequent aliquots looking for cardiac decompensation. A recent study of the long-term benefit of routine plasma expansion in the preterm infant showed no significant benefit to outcome at 2 years,[98] in contrast to a smaller earlier study.[97]

Inotropes

Poor blood pressure response to plasma expanders frequently leads to the use of inotropes. Both dopamine and dobutamine are effective in increasing blood pressure in the preterm newborn, though dopamine performs this function more consistently.[58, 59, 143, 144]

The mechanism of action of inotropes in the preterm newborn is not as clearly documented as in the adult. Underlying this is the relatively poor understanding of the pre- and post-natal maturation of the autonomic and endocrine cardiovascular control systems in the preterm infant. Catecholamine receptors are anatomically present at approximately 24 weeks' gestation in the preterm human, though their ability to function is not well established; dopaminergic receptors become functional in different organs at different gestations in the pig.[145, 146] A maturational effect in dopamine receptor activity has been postulated in the human preterm:[110, 111, 147] whereas in adults incremental doses of dopamine produce first tachycardia (β receptors) followed by peripheral vasoconstriction (α receptors), in the preterm infant this order of sensitivity is reversed, so that a rise in mean blood pressure (following peripheral vasoconstriction) occurs before tachycardia is induced. Given the differential rates of maturation of different receptors, the same receptors in different tissues and the question of how quickly receptors are able to mature in response to preterm delivery, inotropes may have very different actions in different patients, different organs and at different postnatal ages.

Dopamine

Dopamine is an immediate precursor of epinephrine (adrenaline) and norepinephrine (noradrenaline) and has several well documented cardiovascular effects in mature humans:[148, 149]

- increases cardiac contraction directly by cardiac $\beta 1$ receptors and indirectly by prompting norepinephrine release;
- peripherally vasoconstricts by α_2-adrenergic activity;
- enables dopaminergic receptor-mediated vasodilatation in renal, mesenteric, hepatic, coronary and cerebral circulations;
- has a serotonin-like activity (not as well documented as the above).

In the VLBW infant, sympathetic innervation of the heart is incomplete and receptor sensitivity to catecholamines is reduced,[150] and so the hypertensive effect of dopamine is probably achieved as a result of peripheral vasoconstriction. Poor peripheral vasomotor tone is a common cause of hypotension in the VLBW preterm and the vasoconstrictive properties of dopamine probably explain its success over dobutamine in effecting an increase in blood pressure. The ability of dopamine receptors to mediate vasodilatation of organ blood flow,[151] has not been satisfactorily proven in the VLBW infant,[111] though the case for vasodilatation of renal vessels even in infants of 25 weeks' gestation is strong.[110, 152] In the adult, renal vasodilatation is preserved even in the presence of elevated α-adrenergic activity,[153, 154] though at high doses dopamine's serotonin-like activity may cause vasoconstriction in vascular beds.[155] At low dose (<4 μg/kg/min), dopamine increases urine output independently of increases in systemic blood pressure,[30] though the urine is poorly concentrated as a result of solute washout.[156] Dopamine has a catabolic effect on tissues and has been demonstrated to exacerbate hypoxia in the renal tubules[157] and gut.[158] An opposite effect was observed by Seri, who felt that dopamine could protect against hypoxic tubular damage by virtue of its inhibition of Na^+/K^+ ATPase.[156]

The dose of dopamine required for action varies significantly in preterm infants and animals do not give a reliable dose–response model. Certainly, cardiovascular effects of dopamine can be demonstrated from 1 μg/kg/min,[147] though it is most often effective in the range 5–15 μg/kg/min[144, 159] and doses above this range, probably, give little additional benefit.

Dobutamine

Dobutamine is a mixture of 2 racemic isomers, 1 of which has α-agonist vasoconstrictor properties and the other has both β_1- and β_2-agonist vasodilator properties. These actions are therefore said to cancel out. It is not completely clear, however, whether this is the case in the preterm infant who has variable rates of receptor maturity. Dobutamine acts primarily via β1 activity to increase heart rate and contraction without vasoconstriction. Increasing perfusion improves peripheral oxygenation and offloads the poorly compliant left ventricle. Dobutamine, however, is not as successful as dopamine in increasing blood pressure in the preterm infant, particularly at lower gestations.[59] One can only speculate that this is because the extreme preterm infant has little ability to increase cardiac output by increasing heart rate,[160] and/or that a poor ability to peripherally vasoconstrict is a significant contributor to low blood pressure at these gestations, where the benefit to blood pressure afforded by an increase in peripheral vascular resistance (with dopamine) is more than balanced by the associated reduction in left ventricular output.

Other inotropes

Epinephrine is occasionally of value in managing blood pressure in cases of hypotension poorly responsive to dopamine (though see below regarding steroids). The therapeutic windows for focusing on specific catecholamine receptors are small; the difference in dosage between the primary β_1 ability to increase contractility and secondary α_2 vasoconstriction is often small in neonates and is not documented in the preterm. *Norepinephrine*, with its strong vasoconstrictive α_2 activity, is often considered too potent for use in the VLBW preterm infant.

Studies examining the role of epinephrine and norepinephrine in the VLBW newborn are appearing.[51, 161] Low dose epinephrine/norepinephrine as a final adjunct to dopamine and steroids may be of supplemental benefit, though these drugs have yet to be fully assessed with regard to their effects on afterload, myocardial excitability (reducing compliance) inducible by catecholamine excess, and the vasoconstrictive effects on organ perfusion.

The cardiovascular effects of the newer phosphodiesterase inhibitors, *milrinone* and *enoximone,* have not yet been reported in VLBW preterm infants.[148] Whilst their ability to increase calcium concentration in the sarcoplasmic reticulum (low in the preterm) and to enhance diastolic relaxation (improve compliance) would be useful, their cAMP-induced vasodilatation often produces dramatic falls in blood pressure and so they would probably only be of benefit as part of combination therapy.

The indiscriminate use of inotropes should be guarded against. These agents increase blood pressure by several mechanisms, all of which can produce effects opposite to those desired (and these may not be immediately apparent to the unwary):

- the immature myocardium, with its poor sarcomere concentration and high water content, is poorly compliant;
- catecholamines can reduce stroke volume by reducing diastolic filling time (tachycardia) and reducing ventricular compliance (increased resting contractile state);[67]
- peripheral vasoconstriction increases cardiac afterload and so may reduce output of the poorly compliant left ventricle;[58]
- catecholamines may mask hypovolaemia by increasing blood pressure and inducing urine output, creating a spiral of increasing catecholamine use and declining circulating blood volume.[148]

Just as an infant with inadvertent positive end expiratory pressure can be helped initially by an increase in the ventilator pressures which are creating the problem, so too can inotropes temporarily improve a situation which they are creating.

Corticosteroids

Corticosteroids increase maturity and numbers of α- and β-adrenergic receptors and are necessary for their optimal function.[162] The action of steroids in improving blood pressure appears to be as a result of increasing vascular reactivity[163] and accelerating elastin deposition in arterial vessels.[16] Their action is not dependent on mineralocorticoid action or direct increases in cardiac output.[164–166] Steroids have increased response to inotropes when given to stressed critically ill adults in whom high cortisol levels were considered inappropriately low for the degree of illness.

Antenatal steroids have been associated with stabilization of blood pressure postnatally, independent of improvements in respiratory function:[60, 167] this effect has been confirmed in animals.[163, 168, 169] Although there is little evidence of cortisol deficiency in response to stress in preterm infants,[170] relative receptor immaturity/insensitivity may reduce the effectiveness of cortisol in the preterm infant.[171] Low cortisol production has been associated with low mean blood pressure in preterm neonates,[170] and supplemental corticosteroids have been anecdotally associated with improvements in blood pressure control,[172, 173] even at relatively low doses.[174] In a randomized trial, hydrocortisone was effective in raising blood pressure in VLBW infants, though compared with dopamine the rise in blood pressure was delayed and hydrocortisone was not as effective as dopamine in reaching the target blood pressure (though the hydrocortisone group were of significantly lower birth weight and had a lower starting blood pressure).[50] Hypertension was seen later in 14% of the hydrocortisone-treated group, but no other significant side effects were noted. Supplemental corticosteroids are a valuable adjunct to the treatment of resistant hypotension, though the dose required needs further assessment.

WHAT IS AN ADEQUATE BLOOD PRESSURE IN THE PRETERM NEWBORN?

Disappointingly, the research base is not yet available to answer this question. The 'rules of thumb' are too inflexible and are not supported by strong evidence. Observational studies of blood pressure have not provided a satisfactory, unbiased reference of blood pressure in relation to outcome. There are no adequate tools with which to measure real-time cellular oxygen requirements and therefore we cannot ensure that the basic definition of adequacy of perfusion (enough oxygen) is fulfilled.[175] Cardiovascular feedback mechanisms are immature and as yet there is inadequate knowledge of the speed of postnatal maturation at different gestations.

However, it is known that cardiovascular instability can compromise blood flow to all organs and that any of the components of the cardiovascular system can be responsible for this instability in the preterm infant. Immature cardiovascular and autonomic feedback mechanisms may be unable to respond adequately to such stresses, particularly during periods of hypoxia to which preterm infants are all too frequently susceptible. Intensive care is the support of body systems that are compromised, supporting one system to enable its recovery (or maturation), without compromise to other organs. A 'survival of the fittest' approach to blood pressure (no support in any infant)[52] is untenable with current data. A knowledge of the physiology of the preterm cardiovascular system, and the cardiovascular effects of hypertensive agents in the preterm, as outlined in this chapter, should enable the clinician to come to a global assessment of the adequacy of perfusion that will safeguard individual organ perfusion and will not leave the infant too susceptible to immature cardiovascular feedback mechanisms. The prospect of increased understanding of cellular energy metabolism and the maturation of cardiovascular control is an exciting one.

REFERENCES

1. Heitmiller ES, Zhaka KG and Roger MC. Developmental physiology of the cardiovascular system. In: Rogers MC (ed) *Textbook of Pediatric Intensive Care.* Baltimore: Williams and Wilkins, 1992, pp 383–422.
2. Friedman WF. The intrinsic physiologic properties of the developing heart. *Prog Cardiovasc Dis* 1972;**15**: 87–111.
3. Sheldon CA, Friedman WF and Sybers HD. Scanning electron microscopy of fetal and neonatal lamb cardiac cells. *J Mol Cell Cardiol* 1976;**8**: 853–862.
4. Emery JL and MacDonald MS. The weight of the ventricles in the later weeks of intra-uterine life. *Br Heart J* 1960;**22**: 563–570.
5. Rein AJJT, Sanders SP, Colan SD, Parness IA and Epstein M. Left ventricular mechanics in the normal newborn. *Circulation* 1987;**76**: 1029–1036.
6. Emery JL and Mithal A. Weights of cardiac ventricles at and after birth. *Br Heart J* 1961;**23**: 313–316.
7. Van Hare GF, Hawkins JA, Schmidt KG and Rudolph AM. The effects of increasing mean arterial pressure on left ventricular output in newborn lambs. *Circ Res* 1990;**67**: 78–83.
8. Hawkins J, Van Hare GF, Schmidt KG and Rudolph AM. Effects of increasing afterload on left ventricular output in fetal lambs. *Circ Res* 1989;**65**: 127–134.
9. Reed KL, Sahn DJ, Scagnelli S *et al.* Doppler echocardiographic studies of diastolic function in the human fetal heart: Changes during gestation. *J Am Coll Cardiol* 1986;**8**: 391–395.
10. Areias JC, Meyer R, Scott WA and Goldberg SJ. Serial echocardiographic and Doppler evaluation of left ventricular diastolic filling in full-term neonates. *Am J Cardiol* 1990;**66**: 108–111.
11. Romero TE and Friedman WF. Limited left ventricular response to volume overload in the neonatal period: a comparative study with the adult animal. *Pediatr Res* 1979;**13**: 910–915.
12. Baylen BG, Ogata H, Ikegami M *et al.* Left ventricular performance and contractility before and after volume infusion: A comparative study of preterm and full-term newborn lambs. *Circulation* 1986;**73**: 1042–1049.
13. Lee LA, Kimball TR, Daniels SR, Khoury P and Meyer RA. Left ventricular mechanics in the preterm infant and their effect on the measurement of cardiac performance. *J Pediatr* 1992;**120**: 114–119.
14. Kitanaka T, Alonso JG, Gilbert RD, Siu BL, Clemons GK and Longo LD. Fetal responses to long-term hypoxemia in sheep. *Am J Physiol – Regulatory Integrative and Comparative Physiology* 1989;**256**: 25/6 R1348–R1354.
15. Dawes GS. The control of fetal heart rate and its variability in lambs. In: Kunzel W (ed) *Fetal Heart Rate Monitoring.* Berlin: Springer Verlag, 1985, pp 184–190.
16. Bendeck MP, Keeley FW and Langille BL. Perinatal accumulation of arterial wall constituents: Relation to hemodynamic changes at birth. *Am J Physiol* 1994;**267**: H2268–H2279.

17. Brace RA. Regulation of blood volume in utero. In: Hansen MA, Spencer JAD and Rodeck CH (eds) *The Circulation.* Cambridge: Cambridge University Press, 1993, pp 75–99.
18. Robinson RB. Autonomic receptor-effector coupling during post-natal development. *Cardiovasc Res* 1996;**31**: E68–E76.
19. Papp JG. Autonomic responses and neurohumoral control in the human early antenatal heart. *Basic Res Cardiol* 1988;**83**: 2–9.
20. Padbury JF, Polk DH, Newnham JP and Lam RW. Neonatal adaptation: Greater sympathoadrenal response in preterm than full-term fetal sheep at birth. *Am J Physiol – Endocrinology and Metabolism* 1985;**11**: E443–E449.
21. Greenough A, Nicolaides KH and Lagercrantz H. Human fetal sympathoadrenal responsiveness. *Early Hum Develop* 1990;**23**: 9–13.
22. Demarini S and Donnelly M. Heart rate increases in very low birthweight infants during the first month of life: A trend opposite to comparable fetal heart rate. *Pediatr Res* 1994;**37**: 201A(Abstract).
23. Lagercrantz H, Edwards D, Henderson-Smart D, Hertzberg T and Jeffery H. Autonomic reflexes in preterm infants. *Acta Paed Scand* 1990;**79**: 721–728.
24. Drouin E, Gournay V, Calamel J, Mouzard A and Roze JC. Assessment of spontaneous baroreflex sensitivity in neonates. *Arch Dis Child* 1997;**76**: F108–F112.
25. Walker AM. Circulatory transition at birth and the control of the neonatal circulation. In: Hansen MA, Spencer JAD and Rodeck CH (eds) *The Circulation.* Cambridge: Cambridge University Press, 1993, pp 160–196.
26. Blanco CE, Dawes GS, Hanson MA and McCooke HB. Carotid baroreceptors in fetal and newborn sheep. *Pediatr Res* 1988;**24**: 342–346.
27. Patton DJ and Hanna BD. Maturation postnatalie de la maitrise de la frequence cardiaque chez les procelets nouveau-nez (Postnatal maturation of baroreflex heart rate control in neonatal swine). *Can J Cardiol* 1994;**10**: 233–238.
28. Bossaert LL, Demey HE, De Jongh R and Heytens L. Haemodynamic monitoring: Problems, pitfalls and practical solutions. *Drugs* 1991;**41**: 857–874.
29. Winberg P and Ergander U. Relationship between heart rate, left ventricular output, and stroke volume in preterm infants during fluctuations in heart rate. *Pediatr Res* 1992;**31**: 117–120.
30. Cuevas L, Yeh TF, John EG, Cuevas D and Plides RS. The effect of low-dose dopamine infusion on cardiopulmonary and renal status in premature newborns with respiratory distress syndrome. *Am J Dis Child* 1991;**145**: 799–803.
31. Heaf DP, Belik J, Spitzer AR *et al.* Changes in pulmonary function during the diuretic phase of respiratory distress syndrome. *J Pediatr* 1982;**101**: 103–107.
32. Walker AM. Physiological control of the fetal cardiovascular system. In: Beard RW and Nathanielsz PW (eds) *Fetal Physiology and Medicine.* New York: Marcel Dekker, 1984, pp 287–316.
33. Lyon AJ, Pikaar MS, Badger P and McIntosh N. Temperature control in very low birthweight infants during the first five days of life. *Arch Dis Child* 1997;**76**: F47–F50.

34. Martinussen M, Brubakk AM, Vik T and Yao AC. Mesenteric blood flow velocity and its relation to transitional circulatory adaptation in appropriate for gestational age preterm infants. *Pediatr Res* 1996;**39**: 275–280.
35. Manz F, Kalhoff H and Remer T. Renal acid excretion in early infancy. *Pediatr Nephrol* 1997;**11**: 231–243.
36. Perlman J and Thach B. Respiratory origin of fluctuations in arterial blood pressure in premature infants with respiratory distress syndrome. *Pediatrics* 1988;**81**: 399–403.
37. Rennie JM. Cerebral blood flow velocity variability after cardiovascular support in premature babies. *Arch Dis Child* 1989;**64**: 897–901.
38. Diprose GK, Evans DH, Archer LNJ and Levene MI. Dinamap fails to detect hypotension in very low birthweight infants. *Arch Dis Child* 1986;**61**: 771–773.
39. Smolich JJ, Soust M, Berger PJ and Walker AM. Indirect relation between rises in oxygen consumption and left ventricular output at birth in lambs. *Circ Res* 1992;**71**: 443–450.
40. Saigal S, Rosenbaum P, Stoskopf B *et al.* Comprehensive assessment of the health status of extremely low birth weight children at eight years of age: Comparison with a reference group. *J Pediatr* 1994;**125**: 411–417.
41. Saigal S, Feeny D, Rosenbaum P, Furlong W, Burrows E and Stoskopf B. Self perceived health status and health related quality of life of extremely low birthweight infants at adolescence. *JAMA* 1996;**276**: 453–459.
42. Hanson MA. The control of heart rate and blood pressure in the fetus: theoretical considerations. In: Hansen MA, Spencer JAD and Rodeck CH (eds) *The Circulation*. Cambridge: Cambridge University Press, 1993, pp 1–22.
43. Versmold HT, Kitterman JA, Phibbs RH *et al.* Aortic blood pressure during the first 12 hours of life in infants with birth weight 610 to 4,220 grams. *Pediatrics* 1981;**67**: 607–613.
44. Watkins AMC, West CR and Cooke RWI. Blood pressure and cerebral haemorrhage and ischaemia in very low birthweight infants. *Early Hum Dev* 1989;**19**: 103–110.
45. Bada HS, Korones SB, Perry EH *et al.* Mean arterial blood pressure changes in premature infants and those at risk for intraventricular hemorrhage. *J Pediatr* 1990;**117**: 607–614.
46. Hegyi T, Carbone MT, Anwar M *et al.* Blood pressure ranges in premature infants. I. The first hours of life. *J Pediatr* 1994;**124**: 627–633.
47. Hegyi T, Anwar M, Carbone MT *et al.* Blood pressure ranges in premature infants: II. The first week of life. *Pediatrics* 1996;**97**: 336–342.
48. Cunningham S, Symon AG, Elton RA and McIntosh N. Mean blood pressure in the very low birthweight and its relation to long term outcome. 1998 (in press)
49. Gill AB and Weindling AM. Echocardiographic assessment of cardiac function in shocked very low birthweight infants. *Arch Dis Child* 1993;**68**: 17–21.
50. Bourchier D and Weston PJ. Randomised trial of dopamine compared with hydrocortisone for the treatment of hypotensive very low birthweight infants. *Arch Dis Child* 1997;**76**: F174–F178.

51. Campbell ME and Byrne PJ. Does intravenous epinephrine by infusion improve outcome in ELBW infants (<750g)? *Pediatr Res* 1997;**40**: 142A(Abstract).
52. Moise AA, Wearden ME, Welty SE, Kozinetz CA and Hansen TN. Treatment of hypotension in a 24 week premature infant: A national survey. *Pediatr Res* 1993;**33**: 226A(Abstract)
53. Barr PA, Bailey PE, Sumners J and Cassady G. Relation between arterial blood pressure and blood volume and effect of infused albumin in sick preterm infants. *Pediatrics* 1977;**60**: 282–289.
54. Kopelman AE. Blood pressure and cerebral ischemia in very low birth weight infants. *J Pediatr* 1990;**116**: 1000–1002.
55. Szymonowicz W, Yu VYH, Walker A and Wilson F. Reduction in periventricular haemorrhage in preterm infants. *Arch Dis Child* 1986;**61**: 661–665.
56. Miall-Allen VM, De Vries LS and Whitelaw AGL. Mean arterial blood pressure and neonatal cerebral lesions. *Arch Dis Child* 1987;**62**: 1068–1069.
57. Puccio VF, Nahum L, Massone ML, Tassara GB and Soliani M. Arterial blood pressure and cerebral hemorrhage in the critically ill premature infants. *J Perinat Med* 1994;**22** (**Suppl**): 93–96.
58. Roze JC, Tohier C, Maingueneau C, Lefevre M and Mouzard A. Response to dobutamine and dopamine in the hypotensive very preterm infant. *Arch Dis Child* 1993;**69**: 59–63.
59. Klarr JM, Faix RG, Pryce CJE and Bhatt-Mehta V. Randomized, blind trial of dopamine versus dobutamine for treatment of hypotension in preterm infants with respiratory distress syndrome. *J Pediatr* 1994;**125**: 117–122.
60. Moise AA, Wearden ME, Kozinetz CA, Gest AL, Welty SE and Hansen TN. Antenatal steroids are associated with less need for blood pressure support in extremely premature infants. *Pediatrics* 1995;**95**: 845–850.
61. Tyszczuk L, Meek J, Elwell C, Wyatt J and Reynolds EOR. Cerebral blood flow measured by near infrared spectroscopy in hypotensive preterm infants. *Early Hum Dev* 1996;**45**: 133A(Abstract)
62. Levene M, Chiswick M, Field D *et al.* Development of audit measures and guidelines for good practice in the management of neonatal respiratory distress syndrome. *Arch Dis Child* 1992;**67**: 1221–1227.
63. Cunningham S, Symon AG, Elton RA and McIntosh N. Gestational age as a lower limit for mean blood pressure. *Early Hum Dev* 1994;**36**: 232–233(Abstract).
64. D'Souza SW, Janakova H, Minors D *et al.* Blood pressure, heart rate, and skin temperature in preterm infants: Associations with periventricular haemorrhage. *Arch Dis Child* 1995;**72**: F162–F167.
65. Kuban KCK, Epi SM and Volpe JJ. Intraventricular hemorrhage: An update. *J Intensive Care Med* 1993;**8**: 157–176.
66. Cooke RWI. Annual audit of neonatal morbidity in preterm infants. *Arch Dis Child* 1992;**67**: 1174–1176.
67. Bryan-Brown CW. Blood flow to organs: Parameters for function and survival in critical illness. *Crit Care Med* 1988;**16**: 170–178.

68. Cronin CM and Milley JR. Splanchnic blood flow, oxygen delivery and oxygen consumption in hypotensive newborn piglets. *Biol Neonate* 1992;**61**: 374–380.
69. ONeill JT, Golden SM, Franklin GA and Alden ER. Cerebral vascular response to hemorrhagic hypotension in newborn lambs: The influence of developing anemia. *Proc Soc Exp Biol Med* 1994;**205**: 132–139.
70. Rosenberg AA, Harris AP, Koehler RC *et al.* Role of O_2-hemoglobin affinity in the regulation of cerebral blood flow in fetal sheep. *Am J Physiol* 1986;**251**: H56–H62.
71. Tweed WA, Cote J, Wade JG *et al.* Preservation of fetal brain blood flow relative to other organs during hypovolemic hypotension. *Pediatr Res* 1982;**16**: 137–140.
72. Aperia A and Herin P. Effect of arterial blood pressure reduction on renal hemodynamics in the developing lamb. *Acta Physiol Scand* 1976;**98**: 387–394.
73. Tuor UI and Grewal D. Autoregulation of cerebral blood flow: Influence of local brain development and postnatal age. *Am J Physiol* 1994;**267**: H2220–H2228.
74. Anwar M, Agarwal R, Rashduni D and Weiss HR. Effects of hemorrhagic hypotension on cerebral blood flow and perfused capillaries in newborn pigs. *Can J Physiol Pharmacol* 1996;**74**: 157–162.
75. Tweed A, Cote J, Lou H *et al.* Impairment of cerebral blood flow autoregulation in the newborn lamb by hypoxia. *Pediatr Res* 1986;**20**: 516–519.
76. Jorch G and Jorch N. Failure of autoregulation of cerebral blood flow in neonates studied by pulsed Doppler ultrasound of the internal carotid artery. *Eur J Pediatr* 1987;**146**: 468–472.
77. Van de Bor M and Walther FJ. Cerebral blood flow velocity regulation in preterm infants. *Biol Neonate* 1991;**59**: 329–335.
78. Gunn AJ, Parer JT, Mallard EC, Williams CE and Gluckman PD. Cerebral histologic and electrocorticographic changes after asphyxia in fetal sheep. *Pediatr Res* 1992;**31**: 486–491.
79. Mallard EC, Williams CE, Johnston BM, Gunning MI, Davis S and Gluckman PD. Repeated episodes of umbilical cord occlusion in fetal sheep lead to preferential damage to the striatum and sensitize the heart to further insults. *Pediatr Res* 1995;**37**: 707–713.
80. Szymonowicz W, Walker AM, Cussen L, Cannata J and Yu VYH. Developmental changes in regional cerebral blood flow in fetal and newborn lambs. *Am J Physiol* 1988;**254**: 23/1 H52–H58.
81. Low JA, Froese AB, Galbraith RS, Smith JT, Sauerbrei EE and Derrick EJ. The association between preterm newborn hypotension and hypoxemia and outcome during the first year. *Acta Paediatr Int J Paediatr* 1993;**82**: 433–437.
82. Lou HC, Skov H and Henriksen L. Intellectual impairment with regional cerebral dysfunction after low neonatal cerebral blood flow. *Acta Paediatr Scand* 1989;**78 (Suppl)**: 72–82.
83. Greisen G. Ischaemia of the preterm brain. *Biol Neonate* 1992;**62**: 243–247.
84. Greisen G. Cerebral blood flow in preterm infants during the first week of life. *Acta Paed Scand* 1986;**75**: 43–51.

85. Pryds O, Greisen G, Lou H and Friis-Hansen B. Heterogeneity of cerebral vasoreactivity in preterm infants supported by mechanical ventilation. *J Pediatr* 1989;**115**: 638–645.
86. Altman DI, Powers WJ, Perlman JM, Herscovitch P, Volpe SL and Volpe JJ. Cerebral blood flow requirement for brain viability in newborn infants is lower than in adults. *Ann Neurol* 1988;**24**: 218–226.
87. Funato M, Tamai H, Noma K *et al.* Clinical events in association with timing of intraventricular hemorrhage in preterm infants. *J Pediatr* 1992;**121**: 614–619.
88. Szymonowicz W, Yu VYH and Wilson FE. Antecedents of periventricular haemorrhage in infants weighing 1250 g or less at birth. *Arch Dis Child* 1984;**59**: 13–17.
89. Thorburn RJ, Lipscomb AP, Stewart AL *et al.* Timing and antecedents of periventricular haemorrhage and of cerebral atrophy in very preterm infants. *Early Hum Dev* 1982;**7**: 221–238.
90. Leviton A, Pagano M, Kuban KCK, Krishnamoorthy KS, Sullivan KF and Allred EN. The epidemiology of germinal matrix hemorrhage during the first half day of life. *Dev Med Child Neurol* 1991;**33**: 138–145.
91. Perlman JM, Goodman S, Kreusser KL and Volpe JJ. Reduction in intraventricular hemorrhage by elimination of fluctuating cerebral blood-flow velocity in preterm infants with respiratory distress syndrome. *N Engl J Med* 1985;**312**: 1353–1357.
92. Perry EH, Bada HS, Ray JD, Korones SB, Arheart K and Magill HL. Blood pressure increases, birth weight-dependent stability boundary, and intraventricular hemorrhage. *Pediatrics* 1990;**85**: 727–732.
93. McDonald MM, Koops BL, Johnson ML *et al.* Timing and antecedents of intracranial hemorrhage in the newborn. *Pediatrics* 1984;**74**: 32–36.
94. Perlman JM, McMenamin JB and Volpe JJ. Fluctuating cerebral blood-flow velocity in respiratory-distress syndrome. Relation to the development of intraventricular hemorrhage. *N Engl J Med* 1983;**309**: 204–209.
95. Milligan DWA. Failure of autoregulation and intraventricular haemorrhage in preterm infants. *Lancet* 1980;**1**: 896–898.
96. Miall-Allen VM, De Vries LS, Dubowitz LMS and Whitelaw AGL. Blood pressure fluctuation and intraventricular hemorrhage in the preterm infant of less than 31 weeks' gestation. *Pediatrics* 1989;**83**: 657–661.
97. Beverley DW, Pitts-Tucker TJ, Congdon PJ *et al.* Prevention of intraventricular haemorrhage by fresh frozen plasma. *Arch Dis Child* 1985;**60**: 710–713.
98. Tin W, Wariyar U and Hey E. Randomised trial of prophylactic early fresh frozen plasma or gelatin or glucose in preterm babies: outcome at 2 years. *Lancet* 1996;**348**: 229–232.
99. Van de Bor M. Renal blood flow velocity in non-distressed preterm infants during the first 72 hours of life. *Biol Neonate* 1995;**67**: 346–351.
100. Ekblad H, Kero P and Korvenranta H. Renal function in preterm infants during the first five days of life: Influence of maturation and early colloid treatment. *Biol Neonate* 1992;**61**: 308–317.

101. Jose PA, Harmati A and Fildes R. Postnatal maturation of renal blood flow. In: Polin RA and Fox WW (eds) *Fetal and Neonatal Physiology*. Philadephia: Saunders, 1992, pp 1196–1200.
102. Seikaly MG and Arant BS Jr. Development of renal hemodynamics: Glomerular filtration and renal blood flow. *Clin Perinatol* 1992;**19**: 1–13.
103. Vanpee M, Ergander U, Herin P and Aperia A. Renal function in sick, very low-birth-weight infants. *Acta Paediatr Int J Paediatr* 1993;**82**: 714–718.
104. Guignard JP, Torrado A, Mazouni SM and Gautier E. Renal function in respiratory distress syndrome. *J Pediatr* 1976;**88**: 845–850.
105. Spitzer AR, Fox WW, Delivoria-Papadopoulos M. Maximum diuresis – a factor in predicting recovery from respiratory distress syndrome and the development of bronchopulmonary dysplasia. *J Pediatr* 1981;**98**: 476–479.
106. Bhat R, John E, Diaz-Blanco J, Ortega R, Fornell L and Vidyasagar D. Surfactant therapy and spontaneous diuresis. *J Pediatr* 1989;**114**: 443–447.
107. Lucking SE, Williams TM and Mickell JJ. Organ blood flow and cardiovascular effects of high-frequency oscillation versus conventional ventilation in dogs with right heart failure. *Crit Care Med* 1989;**17**: 158–162.
108. Kinsella JP, Gerstmann DR, Gong AK, Taylor AF and DeLemos RA. Ductal shunting and effective systemic blood flow following single dose surfactant treatment in the premature baboon with hyaline membrane disease. *Biol Neonate* 1991;**60**: 283–291.
109. Miller FC, Read JA, Cabal L and Siassi B. Heart rate and blood pressure in infants of pre-eclamptic mothers during the first half hour of life. *Crit Care Med* 1983;**11**: 532–535.
110. Seri I, Rudas G, Bors Z, Kanyicska B and Tulassay T. Effects of low-dose dopamine infusion on cardiovascular and renal functions, cerebral blood flow, and plasma catecholamine levels in sick preterm neonates. *Pediatr Res* 1993;**34**: 742–749.
111. Barrington KJ and Seri I. Circulatory effects of dopamine in neonates [2]. *J Pediatr* 1995;**127**: 843–844.
112. Barrington KJ, Finer NN and Chan WKY. A blind, randomized comparison of the circulatory effects of dopamine and epinephrine infusions in the newborn piglet during normoxia and hypoxia. *Crit Care Med* 1995;**23**: 740–748.
113. Ascuitto RJ, Ross-Ascuitto NT, Ramage D, McDonough KH and Kadowitz PJ. Acetylcholine-induced coronary vasoconstriction and negative inotropy in the neonatal pig heart. *Pediatr Res* 1992;**32**: 236–242.
114. Coombs RC, Morgan MEI, Durbin GM, Booth IW and McNeish AS. Abnormal gut blood flow velocities in neonates at risk of necrotising enterocolitis. *J Pediatr Gastroenterol Nutr* 1992;**15**: 13–19.
115. Nowicki PT, Hansen NB and Menke JA. Intestinal blood flow and oxygen uptake in the neonatal piglet during reduced perfusion pressure. *Am J Physiol – Gastrointestinal and Liver Physiology* 1987;**252**: 15/2 G190–G194.
116. Nowicki PT and Miller CE. Autoregulation in the developing postnatal intestinal circulation. *Am J Physiol – Gastrointestinal and Liver Physiology* 1988;**254**: 17/2 G189-G193.

117. Buckley NM, Brazeau P and Frasier ID. Intestinal and femoral blood flow autoregulation in developing swine. *Biol Neonate* 1986;**49**: 229–240.
118. Gosche JR, Harris PD and Garrison RN. Age-related differences in intestinal microvascular responses to low-flow states in adult and suckling rats. *Am J Physiol – Gastrointestinal and Liver Physiology* 1993;**264**: G447–G453.
119. Hoang TV, Choe EU, Burgess RS, Cork RC, Flint LM and Ferrara JJ. Characterization of alpha-adrenoceptor activity in the preterm piglet mesentery. *J Pediatr Surg* 1996;**31**: 1659–1662.
120. Hentschel R, Hensel D, Brune T, Rabe H and Jorch G. Impact on blood pressure and intestinal perfusion of dobutamine or dopamine in hypotensive preterm infants. *Biol Neonate* 1995;**68**: 318–324.
121. Leidig E. Doppler analysis of superior mesenteric artery blood flow in preterm infants. *Arch Dis Child* 1989;**64**: 476–480.
122. Clyman RI. Developmental physiology of the ductus arteriosus. In: Long WA (ed) *Fetal and Neonatal Cardiology*. Philadelphia: WB Saunders, 1990, pp 64–75.
123. Waffarn F, Siassi B, Cabal LA and Schmidt PL. Effect of antenatal glucocorticoids on clinical closure of the ductus arteriosus. *Am J Dis Child* 1983;**137**: 336–338.
124. Evans N and Iyer P. Longitudinal changes in the diameter of the ductus arteriosus in ventilated preterm infants: Correlation with respiratory outcomes. *Arch Dis Child* 1995;**72**: F156–F161.
125. Skelton R, Evans N and Smythe J. A blinded comparison of clinical and echocardiographic evaluation of the preterm infant for patent ductus arteriosus. *J Pediatr Child Health* 1994;**30**: 406–411.
126. Baylen BG, Ogata H, Oguchi K *et al.* The contractility and performance of the preterm left ventricle before and after early patent ductus arteriosus occlusion in surfactant-treated lambs. *Pediatr Res* 1985;**19**: 1053–1058.
127. Mellander M and Larsson LE. Effects of left-to-right ductus shunting on left ventricular output and cerebral blood flow velocity in 3-day-old preterm infants with and without severe lung disease. *J Pediatr* 1988;**113**: 101–109.
128. Evans N and Iyer P. Change in blood pressure after treatment of patent ductus arteriosus with indomethacin. *Arch Dis Child* 1993;**68**: 584–587.
129. Morrow WR, Taylor AF, Kinsella JP, Lally KP, Gerstmann DR and DeLemos RA. Effect of ductal patency on organ blood flow and pulmonary function in the preterm baboon with hyaline membrane disease. *Crit Care Med* 1995;**23**: 179–186.
130. Kimball TR, Ralston MA, Khoury P, Crump RG, Cho FS and Reuter JH. Effect of ligation of patent ductus arteriosus on left ventricular performance and its determinants in premature neonates. *J Am Coll Cardiol* 1996;**27**: 193–197.
131. Ratner I, Perlmuter B, Toews W and Whitfield J. Association of low systolic and diastolic blood pressure with significant patent ductus arteriosus in the very low birth weight infant. *Crit Care Med* 1985;**13**: 497–500.
132. Studer RK, Morgan J, Penkoske M and Potchen EJ. Regional vascular volume and extravascular accumulation of labeled protein during plasma volume expansion. *Am J Physiol* 1973;**224**: 669–704.

133. Kluckow M and Evans N. Early determinants of right and left ventricular output in ventilated preterm infants. *Arch Dis Child* 1996;**74**: F88–F94.
134. Maayan C, Eyal F, Mandelberg A *et al.* Effect of mechanical ventilation and volume loading on left ventricular performance in premature infants with respiratory distress syndrome. *Crit Care Med* 1986;**14**: 858–860.
135. Bauer K, Linderkamp O and Versmold HT. Systolic blood pressure and blood volume in preterm infants. *Arch Dis Child* 1993;**69**: 521–522.
136. Brown EG, Krouskop RW, McDonnell FE and Sweet AY. Blood volume and blood pressure in infants with respiratory distress. *J Pediatr* 1975;**87**: 1133–1138.
137. Bauer K, Linderkamp O and Versmold HT. Short-term effects of blood transfusion on blood volume and resting peripheral blood flow in preterm infants. *Acta Paediatr* 1993;**82**: 1029–1033.
138. Lay KS, Bancalari E, Malkus H *et al.* Acute effects of albumin infusion on blood volume and renal function in premature infants with respiratory distress syndrome. *J Pediatr* 1980;**97**: 619–623.
139. Kempley ST and Gamsu HR. Arterial blood pressure and blood flow velocity in major cerebral and visceral arteries: II – Effects of colloid infusion. *Early Hum Dev* 1993;**35**: 25–30.
140. Emery EF, Greenough A, Gamsu HR. Randomised controlled trial of colloid infusions in hypotensive preterm infants. *Arch Dis Child* 1992;**67**: 1185–1188.
141. Bignall S, Bailey PC, Bass CA, Cramb R, Rivers RPA and Wadsworth J. The cardiovascular and oncotic effects of albumin infusion in premature infants. *Early Hum Dev* 1989;**20**: 191–201.
142. Igarashi H, Shiraishi H, Endoh H and Yanagisawa M. Left ventricular contractile state in preterm infants: Relation between wall stress and velocity of circumferential fiber shortening. *Am Heart J* 1994;**127**: 1336–1340.
143. Martinez AM, Padbury JF and Thio S. Dobutamine pharmacokinetics and cardiovascular responses in critically ill neonates. *Pediatrics* 1992;**89**: 47–51.
144. Greenough A and Emery EF. Randomized trial comparing dopamine and dobutamine in preterm infants. *Eur J Pediatr* 1993;**152**: 925–927.
145. Gootman N, Buckley BJ and Gootman PM. Maturational related differences in regional circulatory effects of dopamine in swine. *Dev Pharmacol Ther* 1983;**6**: 9–22.
146. Pearson RJ, Barrington KJ, Jirsch DW and Cheung PY. Dopaminergic receptor-mediated effects in the mesenteric vasculature and renal vasculature of the chronically instrumented newborn piglet. *Crit Care Med* 1996;**24**: 1706–1712.
147. Padbury JF, Agata Y, Baylen BG *et al.* Dopamine pharmacokinetics in critically ill newborn infants. *J Pediatr* 1987;**110**: 293–298.
148. Kulka PJ and Tryba M. Inotropic support of the critically ill patient: A review of the agents. *Drugs* 1993;**45**: 654–667.
149. Driscoll DJ. Use of inotropic and chronotropic agents in neonates. *Clin Perinatol* 1987;**14**: 931–949.
150. Padbury JF, Ludlow JK, Ervin MG *et al.* Thresholds for physiological effects of plasma catecholamines in fetal sheep. *Am J Physiol – Endocrinology and Metabolism* 1987;**252**: 15/4 E530–E537.

151. Ferrara JJ, Dyess DL, Peoples GL *et al.* Effects of dopamine and dobutamine on regional blood flow distribution in the neonatal piglet. *Ann Surg* 1995;**221**: 531–542.
152. Abbasi S, Seri I, Wood DC and Gerdes JS. Evidence for functional maturity of the renal vascular dopamine receptors in extremely low birthweight neonates. *Pediatr Res* 1997;**41**: 134A(Abstract)
153. Goldberg LI and Raifer SI. Dopamine receptors: applied clinical cardiology. *Circulation* 1985;**72**: 245–248.
154. Schaer GL, Fink MP and Parillo JE. Norepinephrine alone versus norepinephrine plus low dose dopamine: enhanced renal blood flow with combination pressure therapy. *Crit Care Med* 1985;**13**: 492–501.
155. Bhatt-Mehta V and Nahata MC. Dopamine and dobutamine in pediatric therapy. *Pharmacotherapy* 1989;**9**: 303–314.
156. Seri I. Cardiovascular, renal, and endocrine actions of dopamine in neonates and children. *J Pediatr* 1995;**126**: 333–344.
157. Duke GJ and Bersten AD. Dopamine and renal salvage in the critically ill patient. *Anaesth Intensive Care* 1992;**20**: 277–302.
158. Segal JM, Phang PT and Walley KR. Low-dose dopamine hastens onset of gut ischemia in a porcine model of hemorrhagic shock. *J Appl Physiol* 1992;**73**: 1159–1164.
159. Gill AB and Weindling AM. Randomised controlled trial of plasma protein fraction versus dopamine in hypotensive very low birthweight infants. *Arch Dis Child* 1993;**69**: 284–287.
160. McIntosh N. Hypotension associated with pancuronium use in the newborn. *Lancet* 1985; **ii**: 279 (letter)
161. Derleth DP. Clinical experience with norepinephrine infusions in critically ill newborns. *Pediatr Res* 1997;**41**: 145A(Abstract)
162. Haigh RM and Jones CT. Effect of glucocorticoids on alpha1-adrenergic receptor binding in rat vascular smooth muscle. *J Mol Endocrinol* 1990;**5**: 41–48.
163. Wood CE, Cheung CY and Brace RA. Fetal heart rate, arterial pressure, and blood volume responses to cortisol infusion. *Am J Physiol – Regulatory Integrative and Comparative Physiology* 1987;**253**: 22/6 R904–R909.
164. Grunfeld JP. Glucocorticoids in blood pressure regulation. *Hormone Res* 1990;**34**: 111–113.
165. Grunfeld JP and Eloy L. Role of glucocorticoids in blood pressure regulation. *Kidney Int* 1988;**34**: S49–S51.
166. Grunfeld JP and Eloy L. Glucocorticoids modulate vascular reactivity in the rat. *Hypertension* 1987;**10**: 608–618.
167. Garland JS, Buck R and Leviton A. Effect of maternal glucocorticoid exposure on risk of severe intraventricular hemorrhage in surfactant-treated preterm infants. *J Pediatr* 1995;**126**: 272–279.
168. Padbury JF, Polk DH, Ervin MG, Berry LM, Ikegami M and Jobe AH. Postnatal cardiovascular and metabolic responses to a single intramuscular dose of betamethasone in fetal sheep born prematurely by cesarean section. *Pediatr Res* 1995;**38**: 709–715.

169. Stein HM, Martinez A, Blount L, Oyama K and Padbury JF. The effects of corticosteroids and thyrotropin-releasing hormone on newborn adaptation and sympathoadrenal mechanisms in preterm sheep. *Am J Obstet Gynecol* 1994;**171**: 17–24.
170. Arnold JD, Bonacruz G, Leslie GI, Veldhuis JD, Milmlow D and Silink M. Cortisol production rate is related to mean arterial blood pressure in neonates. *Pediatr Res* 1997;**41**: 138A(Abstract).
171. Korte C, Styne D, Merritt TA, Mayes D, Wertz A and Helbock HJ. Adrenocortical function in the very low birth weight infant: Improved testing sensitivity and association with neonatal outcome. *J Pediatr* 1996;**128**: 257–263.
172. Fauser A, Pohlandt F, Bartmann P and Gortner L. Rapid increase of blood pressure in extremely low birth weight infants after a single dose of dexamethasone. *Eur J Pediatr* 1993;**152**: 354–356.
173. Helbock HJ, Insoft RM and Conte FA. Glucocorticoid-responsive hypotension in extremely low birth weight newborns. *Pediatrics* 1993;**92**: 715–717.
174. Derleth DP. Blood pressure in low birth weight infants after dexamethasone. *Eur J Pediatr* 1994;**153**: 211.
175. Yoxall CW and Weindling AM. The measurement of peripheral venous oxyhemoglobin saturation in newborn infants by near infrared spectroscopy with venous occlusion. *Pediatr Res* 1996;**39**: 1103–1106.
176. Kitterman JA, Phibbs RH and Tooley WH. Aortic blood pressure in normal newborn infants during the first 12 hours of life. *Pediatrics* 1969;**44**: 959–968.
177. Bucci G, Scalamandre A, Savignoni PG, Mendicini M and Bucci SP. The systemic systolic blood pressure of newborns with low weight: a multiple regression analysis. *Acta Paediat Scand* 1972;**229 (Suppl)**: 1–22.
178. Moscoso P, Goldberg RN, Jamieson J and Bancalari E. Spontaneous elevation in arterial blood pressure during the first hours of life in the very-low-birth-weight infant. *J Pediatr* 1983;**103**: 114–117.
179. Adams MA, Pasternak JF, Kupfer BM and Gardner TH. A computerized system for continuous physiologic data collection and analysis: Initial report on mean arterial blood pressure in very low-birth-weight infants. *Pediatrics* 1983;**71**: 23–30.
180. Kollée LAA, Schölls WA and Peer PGM. Non invasive blood pressure measurement in the neonate. Rolfe, P (ed); **1(2)**: 69–73, 1986. Oxford, Butterworth & Co. Proceedings of International Conference on Fetal and Neonatal Physiological Measurements.
181. Tan KL. Blood pressure in very low birth weight infants in the first 70 days of life. *J Pediatr* 1988;**112**: 266–270.
182. Shortland DB, Evans DH and Levene MI. Blood pressure measurements in very low birth weight infants over the first week of life. *J Perinat Med* 1988;**16**: 93–97.
183. Spinazzola RM, Harper RG, de Soler M and Lesser M. Blood pressure values in 500 to 750 gram birthweight infants in the first week of life. *J Perinatol* 1991;**11**: 147–151.

184. Low JA, Froese AB, Smith JT, Galbraith RS, Sauerbrei EE and Karchmar EJ. Blood pressure and heart rate of the preterm newborn following delivery. *Clin Invest Med* 1991;**14**: 183–187.
185. Powell PJ, Assassa P, Ellis A, Hollis S and Robinson MJ. Normal blood pressure measurements in very low birthweight babies. *Early Hum Dev* 1992;**30**: 84A(Abstract).
186. Greenough A and Emery EF. Systolic blood pressure levels of ventilated, very preterm infants. *Br J Intensive Care* 1993;**1**: 130–136.

5

Nutrition and the Brain

Forrester Cockburn

All plants and animals require a supply of basic nutrients if growth and development to the final adult form and size, determined by their genetic endowment, is to be achieved. Plants can utilize simple elements, water and gases under the influence of the warmth and light of the sun but herbivores require a supply of more complex nutrients synthesized by plants, whilst carnivores require a supply of very complex nutrients synthesized by herbivores to achieve their genetic potential.

The feature which differentiates man from other animals is the size, complexity and ingenuity of his brain. Processes of evolution which have allowed the survival of Homo sapiens, and the growth and continuing development of the human brain, must relate to the supply of nutrients reaching the brain cells and to genetic (DNA) adaptations. As most of the brain's growth is achieved during the first 3 years of life, nutrient supply during intrauterine development and the first 2 postnatal years must have a major influence on the structure, quality and function of that organ.

What evidence is there that nutritional 'deficiencies' during early life affect brain growth and development? In order to know what constitutes a 'deficiency' of one or more nutrients for growing brain cells, knowledge would be needed of the 'ideal' composition of every element of this cell from membrane to nucleolus. There can be no simple answer to the question, 'What is the ideal chemical structure and composition of, for example, a motor neurone?' As the evolution of the brain of Homo sapiens will have been determined in part by variations in the supply of nutrients, future beneficial and detrimental evolution of brain function may also be determined by changes in the food ingested by mothers and infants.

FETAL BRAIN GROWTH

Embryogenesis in the human has been arbitrarily defined as occurring between 20 and 60 days post-conception. Neural crest elements appear in the human conceptus before 20 days and changes in brain structure continue well beyond 60 days and even well after birth. The prolonged intrauterine and postnatal growth and development of the human infant brain differentiates it from central nervous system development in other animals and also makes the human brain more susceptible to a variety of insults over a longer period of time.

Dysmorphogenesis of the developing brain could result from a wide range of potential nutrient imbalances affecting a very complex range of genetic/environmental interactions. Chromosomal and gene mutation abnormalities act during all phases of pre- and post-natal life and can cause isolated or multiple brain anomalies. Regulatory (master) genes code for polypeptides that are active in cell nuclei and modify the array of transcribed genes from the totipotent cells of the 2–8 cell embryo to the specialized cell populations of later brain development. Proliferation and differentiation of brain cells is largely mediated by growth and transcription factors. Transcription factors, controlled by regulatory genes, promote a cascade of temporally and spacially organized events that cause the formation of, for example, the neural tube, diencephalon, mesencephalon and corpus callosum.

It is at about 18 days post conception when the total fetal length is 1.5 mm that the neural crest first becomes evident.[1] Between 21 and 24 days the spinal cord and neural tube are formed and closed. At 30 days the cerebellum and at 32 days the cerebral hemispheres first appear. By 37 days the neurohypophysis is identified and links with the developing endocrine system are evident. At 41 days the olfactory bulb with its sensory links has appeared. The first appearance of the cortical plate occurs at 52 days when the embryo is 25 mm long. This complex sequence of events is controlled by regional differences in molecular composition which in turn is determined by regional gene expression. Abnormal transcription regulation can cause profound errors of brain embryogenesis and is involved in disorders such as schizencephaly and holoprosencephaly; the PAX 6 gene is essential for brain development.[2, 3] The craniosynostoses found in Crouzon's and Apert's disorders are associated with fibroblast growth factor receptor defects.[4, 5] Cell replication, programmed cell death (apoptosis) induction and intercellular communication, cell migration and movement of contiguous cell populations are all in part determined by regulatory genes and their transcription factors. Nutritional and metabolic disorders present at critical stages of embryogenesis have the potential to interfere with the developmental changes controlled and influenced by the regulatory genes.

The X-linked metabolic disorder pyruvate dehydrogenase deficiency is associated with gross cerebral atrophy and corpus callosum agenesis.[6] Septo-optic dysplasia and Leigh's encephalopathy are also disorders associated with mitochondrial energy defects. It is possible that other events such as intrauterine ischaemia associated with vascular events and hypoxia could result in the same type of anatomical defect.

Most neurones have formed by 22 weeks' gestation and have migrated from their area of origin in the subendymal regions to the cortical surface. During the second half of pregnancy these cells develop complex arborizations and after birth there is a very rapid increase in the numbers of synaptosomes.[7–10] Synaptosomes are largely comprised of phospholipid membrane and the protein/peptide structures essential for neurotransmission. Maternal infections, physical insults and metabolic disorders, such as diabetes mellitus, phenylketonuria and maternal ingestion of teratogens (e.g. alcohol), increase the risk of congenital brain anomaly by affecting early developmental processes. The role of maternal malnutrition in altering the composition and structure of the developing fetal brain and its membranes is less clear.

MINERAL AND VITAMIN DEFICIENCIES

Severe zinc deficiency states can adversely influence transcriptions through effects on zinc-dependent nucleoprotein enzyme systems. Severe zinc deprivation during embryonic and fetal development in the rat has profound effects on virtually all derivatives of the neural tube and associated structures including the brain, spinal cord, eyes and olfactory tract.[11, 12] Deficiencies of manganese, copper, iron, selenium and iodine have been shown to affect the developing brain.[13–16]

Folic acid is important in neurogenesis, cell growth and myelination. Reduced DNA found in the brain tissue of rats born to folate-deficient mothers is probably due to the important role of folate in DNA and RNA metabolism.[17–20] Normal closure of the neural tube in man occurs between days 21 and 24. Folate deficiency before and during this stage of development results in neural tube defects. Individual mothers heterozygous for mutations in the genes for the common thermo-labile variant of 5,10-methylene tetrahydrofolate reductase (MTHFR) have increased blood concentrations of homocysteine when their dietary folate intakes are marginal. In some European populations the MTHFR defect is found in 5–7% of the population. Improving maternal dietary intakes of folate significantly reduces the incidence of neural tube defects and possibly other central nervous system defects.[17, 18]

Vitamin B_1 (thiamine) deficiency is relatively common in the developing world. Chronic alcoholism results in thiamine deficiency and the fetal defects associated with maternal alcohol ingestion may be mediated through thiamine deficiency.[19] Pyridoxine (vitamin B_6) deficiency studies in rats have shown that maternal deficiency can adversely affect cerebellar development.[20, 21] Maternal niacin and vitamin A deficiencies in animals have also been shown adversely to affect brain development.[22, 23]

Although it is possible to demonstrate that deficiencies or excesses of individual nutrients in pregnant animal studies have significant adverse effects on fetal brain development, it is not easy to identify parallel changes in human pregnancy. In reality it would be rare for women to have isolated nutrient deficiency states. It is more likely that within population subgroups there are young women with a suboptimal nutrient status for a range of nutrients, the combined effects of which could adversely affect brain growth and development of the fetus.

MALNUTRITION

Well nourished women of average size in the UK gain 11–13 kg during pregnancy[24] and the weight gained is proportional to the women's height.[25] The nutritional status of the mother before pregnancy, particularly when she is not yet fully grown herself, strongly influences fetal growth. It is only when there is evidence of severe pre-pregnancy and pregnancy undernutrition that head circumference is significantly reduced.[26] Combined pre- and post-natal malnutrition significantly reduces brain cell numbers permanently in humans.[27]

The developing brain of the newborn human infant and rat utilizes a mixture of glucose, ketone bodies and possibly fatty acids for their energy supply. After birth, under normal circumstances in both species, there is a gradual transition to the utilization of glucose alone through postnatal change in the pyruvate dehydrogenase complex (PDH) activities. In the brains of non-precocial species (e.g. guinea-pig), PDH is fully active prenatally.[28] Up until the time of birth, the energy supply is dependent upon maternal–placental supply whilst after birth, milk provides the energy. Different mammalian milks contain very different quantities and qualities of fats and carbohydrates.[29] It is likely that the enzymatic activities of mitochondria, cell membranes and cytoplasm of the newborn of individual species is 'adapted' to the range of substrates supplied by the milk of that species. Cross-species milk feeding will not supply optimal amounts of energy substrates for developing organs.

Effects on Brain Cells

There is a large body of evidence from animal studies to show the effects of pre- and post-natal under-feeding on the anatomical development of the brain.[30] Cerebral neurones are mainly formed at germinal zones in the subependymal layer which surrounds the ventricle and the dentate fascia of the hippocampus, while cerebellar cells originate mainly from the external granular layer. There are large numbers of glial cell precursors scattered throughout the brain.

Different cell types are more susceptible to undernutrition at different stages of brain development and dendritic networks and the number of nerve terminals and synapses per neurone in the cerebral cortex can be affected by both pre- and post-natal dietary restriction.[31–34] Purkinje cells are formed exclusively before birth and are markedly reduced in animals subjected to prenatal undernutrition.[35] Similar observations on cerebellar granular cells have shown that undernutrition decreases their numbers and that a degree of recovery can occur with nutritional enhancement after weaning in the rat. In rats and mice, the formation of astrocytes begins in late fetal life and precedes that of oligodendroglia which largely develop postnatally. In the human, a substantial portion of oligodendrocyte maturation takes place *in utero*. Postnatal malnutrition in rats adversely affects oligodendroglial function and myelination.[36] Myelination in the optic nerve, corpus callosum and pyramidal tracks is delayed in postnatally malnourished rats and although subsequent nutritional rehabilitation can result in some recovery there remains a permanent deficit.[37–39]

Astrocytes and their projections have a major role in guiding neuronal neurite outgrowths (growth cones) to their destinations where they form synapses. For example, there is a structure of astrocytes which predetermines the route for neuronal axons passing through the developing corpus callosum.[40] Populations of astrocytes in different brain regions elaborate differing chemical cues for adjacent neuronal growth cones and growth cones in turn may, by secretion of cytokines, change the chemical cues of adjacent glial cells.[41–43]

Underdevelopment of the glial guidance systems due to malnutrition results in a marked reduction of the number of axons reaching their targets. Astrocytic and oligodendrocytic proliferation in the immediate postnatal period is determined by the normal sequence of gene expression and by the availability of appropriate nutrients. If this time sequence of transcription-regulated activity is disrupted because of nutritional deficit, lack of environmental stimuli from parents or other sensory deprivation, optimal brain development and learning cannot be achieved. However, even late in development, late rehabilitation because of inherent functional plasticity and redundancy of cortical neurones can improve brain function.[44] The essential role of astrocytes in neuronal nutrition and functioning continues during and after completion of brain development and maturation. Maintenance of osmotic and electrolytic balance within neurones subject to rapid alternating polarization and depolarization requires astrocytic mediation through chemical shifts involving glutamine/glutamic acid, calcium, taurine and zinc.[45–47]

ALCOHOL AND HYPERPHENYLALANINAEMIA IN PREGNANCY

Prenatal exposure of the human brain to high concentrations of alcohol and phenylalanine can reduce total brain cell numbers and cause neuronal migration defects.[48–50] Mothers with poorly controlled phenylketonuria and who have high blood concentration of phenylalanine during early pregnancy produce infants with microcephaly and brain abnormalities. The anomalies can be prevented in subsequent pregnancies by controlling phenylalanine concentrations. Similarly, the morphological defects found in the brains of infants with fetal alcohol syndrome can be prevented in subsequent pregnancies by alcohol avoidance. The mechanisms of fetal brain damage caused by exposure to alcohol and excessive amounts of phenylalanine are unknown but may be the result of interference with transcription factors, neurotrophins or energy supply.

Malnutrition can distort synaptic transmitter systems and some of the structural and functional changes in the brain are related to early disruption of monoaminergic transmitter systems due to altered availability of amino acid precursors such as phenylalanine, tyrosine,[51] tryptophan[52, 53] and histidine.[54] The increased availability of precursor amino acids such as phenylalanine during early brain development might act by affecting the activity and expression of enzymes and/or receptors involved in the control of catecholamine and serotonin-mediated pathways in later life, i.e. dysfunctional programming.[55–60]

DIETARY FATTY ACIDS AND NEONATAL BRAIN GROWTH

At birth, the average term human infant brain weighs about 350 g. A preterm infant born at 24 weeks has an average brain weight of only 100 g. During the first postnatal year of life (infancy) the term infant brain weight increases by 750 g to a total weight of 1.1 kg. Approximately 47% of this increase in brain weight takes place in the cerebral cortex and 60% of the weight increase in cortex is lipid, predominantly (67%) phospholipid (Table 5.1).

For most normal infants the source of dietary fat is maternal milk but in infants fed formulae it may be vegetable oils and/or other animal milk fats. Infants born preterm may have to depend upon parenteral or enteral lipids from a variety of origins to supply structural lipids for the developing brain. Immaturity of function of the preterm infant's organs, particularly the gastrointestinal tract, liver, lung and vasculature, together with inadequate dietary sources of lipid, can adversely affect the development of the brain. Term infants fed formulae with fatty acid compositions significantly different from maternal milk also incorporate inappropriate combinations of fatty acids into the membranes of their vasculature and brain cells.

After birth there is a rapid increase in the numbers of synaptosomes which are largely comprised of phospholipid membrane and the protein/peptide structures essential for neurotransmission. This specialized phospholipid membrane, like all other body membranes, is comprised of a bimolecular sheet with fatty acids held in the interior of the bilayer and with polar phospholipid head groups on the internal and external faces of the membrane. Animal membranes which form cell surfaces and intracellular organelles such as mitochondria and peroxisomes are predominantly phosphoglycerols and

Table 5.1 Brain growth and lipid content during the first year in the human infant.

	Increase in weight (g)
Brain	750
Cortex	350
Cortex (dry weight)	125
Cortical lipid	75
Cortical phospholipid	50
Cortical docosahexaenoic acid	4

unesterified cholesterol. The major membrane phospholipids contain 2 fatty acids which are hydrophobic and a substituted (amino) alcohol attached to a glycerol phosphate backbone which is hydrophilic. In neuronal membranes, in addition to phosphoglycerols, there are sphingomyelins (phosphosphingolipids) and cerebrosides (glycosphingolipids). Alcohol head groups and the attached fatty acids have major effects on the functions of the membrane.[61] Phosphatidylcholine (PC), phosphatidylethanolamine (PE), phosphatidylserine (PS) and phosphatidylinositol (PI) are the major components of neuronal membranes. PC confers structural stability to the neuronal membrane,[62] while carboxyl groups of PS function as ion exchanges sites.[63]

For nerve cells to fulfil their function of neurotransmission, the peptides and proteins responsible for enzymatic activity and neurotransmission in phospholipid membranes must be inserted into the membrane at the appropriate site and in appropriate numbers. Control of the numbers and siting of the peptides and proteins is dependent not only upon genetic control but also upon the distribution of PS, PE and the type of fatty acid attached to these phospholipids.[63, 64] Incorporation of protein and peptide enzymes into the PS- and PE-rich areas of membrane is critically dependent upon the chain length, degree of unsaturation and molecular configuration of each of the 2 fatty acids attached to the PS and PE moieties. The polyunsaturated fatty acid docosahexaenoic acid (DHA) in neuronal membranes preferentially cross-links with proteins and the degree of unsaturation (6 double-bonds) conveyed by these molecules mediates the activities of the membrane-bound enzymes.[65, 66] The biophysical influence of high concentrations of DHA attached to PS and PE at the inner aspect of the phospholipid bilayer is essential for the rapid and repeated complex biochemical activities which allow neurotransmission to take place at neuronal synaptosomes. This is particularly important in the retina to allow the rapid conversion of light energy into electrical impulses in retinal photoreceptors.[67, 68]

Where there are deficiencies in the availability of long-chain polyunsaturated fatty acids (LCPUFA) there is substitution with fatty acids of similar chain length and desaturation. Insertion of the substituted LCPUFA can render membranes metabolically unstable and more permeable to water and electrolytes.[69] From Table 5.1 it can be seen that DHA, an n-3 fatty acid, is a particularly prominent component of cerebral cortex phospholipid. Animal studies have shown that in n-3 fatty acid deficiency states there is selective substitution of DHA in neuronal phospholipid membrane by n-6 docosapentaenoic acid (DPA).[70–72] Breastfed preterm and term infants have significantly greater concentrations of DHA in their cerebral cortex phospholipids than infants fed current infant formulae.[73–75]

Myelination, which is predominantly a postnatal process occurring in the first 18 months of postnatal life, is a function of neuroglial cells. Sheaves of myelin layers are wound round the neuronal axon and speed the rates of axonal transmission. The processes of myelination require the deposition of sphingomyelins and cerebrosides with relatively high concentrations of the fatty acids nervonic (C24:1n-9) and lignoceric (C24:0) acids. In infant cerebral white matter, there is, in addition to a reduced DHA content, a significantly lower concentration of nervonic (C24:1n-9) and lignoceric (C24:0) acids in formula-fed infants when compared to breastfed infants during the first 3–6 months of life.[76]

There is now a balance of evidence which shows that human milk conveys significant advantage to preterm and term infants' visual and cognitive functions when compared with those of infants fed standard infant formulae.[77–84]

NEONATAL BRAIN DEVELOPMENT

In fetal life brain anatomy, whilst affected by nutritional aberration, is largely determined by genomic guidance. After birth, human attributes such as motor coordination of finger movements, self awareness, memory, thought processes, speech, language and socialization are vulnerable to nutritional disorders and the quality of maternal care.[85–87]

The intercellular communications which subserve these complex activities require the integration of many neurobiological components. That every child has a completely different 'personality' by the age of 2–3 years is a result of differences in learning. The learning process is the result of serial neurochemical reactions which establish pathways and linkages between neurones and various glial cell types. At an early stage of brain development links are made with a variety of organs, including skin, vasculature, gut, hypothalamus, endocrine organs and the autonomic nervous systems, as well as with the organs of vision, hearing and olfaction.

Cerebral cortical 'control' of some autonomic and other brain stem responses are determined by early rearing practices. In order that intellectual and emotional functions are robust, there must be well modulated development of learned responses (behaviour). Not only must the basic neurones and connections be in the correct anatomical position, but the temporally sequenced electrophysiological stimuli (visual, auditory, nutritive and caring) must be appropriate and consistent.

Electrophysiological signals, when repetitive or prolonged, stimulate glial proliferation, direct and guide axonal growth cones to their destination and selectively reinforce synaptic pathways.[88, 89] Transduction of electrophysiological signals in neurochemical switches may involve a wide range of metabolic events such as phosphorylation–dephosphorylation, calcium mobilization, neurotransmitter release, cytokine activation, increase or decrease in cell membrane receptors for a variety of chemical messengers and nutrients and induction of enzyme activities. As the environmental stimuli and the resultant electrophysiological signals become more complex, more regions, particularly the frontal and prefrontal cortical regions, are affected by patterned combinations of electrical and neurochemical stimuli. This individual yet diverse input of signals to the infant brain enriches neuronal interconnections which allow and 'encourage' the brain to receive, assimilate, interpret, transform and retain information, i.e. to think, to learn and to develop a mind.

After birth, the number of dendrites and their distribution are not only dependent upon a supply of appropriate nutrients and the genetic control systems but also on sensory and other stimuli. Hubel[90] demonstrated that deprivation of visual stimuli in cats and monkeys resulted in anatomical defects within the visual cortex; he writes 'It seems conceivable that early starvation of social interaction, such as contacts with mother, may lead to mental disturbances that have their counterpart in actual structural abnormalities in the brain.' There is increasing evidence that the developing human infant brain requires visual, aural and emotional stimuli as well as good nutrition properly to develop the pathways which subserve and integrate normal brain development and function. Sensory input to the normal term human infant is largely dependent upon the mother's physical, intellectual and emotional state and on the family and social support she receives. Psychological research suggests both that there is a period which is most important in the development of emotional regulation and that the age at which the infant is capable of regulating emotional expression may differ for each of the discreet emotions.[91] The primary care giver, usually the mother, supplies the 'experience' required for the experience-dependent maturation of a structural system responsible for the regulation of the infant's socioemotional function. By providing well-modulated stimulation, the mother facilitates the growth of connections between cortical limbic and subcortical limbic structures that neurobiologically mediate self-regulatory functions. Schore[92] argues that early relational experiences directly influence the emergence of a frontal limbic system in the right hemisphere which can adaptively autoregulate both positive and negative affect in response to changes in the socioemotional environment. He further argues that failure of the mother and infant to develop this type of affect regulation and cortical and subcortical limbic structures can result in the developmental psychopathology that underlines various forms of psychiatric disorders. The move from breast to artificial feeding may have both long- and short-term effects. It would appear prudent to encourage mothers to breastfeed their infants and to give them the visual, aural, tactile and emotional stimuli they require during the first 2 years of life whilst neuronal membranes are forming and making inter-neuronal connections.

Poor nutrition is often associated with an impoverished social environment, a combination which will inevitably limit brain development and capability.

REFERENCES

1. O'Rahilly R and Müller F. *The Embryonic Human Brain: An Atlas of Developmental Stages*. New York: Wiley-Liss, 1994.
2. Norman MG, McGillivray B, Kalousek DK, Hill A and Poskitt K. *Congenital Malformations of the Brain: Pathological, Embryological, Clinical, Radiological and Genetic Aspects*. New York: Oxford University Press, 1995, pp 386–400.
3. Strachan T and Read AP. PAX genes. *Curr Opin Genet Dev* 1994;**4**: 427–438.
4. Oldridge M, Wilkie AOM, Slaney SF *et al.* Mutations in the third obulin immunoglobulin domain of the fibreblast growth factor receptor-2 gene in Crouzon syndrome. *Hum Mol Genet* 1995;**4**: 1077–1082.
5. Oldridge M, Lunt PW, Zackai EH *et al.* Genotype–phenotype correlation for nucleotide substitutions in the IgII-IgIII links of $FGFR_2$. *Hum Mol Genet* 1997;**6**: 137–143.
6. Brown GK, Otero LJ, LeGris M and Brown RM. Pyruvate dehydrogenase deficiency. *J Med Genet* 1994;31: 875–879.
7. Kostovic I. Zentral Nervensystem. In: Hinrichsen KV (ed) *Human Embryologie*. Berlin: Springer-Verlag, 1990, pp 381–448.
8. Kostovic I. Structural and histochemical re-organisation of the human prefrontal cortex during perinatal and postnatal life. In: Uylings HBM, Van Eden CG, De Bruin JPC, Corner MA and Feenstra MJP (eds) The Prefrontal Cortex. *Prog Brain Res* 1990;**85**: 223–224.
9. Goldman-Rakic PS. Neuronal development and plasticity of association cortex in primates. *Neurol Sci Res Prog Bull* 1992;**20**: 520–532.
10. Kostovic I, Judas M, Petanjek Z and Simic G. Ontogenesis of goal-directed behavior: anatomo-functional considerations. *Int J Psychophys* 1995;**19**: 85–102.
11. Warkany J and Petering HG. Congenital malformation of the central nervous system in rats produced by maternal zinc deficiency. *Teratology* 1972;5: 319–344.

12. Rogers JM, Keen CL and Hurley LS. Zinc, copper and manganese deficiencies in prenatal and neonatal development, with special reference to the central nervous system. In: Gabay S, Harris J and Ho BT (eds) *Metal Ions in Neurology and Psychiatry*. New York: Allan R Liss, 1985, pp 3–34.
13. Rogers JM, Oteiza P and Keen CL. Zinc and manganese deficiencies in prenatal and neonatal development, with special reference to the central nervous system. In: Chan-Palay V and Palay SL (eds) *Nutrition and the Infant Brain*. New York: Wiley-Liss 1990, pp 225–236.
14. Prohaska JR. Functions of trace elements in brain metabolism. *Phys Rev* 1987;**67**: 858–899.
15. Hetzel BS and Mano MT. A review of experimental studies of iodine deficiency during fetal development. *J Nutr* 1989;**119**: 145–151.
16. Yehuda S and Youdim MBH. Brain iron: a lesson from animal models. *Am J Clin Nutr* 1989;**50**: 618–629.
17. Harman DL, Woodside JV, Yarnell JWG *et al.* The common 'thermolabile' variant of methylene, tetrahydrofolate reductase is a major determinant of mild hyperhomocysteinaemia. *Q J Med* 1996;**89**: 571–577.
18. Lucock MD, Wild J, Schorah CJ, Levene MI and Hartley R. The methylfolate axis in neural tube defects. *In vitro* characterisation and clinical investigation. *Biochem Med Metab Biol* 1994;**52**: 101–114.
19. Roecklein B, Levin SW, Comly M and Mukherjee AB. Intrauterine growth retardation induced by thiamine deficiency and pyrithiamine during pregnancy in the rat. *Am J Obstet Gynecol* 1985; **151**: 455–460.
20. Morre DM, Kirksey A and Das GD. Effects of vitamin B6 deficiency on the developing central nervous system of the rat. *J Nutr* 1978;**108**: 1250–1265.
21. Chang SJ, Kirksey A and Morre DM. Effects of vitamin B6 deficiency on morphological changes in dendritic trees of Purkinje cells in developing cerebellum of rats. *J Nutr* 1981;**111(5)**: 848–857.
22. Clausen J. The effect of vitamin A deficiency on myelination in the central nervous system of the rat. *Eur J Biochem* 1969;**7**: 575–582.
23. Butterworth RF. Vitamin deficiencies and brain development. In: (Mal) nutrition and the infant brain. In: Van Gelder NM, Butterworth RF and Drewjan BD (eds) *Neurology and Neurobiology*, vol 58. New York: Wiley-Liss, 1990, pp 207–224.
24. Hytten FE and Leitch I. Weight gain in pregnancy. In: Hytten FE and Leitch I (eds) *The Physiology of Human Pregnancy*. Oxford: Blackwell, 1971, pp 265–285.
25. Rosso P. A new chart to monitor weight gain during pregnancy. *Am J Clin Nutr* 1985;**41**: 644–652.
26. Rosso P. Maternal nutrition and fetal growth: implications for subsequent mental competence. In: Rassin DK, Hayber BH and Drujan B (eds) *Basic and Clinical Aspects of Nutrition and Brain Development*. New York: Allan R Liss 1987, pp 339–357.
27. Winick M. *Malnutrition and Brain Development*. Oxford: Oxford University Press, 1976.

28. Clark JB. The development of the mitochondrial energy system in mammalian brain. In: Van Gelder NM, Butterworth RF and Drewjan BD (eds) *(Mal) Nutrition and the Infant Brain. Neurology and Biology*, vol 58. New York; Wiley-Liss 1990, pp 237–248.
29. Widdowson EM. Milk and the newborn animal. *Proc Nutr Soc* 1984;**43**: 87–100.
30. Lewis PD. Nutrition and anatomical development of the brain. In: Van Gelder NM, Butterworth RF and Drewjan BD (eds) *(Mal) Nutrition and the Infant Brain. Neurology and Neurobiology*. New York; Wiley-Liss 1990, pp 89–109.
31. Cragg BD. The development of cortical synapses during starvation. *Brain* 1972;**95**: 143–150.
32. Gambetti P, Autilio-Gambetti L, Rizzuto N, Shafer B and Phaff L. Synapses and malnutrition: quantitative ultrastructural study of rat cerebral cortex. *Exp Neurol* 1974: **43**: 464–473.
33. Salas M. Effect of early undernutrition on dendritic spine of cortical pyramidal cells in the rat. *Dev Neurosci* 1983;**3**: 119–217.
34. Jones DG and Dyson SE. Influence of protein restriction, rehabilitation and changing nutritional states on synaptic development: a quantitative study in rat brain. *Brain Res* 1981;**208**: 97–112.
35. Dobbing J, Hopewell JW and Lynch A. Vulnerability of developing brain: VII permanent deficit of neurons in cerebral and cerebellar cortex following early mild undernutrition. *Exp Neurol* 1971;**32**: 439–447.
36. Sturrock RR, Smart JL and Dobbing J. Effect of undernutrition during the suckling period on the indusium griseum and rostral part of the mouse anterior commissure. *Neuropath Appl Neurobiol* 1977;**3**: 369–375.
37. Wiggins RC, Fuller GN, Brizzee L, Bissel AC and Samorajski T. Myelination of the rat optic nerve during postnatal undernourishment and recovery: a morphometric analysis. *Brain Res* 1984;**308**: 263–272.
38. Wiggins RC, Bissel AC, Durham L and Samorajski T. The corpus callosum during postnatal undernourishment and recovery: a morphometric analysis of myelin and axon relationships. *Brain Res* 1982;**328**: 51–57.
39. Wiggins RC, Delaney AC and Samorajski T. A morphometric analysis of pyramidal tract structures during postnatal undernourishment and recovery. *Brain Res* 1986;**368**: 277–286.
40. Silver J, Lorenz SE, Wahlsten D and Coughlin J. Axonal guidance during development of the great cerebral commissures: descriptive and experimental studies, *in vivo*, on the role of preformed glial pathways. *J Comp Neurol* 1982;**210**: 10–29.
41. Hammarback JA, Palm SL, Furcht LT and Letourneau PC. Guidance of neurite outgrowth by pathways of substratum-adsorbed laminin. *J Neuro Sci Res* 1985;**13**: 231–240.
42. Espinosa de los Monteros A and de Vellis J. Myelin basic protein and transferrin characterised different sub-populations of oligodendrocytes in rat primary glial culture. *J Neuro Sci Res* 1988;**21**: 181–187.

43. Giulian D, Vaca K and Johnson B. Secreted peptides as regulators of neuron–glia and glia–glia interactions in the developing nervous system. *J Neuro Sci Res* 1988;**21**: 487–500.
44. Davenport JW, Gonzalez LM, Carey JC, Bishop SB and Hagquist WW. Environmental stimulation reduces learning deficits in experimental cretinism. *Science* 1976;**191**: 578–579.
45. van Gelder NM. A central mechanism of action for taurine: osmoregulation, by bivalent cations and excitation threshold. *Neurochem Res* 1983;**8**: 687–699.
46. van Gelder NM and Barbeau A. The osmoregulatory function of taurine and glutamic acid. In: Oja SS, Ahtee L, Kontro P and Paasonen MK (eds) *Taurine: Biological Actions and Clinical Perspectives*. New York: Alan R Liss, 1985, pp 149–163.
47. van Gelder NM. Brain taurine content as a function of cerebral metabolic rate: osmotic regulation of glucose derived water production. *Neurochem Res* 1989;**14**: 495–497.
48. Clarren SK, Albord EC, Sumi SM, Streissguth AP and Smith DW. Brain malformations related to prenatal exposure to methanol. *J Pediatr* 1978;**92**: 64–67.
49. Fisch RO, Burke B, Bass J, Ferrara TB and Mastri A. Maternal phenylketonuria-chronology of the detrimental effects in embryogenesis and fetal development: pathological report, survey, clinical application. *Pediatr Pathol* 1986;5: 449–461.
50. Lacey DJ and Terplan K. Abnormal cerebral cortical neurones in a child with maternal PKU syndrome. *J Child Neurol* 1987;**2**: 201.
51. Maher TJ. Modification of synthesis, release and function of catecholaminergic systems by phenylalanine. In: Huether G (ed) *Amino Acid Availability and Brain Function in Health and Disease*. NATO-ASI assay series, Volume H20. Heidelberg: Springer Verlag, 1988, pp 201–206.
52. Lauder JM. Hormonal and humoral influences on brain development. *Psychol Neurol* 1983;**8**: 121–155.
53. Huether G. The influence of increased availability of tryptophan on the formation of tryptamine and cerotonin during early ontogenesis. In: Schlossberger HT, Kochen W, Linzen B and Steinhart H (eds) *Progress in Tryptophan Research*. Berlin: Walter de Gruyter & Co, 1984, pp 613–622.
54. Enwonwu CO. Amino acid availability and control of histaminergic systems in the brain. In: Huether G (ed) *Amino Acid Availability and Brain Function in Health and Disease*. NATO-ASI series, Volume H20. Heidelberg: Springer Verlag, 1988, pp 167–174.
55. Rosengarten H and Freidhoff AS. Enduring changes in dopamine receptor cells of pups from drug administration to pregnant and nursing rats. *Science* 1979;**203**: 1133–1135.
56. Hawryleuicz EJ and Kissane JQ. The effect of protein restriction on brain biogenic amines. In: Parvez H and Parvez S (eds) *Biogenic Amines in Development*. Amsterdam: Elsevier/North-Holland Biomedical Press, 1980, pp 493–517.
57. Huether G. The influence of increased availability of tryptophan on the formation of tryptamine and serotonin during early ontogenesis. In:

Schlossberger HG, Kochen W, Linzen B and Steinhart H (eds) *Progress in Tryptophan Research*. Berlin: Walter de Gruyter & Co, 1984, pp 613–622.

58. Whitaker-Azmitia PM and Azmitia AC. Auto-regulation of fetal serotonergic neuronal development – role of high affinity serotonin receptors. *Neurol Sci* 1986;**67**: 307–312.
59. Wallace J. Neurotransmitters and early embryogenesis. In: Huether G (ed) *Amino Acid Availability and Brain Function in Health and Disease*. NATO-ASI series, Volume H20. Heidelberg: Springer Verlag, 1988, pp 431–440.
60. Maher TJ. Modification of synthesis, release and function of catecholaminergic systems by phenylalanine. In: Huether G (ed) *Amino Acid Availability and Brain Function in Health and Disease*. NATO-ASI series, Volume H20. Heidelberg: Springer Verlag, 1988, pp 201–206.
61. Stubbs CD and Smith AD. The modification of membrane polyunsaturated fatty acid composition in relation to membrane fluidity and function. *Biochim Biophys Acta* 1984;**799**: 89–137.
62. Cullis PR and DeKrui JFFB. Lipid polymorphism and the functional roles of lipids in biological membranes. *Biochim Biophys Acta* 1979;**559**: 339–420.
63. Cook AM, Low E and Ishijimi M. Effect of phosphatidylserine decarboxylase on neuronal excitation. *Nature New Biol* 1972;**239**: 150–151.
64. Fenske DB, Jarrell HC, Guo Y and Hui SW. Effect of unsaturated phosphatidylethanolamine on the chain order profile of bilayers at the onset of the hexagonal phase transition. H^2-NMR study. *Biochemistry* 1990;**29**: 11122–11129.
65. Orlacchio A, Maffei E, Binaglia L and Porcellati G. The effect of membrane phospholipid acyl-chain composition on the activity of brain beta-n-acetyl-D-glucosaminidase. *Biochem J* 1981;**195**: 383–388.
66. Tanaka R. Comparison of lipid effects on K^+-Mg^{2+} activated T-nitrophenyl phosphatase and Na^+-K^+-Mg^{2+} activated adenosine triphosphatase of membrane. *J Neurol Chem* 1969;**16**: 1301–1307.
67. Weidmann T, Pates R, Beach J *et al.* Lipid–protein interactions mediate the photochemical function of rhodopsin. *Biochemistry* 1986;**27**: 64–69.
68. Wood J. Essential fatty acids and their metabolites in signal transductions. *Biochem Soc Trans* 1990;**18**: 755–786.
69. Stubbs CD and Smith AD. Essential fatty acids in membrane: physical properties and function. *Biochem Soc Trans* 1990;**18**: 779–781.
70. Bourre JM, Pascal G, Durand G, Masson M, Dumont O and Piciotti M. Alterations in the fatty composition of rat brain cells (neurones, astrocytes and oligodendrocytes) and of subcellular fractions (myelin and synaptosomes) induced by a diet devoid of n-3 fatty acids. *J Neurochem* 1984;**43**: 342–348.
71. Galli C, Trzechiak HI and Paoletti R. Effects of dietary fatty acids on the fatty acid composition of brain ethanolamine phosphoglyceride: reciprocal replacement of n-6 and n-3 polyunsaturated fatty acids. *Biochim Biophys Acta* 1971;**248**: 449–454.
72. Mohrhauer H and Hollman RT. Alterations of the fatty acid composition of brain lipids by varying levels of dietary essential fatty acids. *J Neurochem* 1963;**10**: 523–530.

73. Farquharson J, Cockburn F, Patrick WJA, Jamieson EC and Logan RW. Infant cerebral cortex phospholipid fatty acid composition and diet. *Lancet* 1992;**340**: 810–813.
74. Farquharson J, Jamieson EC, Abbasi KA, Patrick WJA, Logan RW and Cockburn F. Effect of diet on the fatty acid composition of the major phospholipids of infant cerebral cortex. *Arch Dis Child* 1995;**72**: 198–203.
75. Makrides M, Neumann MA, Byard RW, Simmer K and Gibson RA. Fatty acid composition of brain, retina and erythrocytes in breast- and formula-fed infants. *Am J Clin Nutr* 1994;**60**: 189–194.
76. Farquharson J, Jamieson EC, Logan RW, Patrick WJA, Howatson AG and Cockburn F. Docosahexaenoic acid and nervonic acids in term and preterm infant's cerebral white matter. *Prenat Neonat Med* 1996;**1**: 1–7.
77. Lucas A, Morley R, Cole TJ *et al.* Early diet in preterm babies and developmental status at 18 months. *Lancet* 1990;**1**: 1477–1481.
78. Lucas A, Morley R, Cole TJ, Lister G and Leeson-Payne C. Breast milk and subsequent intelligence quotient in children born preterm. Lancet 1992;**339**: 261–264.
79. Uauy R, Birch E, Birch D and Perano P. Visual and brain function measurements in studies of n-3 fatty acid requirements of infants. *J Pediatr* 1992;**120**: S168–180.
80. Makrides M, Simmer A, Goggin M and Gibson RA. Erythrocyte docosahexaenoic acid correlates with the visual response of healthy term infants. *Pediatr Res* 1993;**33**: 424–427.
81. Jorgensen MH, Hernell O, Lund P, Holmer G and Michaelsen KF. Visual acuity and erythrocyte docosahexaenoic acid status in breast-fed and formula-fed term infants during the first four months of life. Lipids 1996;**31**: 99–105.
82. Birch E, Hoffman D, Hale E, Everett M and Uauy R. Breastfeeding and optimal visual development. *J Pediatr Ophthalmol Strabmismus* 1993;**30**: 33–38.
83. Carlson SE, Werkman SH, Peebles JM and Wilson WM. Long chain fatty acids and early visual and cognitive development of preterm infants. *Eur J Clin Nutr* 1994;**48S**: 27–30.
84. Standing Committee on Nutrition of the British Paediatric Association. Is breast feeding beneficial in the UK? *Arch Dis Child* 1994;**71**: 376–380.
85. Butzer KW. Environment, culture and human evolution. *Am Sci* 1977;**65**: 572–584.
86. Werker JF. Becoming a native listener. *Am Sci* 1989;**77**: 54–59.
87. Cockburn F. The minds of our children. in: Cockburn F (ed) Advances in perinatal medicine. London, Parthenon Publishing, 1997, pp 53–60.
88. Ruoslahti E and Pierschbacher MD. New perspectives in cell adhesion: RGD and integrins. *Science* 1987;**238**: 491–497.
89. Abbott NJ. The milieu is the message. *Nature* 1988;**332**: 490–491.
90. Hubel DH. Effects of deprivation on the visual cortex of cat and monkey. *Harvey-Lecht* 1978;**72**: 1–51.
91. Beuchler S and Izard CE. On the emergence, functions and regulation of some emotion expression in infancy. In: Plutchik R and Kellerman H (eds)

Emotion, Theory, Research and Experience, vol 3. New York: Academic Press, 1983, pp 292–313.

92. Schore AN. *Affect Regulation and the Origin of Self.* New Jersey: Lawrence, Erlbaum Associates, 1994.

6

Development of the Gastrointestinal Tract

Tarja Ruuska and Peter Milla

INTRODUCTION

Survival of the infant born extremely prematurely and health in later life is dependent on the infant's ability to successfully adapt from intra- to extra-uterine life. The extremely limited energy reserves of such infants dictate an urgent need to establish an adequate nutrient intake and there is now a compelling body of evidence that suggests the adequacy of establishment of a nutrient intake will determine both physical health and intellectual development later.[1] Whether an adequate intake can be established by the enteral route is determined by the degree of maturation of the gastrointestinal tract, particularly the function of the fore and mid gut. In addition to digestion, absorption and motor activity, the mucosa must also maintain its integrity and act as a barrier to luminal macromolecules. These functions are all the result not only of the cell types present in the gut but also their distribution, composition and organization. All of these factors have an ontogenic timetable and their development proceeds in different species at specific rates which result in different functional activities appearing at different times during and after gestation. An understanding of the different aspects of the developing gastrointestinal tract, especially during the mid and third trimesters, is essential for both the initial and later successful care of infants born very prematurely. This chapter summarizes current concepts regarding the development of the gut and highlights recent advances in knowledge and the development of investigative tools specifically aimed at the premature neonate.

DEVELOPMENT OF THE GASTROINTESTINAL TRACT

The structure and function of the gut results from a complex interplay between various cell types and components which are regulated by growth factors and hormones, immune and neural inputs. The gut develops from 3 germ layers: the endoderm which supplies the epithelial cells of the mucosa and the origin of the neural components; the splanchnic mesoderm giving the mesenchymal cell types such as the muscle layers and ectoderm. In recent years the importance of the formation of endodermal mesenchymal cell assemblages to generate form and cyto-differentiation of the mucosa[2] and the establishment of the intrinsic nervous system of the gut by neural crest cell migration and differentiation have been appreciated.[3] In both, the formation of the mucosa, enteric neuromusculature, adhesive and other interactions between cells and extracellular microenvironment are crucial. The extracellular microenvironment consists of a labile and developmentally regulated group of interacting molecules. Some of these will be located at the interface between epithelial- and mesenchymal-derived cells, especially the epithelial extracellular matrix interface, where they are capable of directing specific cell behaviour. Their regulation plays a key role in the maintenance of the morphology and function of the mucosa of the gut. Another group of interacting molecules are associated with the extracellular matrix of the muscle coats of the gut and are implicated in the morphogenetic steps in the migration, homing and differentiation of both neural and smooth muscle cells.

Three major phases of development of the human gastrointestinal tract occur:

- an early period of proliferation and morphogenesis;
- an intermediate period of differentiation when many different and distinctive cell types appear; and
- a later period of maturation resulting in a bowel capable of transporting, digesting and absorbing nutrients.

The gastrointestinal tract first appears at 4 weeks' gestation as a tube of stratified epithelium which extends from the mouth to the cloaca and can be divided into 3 distinct parts:

- the fore gut (oesophagus, stomach, proximal duodenum, liver and pancreas);

- mid gut (small intestine through to the proximal two-thirds of the transverse colon); and
- hind gut.

In recent years great advances have been made in understanding the development of the small intestinal epithelium and enteric nervous system. These 2 areas are considered further.

Small Intestinal Mucosa

The functional element of digestion and absorption by the small intestinal mucosa is the crypt villous unit. This consists of a layer of simple columnar epithelium in direct contact with the luminal content. It is supported by an extracellular matrix and connective tissue layer – the lamina propria. A variety of elements are present in the lamina propria, including blood and lymph vessels, nerve fibres, immunocytes, smooth muscle cells and fibroblasts.

Initially, the primitive gut is lined with a simple stratified epithelium and in the area that becomes the small intestine, rudimentary villi appear at about 8 weeks' gestation. At this stage the epithelial cells have short irregular microvilli and the highly polarized well-developed columnar cell is not yet present. Between 9 and 12 weeks' gestation these primitive villi elongate and crypts are formed. By 14 weeks' gestation the simple stratified epithelium is replaced by the complex columnar epithelium with well developed crypts and villi.[4, 5] This process, like many others in the gastrointestinal tract, proceeds in a cranio-caudal direction. By this time the small intestinal epithelial layer is composed of 4 differentiated cell types: absorptive enterocytes, goblet, endocrine and Paneth cells. The absorptive enterocytes represent the main cell type and account for some 90% of cells in the epithelial layer. These cells are characterized by an apical brush border which faces the lumen and carries a large number of different integral membrane-bound digestive hydrolases and nutrient transporters. The folding of the apical membrane into microvilli dramatically amplifies the apical surface, thus facilitating absorption. Goblet cells are filled with mucous granules in their apical cytoplasm and various endocrine cells are characterized by basally located secretory granules containing polypeptide hormones. Paneth cells located in the base of the crypts contain large supernuclear granules of lysozyme, immunoglobulins and defensin-related gene products. Thus, the small intestinal epithelium is a highly differentiated structure whose constituent cells display complex morphological specialization suitable for the digestion and absorption of nutrients and secretion of fluid to facilitate that process. The goblet cells appear to play a protective role, the endocrine cells are involved in the regulation of intestinal absorption and secretion and motility and the Paneth cells in the regulation of the intestinal microflora.

The small intestine has an enormous proliferative and differentiation capacity. Cell division is confined to the crypts and there is a resident stem cell population located near the base of the crypts. The 4 different epithelial cell lineages are derived from a common pluripotent crypt stem cell. Following division of the stem cell, cell differentiation occurs bidirectionally with migration of the enterocytes, goblet and endocrine cells up the crypt towards the apex of the villous, whilst Paneth cells differentiate towards the bottom of each crypt. Each villous is surrounded by several crypts and is composed of cells migrating out of them.[6, 7] The functional maturation of the cells is characterized either by a progressive increase in the level of specific molecules or by the turning on of specific genes and thus their products at or around the crypt villous junction. At the villous tip the epithelial cells exfoliate into the intestinal lumen, the whole process taking 5–6 days in the human. The homeobox gene *Cdx2* has recently been shown to play a key role in this process.[7]

Cytodifferentiation in the Developing Intestine

The conversion of the stratified epithelium into a single-layer, columnar epithelium involves the formation of tight junctions which delineate the apical and basolateral membrane domains. These 2 distinct domains express different molecules which are involved in digestive and absorptive function. On the apical side of the cell, digestive hydrolases and transporter proteins are expressed, whilst on the basolateral side there are ion pumps, particularly the Na^+/K^+-ATPase, which are functionally linked with the apical transporter proteins as well as facilitative transporter proteins to get nutrients out of the enterocyte and into the portal circulation.[8]

There is a clear parallel between morphological and functional differentiation of the mucosa. Concomitant with the formation of villi is the appearance of detectable hydrolase activity. In humans, unlike rodents, α- and β-glucosidases reach 70% and 50%, respectively of adult values by 14 weeks' gestation; thus, for the extremely premature infant there is more than adequate brush border lactase to digest ingested milk. Peptidases seem to follow α-glucosidases in their pattern of development and distribution throughout the gut. Certainly, by 22–24 weeks' gestation the brush border of the intestine possesses an integrated system for the final digestion and absorption of nutrients.

Morphological and functional maturation occurs proximo-distally in a sequential, spatial and temporal pattern. For example, lactase mRNA is expressed regularly over the whole length of the rat's small intestine during the suckling period but after weaning it disappears from the distal ileum.[9, 10] A similar pattern occurs in the human except that the lactase does not disappear but is significantly down-regulated in the distal ileum.[11] The establishment of this proximal–distal gradient during development results from an intrinsic programme for differentiation, the nature of which is in the process of being defined.

Epithelial Mesenchymal Interactions

Close contacts between endodermal and mesenchymal cells in the fetal intestine and between crypt epithelial cells and myofibroblastic cells of the extracellular matrix in the adult organ have been reported; these play an important role in directing morphogenesis, cytodifferentiation and in the maintenance of the steady-state of the stem cell compartment in the mature gut.[12] Each of the intestinal endodermal and mesenchymal tissue components exerts an effect on the development of its associated counterparts and the contacts required to allow expression of the reciprocal permissive interaction.[13]

The basal surface of the intestinal epithelium is in contact with a basement membrane or extracellular matrix which is assembled from a variety of specialized molecules. Over 50 different proteins with many domains and multiple binding sites for other matrix molecules have been described over the last 15 years. It is now clear that extracellular matrix molecules are dynamic effectors in morphogenesis and in the generation and maintenance of epithelial cell polarity.[14] The matrix interacts with cell-surface receptors such as integrins which transduce information from the cell environment to the intracellular component. In the intestine, the subepithelial basement membrane has been shown to contain laminin-1, type IV collagen, nidogen and perlecan.[15] Besides the basement membrane the ground substance of the intestinal stroma comprises many fibrillar collagens (types 1 and 3), fibronectin and tenascin. There are also proteoglycans composed of various types of sulphated glycosaminoglycans and unsulphated hyaluronic acid.[15] It is of interest that isolated intestinal epithelial cells are unable to differentiate when cultured *in vitro* unless they are in close contact with mesenchymally-derived cells. Experimentally, in culture conditions, a precise chronology of events occurs:

1. heterologous cell contacts;
2. polarized basement membrane molecules deposited at the epithelial mesenchymal interface; and
3. epithelial cell polarization and differentiation.[16]

That polarized basement membrane molecules are important has been shown by a number of experiments and observations, including blocking the expression of apical hydrolases by co-culturing intestinal epithelial cells with anti-laminin antibodies. Laminin-2 is restricted to the crypt basement membrane and is first expressed when crypts develop. Tenascin is only found in mature intestine with an increasing gradient from base to the tip of the villous. The latter seems to be concentrated just beneath the epithelial cells and its expression gradient, together with the fact that tenascin disturbs epithelial cell adhesion to the extracellular matrix substrate, suggests that this molecule exerts a physiological role in the shedding of epithelial cells from the villous tip.[17]

Thus, cell interactions between embryonic epithelial (endoderm) and stromal cells (mesenchyme) are a prerequisite for intestinal morphogenesis and differentiation. Recent work has demonstrated the key role of the *Cdx2* homeobox gene in regulating extracellular matrix-induced cell differentiation and the formation of the crypt villous unit.[18, 19]

Development of the Enteric Nervous System

It has been known since the 1950s, following a series of *in ovo* microsurgical ablations of the dorsal neural primordium of chick embryos, that the enteric nervous system arises from the neural crest.[20] The neural crest arises on the dorsal mid line as part of the neural tube which later goes on to form the central nervous system. It gives rise to enteric neurones and their support cells, pigment cells and sympathetic nervous tissue together with the adrenal medulla. More recently, much smaller scale ablations have suggested that the neural crest between somites 3 and 5 is particularly important for enteric nervous system development.[21] The use of cell-labelling techniques in chicken quail chimeric embryos by Le Douarin and Teillet[3] confirmed that the enteric neurones arise from the vagal neural crest and colonize the gut in a rostro-caudal migration. However, some neural crest cells appear to arrive in the hind gut from the lumbosacral level via a caudo-rostral wave of colonisation. More recent studies in mice confirm these avian findings that the gut is colonized largely by vagal neural crest cells but that some cells in the hind gut appear to arrive from a lumbar-sacral origin.[22, 23] The cells from the vagal neural crest arrive at the gut by 2 pathways from the neural crest: a dorso-lateral route in a cell-free extracellular matrix between the epidermis and the somites, and a ventral route percolating through the sclerotomal mesenchyme of the somites. In mice, the neural crest cells reach the fore gut after passing through branchial arches 4 and 6.

The fore gut gives rise to the gut down to the duodenum and, given the compressed scale of the gut compared to the neural axis in these early developmental stages, the vagal neural crest cells require virtually no longitudinal movement to do so. Caudal to this, the neural crest cells that have colonized the fore gut migrate longitudinally within the gut mesenchyme in a caudal direction favouring the region close to the serosal surface. The vanguard of cells colonizing the gut primordium advance at a rate of about 40 μm/h[24] and the cells immediately behind this are found just outside the developing circular muscle layer, i.e. they are already in position to form the myenteric plexus.[25] The cells that form the submucous plexus are not seen until later and it is not clear whether they derive from a secondary migration from local myenteric cells or are a separate wave of immigrants. The sacral neural crest cells migrate ventrally through the adjacent somites before entering the hind gut at the cloaca near the stalk of the allantois. They then migrate rostrally in the gut mesenchyme layer. In humans, the vagal timetable appears to start at around 3–4 weeks gestation and is complete by week 12. The presumed sacral input timetable is unknown. Those vagal neural crest cells that migrate and colonize the gut are committed to become neuroblasts or neuronal support cells (glioblasts). Differentiation into neurones and glial cells appears not to take place until they have reached their final resting places in the gut with no further movement through the gut mesenchyme. Survival in the gut and differentiation into mature cells is strongly influenced by contacts with the microenvironment which consists of other cells in the mesenchyme, neural crest and the extracellular matrix.[26] The extracellular matrix components provide directional clues to migrating neural crest cells and together with neighbouring cells provide some of the signals for crest-cell differentiation. In humans, for example, the appearance of neural crest cells in the gut is preceded by expression of extracellular matrix molecules and these may play a role in migrational cues[27] or promote neuronal growth.[28] Other factors, such as glial-derived neurotropic factor, ensure survival of committed neuroblasts.[29] Several transgenic knockout mouse models and naturally occurring strains of mice with particular genetic abnormalities have provided valuable evidence of some of the factors involved. Lethal spotted[30] and piebald spotted mice[31] have defects in the endothelin signalling pathway which results in an alteration of the microenvironment that the neural crest cells find themselves in. This curtails neural crest migration in the distal colon and is associated with localized over-expression of extracellular matrix molecules.[32]

Intrinsic properties of the neural crest cells are also important for migration, survival and differentiation. Two knockout mouse models[29, 33] and the human condition Hirschsprung's disease, now have known be associated genetic defects,[34, 35] and provide very powerful evidence for these intrinsic properties. The neural crest cells express a transmembrane tyrosine kinase receptor at the cell surface, the *Ret* proto-oncogene. A transgenic knockout model of *Ret* in the mouse[33] shows a total absence of the enteric nervous system, suggesting that normal enteric nervous system migration and/or survival of migrating cells is dependent upon the functional integrity of this tyrosine kinase receptor and its ligand. It is now known that the ligand for the *Ret* tyrosine kinase receptor is glial-derived neurotrophic factor and a knockout model of this gene shows a similar lack of expression of enteric neurons.[29] In Hirschsprung's disease, defects in chromosome 10q11.2,[34, 35] which specify the *Ret* gene, have been found and the defects extend all along the gene. It is of interest that other abnormalities of the *Ret* gene result in multiple endocrine neoplasia type 2A and 2B, but these only occur at specific sites. In multiple endocrine neoplasia type 2B there is an association with hyperplasia of enteric neurones, resulting in enteric ganglioneuromatosis.[36] Abnormalities of *Ret* are found in some 30% of patients with Hirschsprung's disease and in families with Hirchsprung's disease there is incomplete penetrance of the genetic abnormality. Whilst abnormalities of *Ret* appear to account for a moderate proportion of patients with Hirschsprung's disease, other neural crest cell abnormalities such as the provision of glial-derived neurotrophic factor only account for a very small proportion. A series of experiments[37] has suggested that glial-derived neurotrophic factor is required for survival and differentiation of the vagal neural crest cells once they arrive in the gut, and some have suggested that the lumbar–sacral outflow into the gut is largely of cells which will become glial cells producing factor such as glial-derived neurotrophic factor that ensure the survival of the migrating cells once they arrive in the hind gut.

The number of vagal neural crest cells colonizing the gut also seems to be important since gross reduction in number leads to the development of the enteric nervous system at the rostral levels of the gut but a complete absence at caudal levels.[20] However, this information also suggests that perhaps there is some specification of different segment identity for potential enteric neurones before they leave the vagal neural crest and this may be dependent upon the correct microenvironment in the gut primordium during the process of migration and ultimately differentiation. It has been suggested that spatially-restricted differential expression of homeobox-containing regulatory genes along the hind brain may be responsible for this.

Developmental Control Regulatory Genes

Homeobox genes are a group of developmental control genes implicated in the positioning and patterning of organs in the embryo. These evolutionarily conserved genes encode transcription factors which self-regulate their own transcription or the transcription of other downstream effector genes in developing embryos ranging from *Drosophila* to humans. A group of genes which has been extensively studied is the antennapedia class of homeobox genes, the so called 'Hox' genes. Hox genes are evolutionarily highly conserved and derived from a common ancestral cluster and are organized into 4 clusters – A, B, C and D on 4 separate chromosomes in mammals comprising some 38 genes in total.[38] The genes are numbered 1–13 by virtue of their 3′ to 5′ position along each chromosome, the lowest number being at the 3′ end and the highest number at the 5′ end. A given gene may have up to 3 related genes in equivalent positions on the other 3 clusters and such a group of genes has sequence homology with each other and forms a so-called paralogous group.[39] Such paralogues can display equivalent expression domains and may therefore have common functions during development, resulting in some functional redundancy.

It is significant that Hox genes are expressed in precise patterns during early embryogenesis, particularly during critical periods of fate specification within a given morphogenetic field such as a limb. The expression domains of the various groups overlap to differing extents within any particular field, leading to the concept that Hox genes have a combinatorial mode of action.[40] Along the body axis these genes are generally expressed with discrete rostral cut offs which coincide with either existing or emergent anatomical landmarks. It has therefore been suggested that they serve to specify component parts of the vertebrate body plan and this is particularly clear in segmented structures such as the branchial arches and the vertebral column.[41] Significantly, at least in these structures, the rostro-caudal sequence of the cut offs map quite precisely with the 3′ to 5′ sequence of Hox genes within their respective cluster and with the order in which these genes are expressed. This phenomenon is known as spatial and temporal colinearity.[42] However, it is also clear that non-overtly segmented structures, such as limbs or internal organs, are also specified by Hox genes and thus Hox genes could be upstream regulatory genes for the morphogenesis of the embryonal gut, for the migration and maturation of neural crest cells and possibly splanchnic mesoderm.

Hox genes from the 5′ paralogous groups 12 and 13 are known to be involved in patterning of the hind gut.[43] Those from paralogous groups 4 and 5 seem to be particularly good candidates as regulators of gut neuromusculature of at least the fore and mid gut, since they are expressed in the developing hind brain at the level of rhombomeres 6–8 from where a proportion of vagal neural crest cells migrate through the branchial arches into the intestine and differentiate into enteric ganglia.[44] In segmented structures such as the branchial arches, the branchial Hox code defined by the patterns of combinatorial Hox gene expression has been interpreted as a developmental strategy whereby positional specification made axially within the neural tube is transmitted to the periphery via the migrating neural crest and is seen as an integral part of the mechanisms whereby the embryo develops an organ such as a head, face or gut.[45] Preliminary data of the expression of 3′ Hox genes in the gut of developing mouse embryos along the length of the gut primordium show nested expression domains.[46] There is both a spatial and temporal expression pattern in the developing intestine. This is spatially restricted to the mesodermal layer and becomes even more spatially restricted as gestation progresses to the developing longitudinal muscle layer. A few isolated observations of transgenic mouse models suggest that Hox genes do indeed play an important role in gut morphogenesis. A transgenic knockout of *Enx* (*Hox 11L1*)[47] causes increased innervation of the hind gut and over-expression of *Hox A4* is associated with a megacolon.[48] Destruction of *Hox C4* severely affects the morphology of oesophageal smooth muscle while knockout of *Hox D13* affects anal sphincters.[49]

It is clear that this family of genes is important within the genetic hierarchy of gut morphogenesis and delineation of those genes comprising the human gut Hox code and their spatio-temporal patterns of expression is an essential and integral part of understanding the molecular events underlying gut dysmorphogenesis in humans. As discussed above, another group of homeobox containing genes, *Cdx1/Cdx2*, is important in mucosal differentiation and the formation of the crypt/villous unit.[18, 19]

FUNCTIONAL DEVELOPMENT OF THE FORE GUT

Intolerance to feeds evident as regurgitation and vomiting occurs commonly in the very preterm infant and limits the amount of enteral nutrition which can be given. These symptoms are both as a consequence of gastro-oesophageal reflux and of functional gastric outlet obstruction. It is assumed that these phenomena occur as a result of immature gastrointestinal motor activity. Gastrointestinal motor activity occurs as the result of the integrated activity of the gastrointestinal smooth muscle, the enteric nervous system modulated by extrinsic innervation from the central nervous system and the endocrine and paracrine environment of the gut wall. The authors and others have shown that small intestinal, gastric and oeosophageal motor activity develops according to an ontogenic timetable which occurs as a result of the development of these control systems.[50–52] As immature development of the fore gut motor apparatus prejudices the ability to feed preterm infants and may result in considerable morbidity due to aspiration, pneumonia, apnoea and oesophagitis, knowledge of its developmental profile is of value to neonatologists. Over the last 10 years there has been a succession of studies of increasing sophistication of the oeosophagus and the small intestine.

Oesophagus

By 8 weeks' gestation the human fetal oesophagus is identifiable as a hollow epithelium-lined tube with primitive nerve and muscle precursors present. Over the next 8 weeks, maturation of the muscle layers and innervation occurs until fetal swallowing commences at about 16 weeks' gestation. An anatomical study of the developing human oesophagus showed that nerve synapses were present from 10 weeks' gestation but nerve cell size increased from 6 μm at 8 weeks' gestation to a near maximal 20 μm at term and that numbers of cells and nerve density all peaked at around 20 weeks' gestation.

Unfortunately, functional studies of oesophageal motor activity are restricted to premature infants over the age of 30 weeks' gestation. One recent study showed that non-peristaltic motor patterns were common in premature infants between 33 and 37 weeks' post conceptional age, that all infants had a high pressure zone at the lower oesophageal sphincter and that the pressure exerted increased from 3.8 mmHg at 29 weeks' gestation to 18.1 mmHg at term.[50] Observations of the behaviour of the lower oesophageal sphincter showed that both swallow-related and transient lower oesophageal sphincter relaxations occurred and that after 33 weeks' gestation the motor events associated with lower oesophageal sphincter relaxation were similar to those seen in healthy adults. However, the relative preponderance of non-peristaltic pressure wave sequences in the oesophagus of premature infants means that they have poorer acid clearance when reflux episodes occur and thus are more likely to develop oesophagitis. Endoscopic studies of premature infants would seem to indicate that this is indeed the case.

Stomach

The stomach acts as an initial reservoir for feeds and the process of digestion starts in the stomach with the secretion of gastric acid and pepsin. In addition, the stomach secretes mucus and mucoproteins, intrinsic factor and the polypeptide hormones gastrin and somatostatin. Gastrin is important in the regulation of acid secretion but in the neonatal period is often present at high levels. Neonatal hypergastrinaemia, its duration, magnitude and probable mechanisms has been reviewed by Lichtenberger.[53] Somatostatin is important for the modulation of fasting motor activity in the stomach and appears to be present from about 34 weeks' gestation.[54] Early studies of acid secretion showed that full-term infants secrete acid within hours of birth, but only some preterm infants do, but this is not supported by more recent studies (see below).

Gastric Acid Secretion

Gastric acid has a number of different functions. It is required for the protection of the upper gastrointestinal tract against bacteria and it is vital for the initial steps of digestion. On the other hand, under certain circumstances in the presence of acid, a variety of barrier-breaking agents can damage the gastric mucosa.[55] A pH level of <4 is thought to be critical for the development of gastric ulceration.[56]

The parietal cells secrete gastric acid by the proton pump, H^+/K-ATPase, in the oxyntic glands. The majority of the oxyntic glands are found in the fundus and corpus of the stomach. The H^+/K-ATPase is a cellular transporting protein and it is present only in the parietal cells. It is responsible for the extrusion of H^+ from the cell into the gastric lumen in exchange for K^+.[57] Parietal cells and gastric H^+/K-ATPase have been detected from the 13th gestational week[58] but the secretory canaliculi do not develop until at least 16–20 weeks. Studies in preterm and term infants show that gastric H^+/K-ATPase is expressed in the parietal cells of the youngest infants (24 weeks) studied and increases with gestational and postnatal age (Grahnquist and Ruuska, unpublished data).

The secretion of gastric acid is regulated by both extrinsic and intrinsic neural control mechanisms, the vagus nerve and the enteric nerve plexuses of the stomach, and hormones released locally into the stomach and/or in other parts of the gastrointestinal tract. These mechanisms cause stimulation of the parietal cells to secrete HCl by histamine, gastrin and acetylcholine.

Gastric pH in newborns
Acidity of the stomach in the newborn human infant, especially in the preterm, has been much debated. Study of preterm and term infants has shown that the gastric contents of those born by elective caesarean section has a neutral pH[54] but acidity increases very soon after birth. Preterm infants have been shown to secrete acid from their first day of life and are able to keep gastric pH levels below 4, but there are no great variations in the acidity of the stomach during the first 10 days of life. No real differences have been demonstrated between infants born before or after 34 weeks' gestation.[54] In addition, it has been shown that in healthy newborns a protein hydrolysate test meal induced an acid secretory response that is qualitatively similar but weaker than the response in older infants or adults.[59] The authors' studies with 24-hour pH monitoring have confirmed these findings, namely a gastric pH level <4 for $>50\%$ of the time was seen in $>40\%$ of infants born between 25 and 41 weeks' gestation.[60]

Mucosal Defence

Mechanisms of gastroprotection are complex and multifactorial. Protection of the stomach is achieved by at least 2 mechanisms: preserving the existing cells or replacing the lost tissue. Preservation of existing cells occurs by anatomic defence mechanisms and the physicochemical properties of the mucosa, of which hydrophobicity is the most important. After superficial damage to the gastrointestinal tract mucosa, rapid epithelial restitution usually occurs, but stress may depress epithelial proliferation.

Anatomical defence mechanisms
Adequate blood flow is essential for all of the protective mechanisms of the gastrointestinal tract. The mucosal microcirculation is crucial; mucosal blood flow increases by 100% 15 min after damage.[61] A gastric mucosal barrier of the bicarbonate-rich mucus layer overlies the epithelial cells of the gastric mucosa. This layer neutralizes H^+ to maintain the pH of epithelial cells at a near neutral level.

Gastric hydrophobicity
One of the protective factors of the gastric mucosa against acid is the hydrophobicity of the mucosa. This is believed to be due to a surfac-

tant-like material consisting of phospholipids and surfactant proteins and which is very similar to the surfactant of pulmonary epithelium. Gastric surfactant has been shown in animal studies to protect the gastric mucosa against damage caused by acid and drugs.[62] Exogenously-administered surface-active phospholipids have also been shown to have this ability.[63] In addition, it is known that the excessive sensitivity of gastric mucosa to luminal acid disappears at the same time as hydrophobicity of the stomach appears in developing mammals, i.e. between the first and third weeks of life.[64]

The authors and others have shown that gastric mucosal damage is very common in neonates under stress.[65] In preterm infants it therefore seems likely that gastric surfactant may play a role in gastroprotection. It can be assumed that gastric surfactant develops concurrently with pulmonary surfactant but very little is known about this in human neonates. The authors' preliminary data derived from ultrastructural studies shows that gastric surfactant can be detected in preterm infants from at least 28 weeks' gestation onwards (Figures 6.1 and 6.2). It is probable that the amount of surfactant in very preterm infants is low, and this makes neonates prone to gastric mucosal damage.

Stress-induced mucosal damage

Stress-induced gastric mucosal damage can be seen in 80% of adults and children treated in intensive care units. As neonates in intensive care usually have several risk factors for stress ulceration, such as asphyxia, hypotension and hypothermia, have received drugs which potentiate stress-induced damage, including indomethacin, tolazoline and corticosteroids, and have poorly developed defence factors, it can be appreciated that this patient group might be at high risk for gastric mucosal damage. The authors' prospective study of 88 infants[60] admitted to a neonatal intensive care unit showed 80% to have gastric mucosal damage; 55 infants were born between 24 and 32 weeks' gestation and 22% of these had oesophagitis, 13% mild gastritis, 25% haemorrhagic gastritis and 27% ulcers. In an older age group (33–41 weeks' gestation), endoscopy showed oesophagitis in 12%, mild gastritis in 12%, haemorrhagic gastritis in 57% and ulcers in 18%.[60] Only 20% of these infants, however, had symptoms and signs of bleeding.

Gastric Function

Studies of gastric function show that in the very preterm infant gastric emptying is poor and that in the fasting state pressure generated in the gastric antrum at about 26–27 weeks' gestation is as low as 5 mmHg

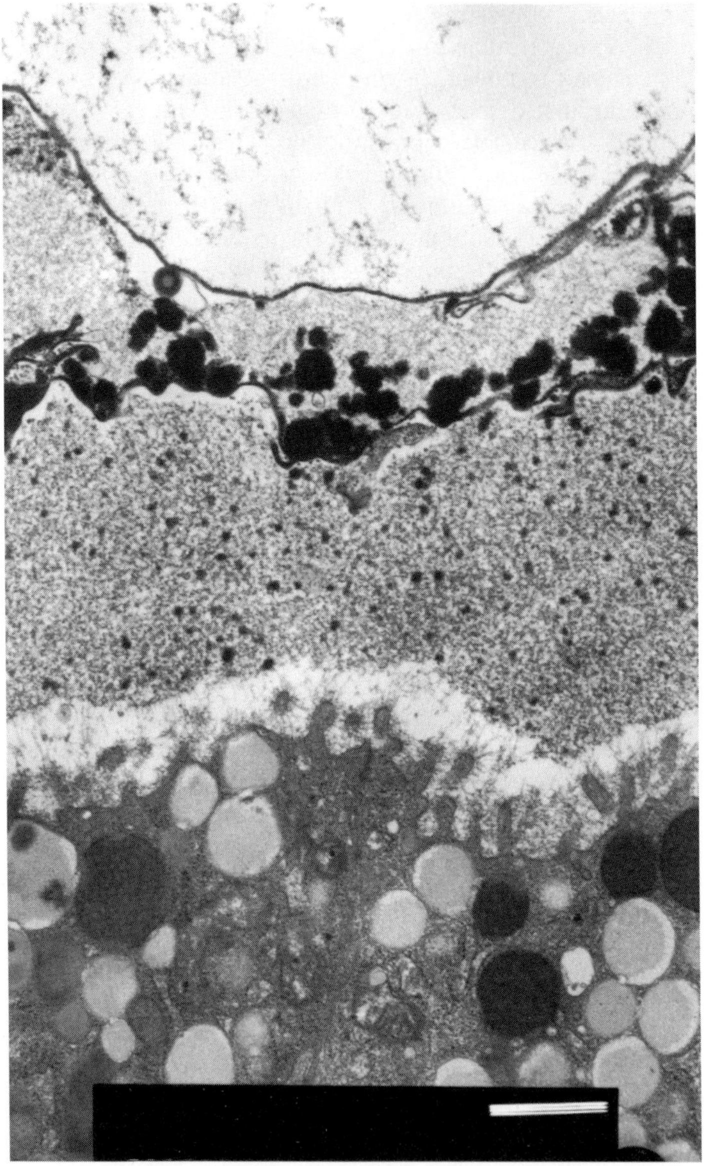

Figure 6.1 Electron micrograph of gastric biopsy of a neonate showing mucosal layer with phospholipid lining and surfactant-like lamellar bodies. Tannic acid staining. Bar = 1 μm.

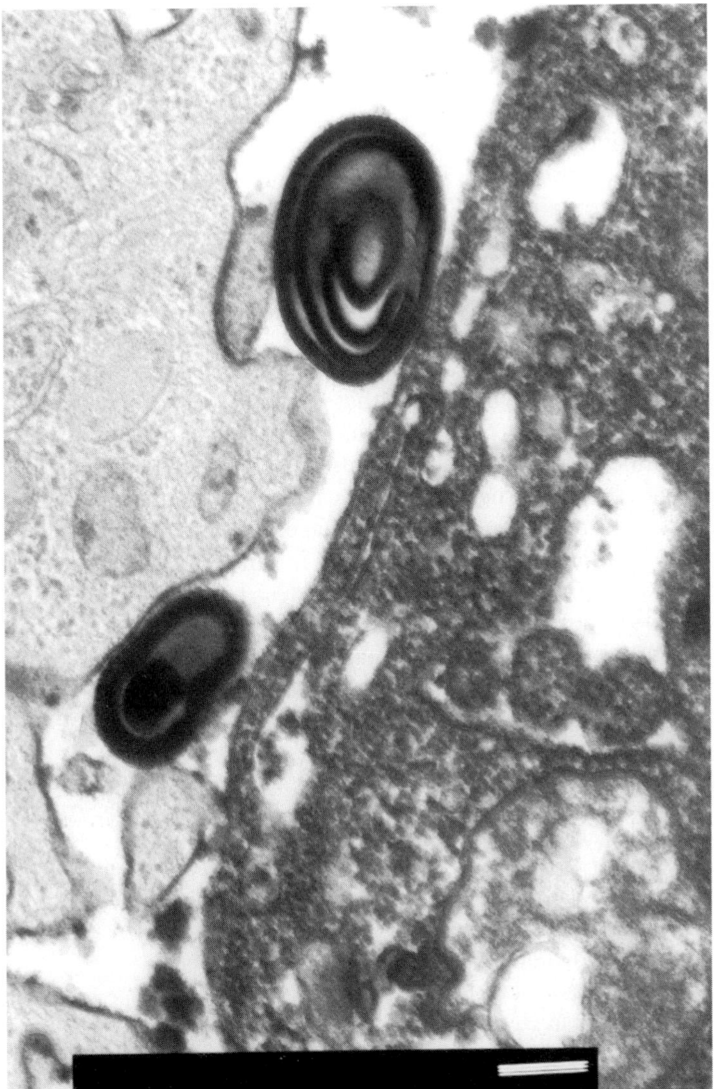

Figure 6.2 Higher power view of lamellar bodies in the gastric mucosal layer of a neonate. Tannic acid staining. Bar = 200 nm.

(approximately 0.7 kPa) as compared with levels of 30 mmHg (4 kPa) by term. Paradoxically, studies of gastric emptying have shown that there is no association between longer half-emptying times with increasing prematurity; however, such studies have been limited to infants able to tolerate relatively large amounts of feed (30 ml/kg/feed or more).[66] In healthy premature infants, human milk empties faster than an adapted milk formula containing 0.7 kcal/ml and having the same casein to whey ratio as human milk.[67] Siegel *et al* observed the effects of altering the carbohydrate source of glucose, lactose and polycose, and fat source of long chain (LCT) and medium chain triglyceride (MCT), on gastric emptying profiles.[68] The inhibition produced by LCT was much greater than that of MCT; alterations in carbohydrate source in contrast had minimal effects on gastric emptying rate. Others have shown that posture, volume and feeding temperature appear to have little effect on gastric emptying but a number of pathological conditions are clearly associated with delayed gastric emptying, including cardiovascular disease, respiratory distress syndrome and gastro-oesophageal reflux. In a study of the emptying of different formulas in older infants with gastro-oesophageal reflux, it was clearly shown that the fastest half emptying times were obtained with human milk and a whey protein hydrolysate.[69] It is no surprise to neonatologists that human milk is tolerated by premature infants best but in its absence, a whey protein peptide hydrolysate containing some MCT might also be considered.

Small Intestinal and Colonic Motor Activity

Over the last 10 years there have been a number of studies of the development of small intestinal motor function and all have identified 4 stages of development of fasting motor activity:[51, 52]

1. a disorganized stage;
2. clusters of phasic activity;
3. prolonged phasic activity; and
4. a regular cyclical migrating motor complex pattern.

These data are summarized in Table 6.1 and Figure 6.3.

It seems clear that the development of intestinal motor activity changes towards a more mature pattern with increasing post-conceptional age. The initiation of clustered phasic activity which then becomes more prolonged may be humorally mediated since the secretion of a number of polypeptide hormones involved in motor activity occurs at this gestational age.70 Propagation and the subsequent shortening of the duration of prolonged phasic contraction with emergence

Table 6.1 Stages of fasting motor activity.

Pattern	Gestational age (weeks)	Complex length (min)	Complex interval (min)	Propagation velocity (cm/min)
Random	28–32	0	0	0
Clustered phasic	30–35	1–20	4–35	0–5
Prolonged phasic	34–36	5–40	4–30	1–5
Migrating motor complex	37–42	3–7	18–45	2–7.5

Reproduced with permission from Ref 51.

of migrating motor complex (MMC) activity is, however, much more likely to be caused by the development of inhibitory networks in the enteric nervous system and their interface with the central nervous system. In animal studies, similar patterns have been observed and the increase in cycle length of the MMC has been associated with the development of serotinergic neurons in the proximal small intestine.71 There are also similarities between these gestationally determined changes and the effects of total vagotomy on adult patterns of fasting activity. This, together with observations of the timing of maturation events determined by the central nervous system and the correlation between cyclical timing of the electrical activity in the enteric and central nervous systems of animals, suggests that not only do events in the enteric nervous system determine the nature of the pattern of fasting motor activity but also that central control systems that may modulate enteric activity develop in parallel.72

In the older child and adult, cyclical fasting motor activity is disrupted after a meal and replaced by continuous activity that promotes mixing and segmentation of the luminal contents. This is required for efficient processing of feeds. There is a modicum of information regarding the development of the motor response to food in the human infant, in particular with the detection of particular motor events and feed factors that determine tolerance to enteral feeds. Bisset *et al*[73] showed that the length of post-prandial activity and the disruption of the cyclical pattern of fasting activity were dependent upon the length of time which the infant had spent taking feed. Berseth and Nordi[74] showed that tolerance to enteral feeds was closely correlated with the development of a continuous pattern of activity in response to food and the development of cyclical clustered phasic activity in the fasting state. These initial observations have received more support recently since

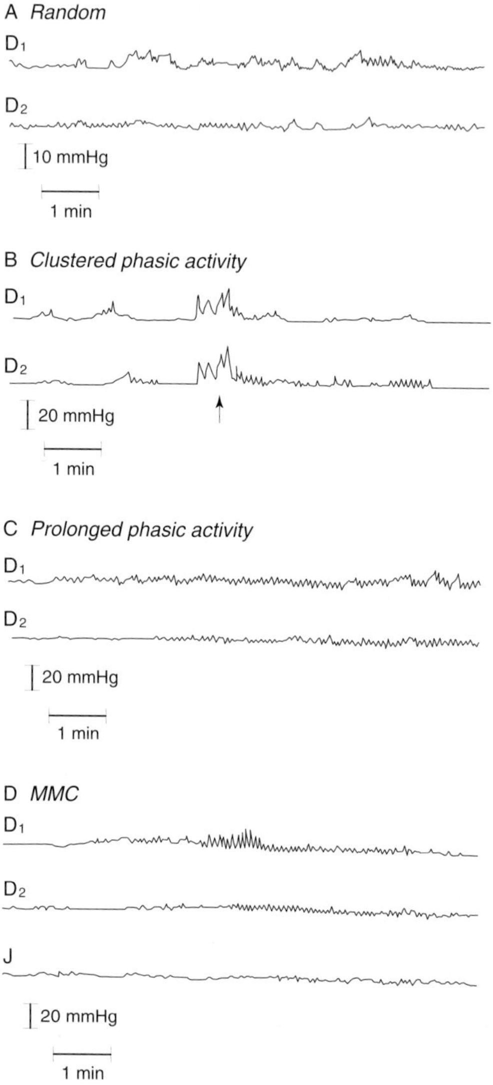

Figure 6.3 Small intestinal pressure recordings at duodenum (D_1 and D_2) and jejunum (J). MMC = migrating motor complex.

the demonstration of the polypeptide hormone response and its effect on motor activity in preterm infants that had been able to tolerate enteral feeds.[75] Thus, post-prandial events appear to be dependent on the nature of the humoral response to food provided that the muscle coats of the gut and the enteric nerves have developed sufficiently to be able to respond to the hormones secreted. The nature of these maturational changes, however, remains poorly explored but increasing knowledge in this area is informing the development of more logical feeding regimens.

INVESTIGATION OF THE NEONATAL GASTROINTESTINAL TRACT

Over the last decade there has been considerable advance in the ability to investigate the function of the upper neonatal gastrointestinal tract. Both oesophageal manometry and 24-hour pH monitoring are possible in preterm infants, though manometry is perhaps mainly a research tool. A number of non-invasive investigations of the stomach and duodenum are now possible, together with the establishment of antroduodenal manometry. Lastly, it is clear that upper gastrointestinal endoscopy is feasible in skilled hands and reveals pathology that would otherwise have been missed.

Oesophagus

Whilst contrast radiology reveals anatomical abnormalities of the oesophagus, its ability to determine function is poor and in up to 60% of cases gastro-oesophageal reflux will be missed. In older children 24-hour pH monitoring is the gold standard to detect gastro-oesophageal reflux and the availability of neonatal pH electrodes now makes this possible in preterm infants.

24-hour pH monitoring
Even in the premature infant, particularly where there is respiratory distress syndrome and the infant is stressed, the majority of gastro-oesophageal reflux is acidic and can be reliably detected by intra-oesophageal pH monitoring.[76] Whilst there are normal ranges for reflux in older children, in the preterm infant, although there is no doubt that gastro-oesophageal reflux occurs, these have yet to be established. Where vomiting occurs, it is not difficult to understand the symptoms that gastro-oesophageal reflux causes; however, in other circumstances, for instance respiratory disorder, the symptoms may be as diverse as recurrent episodes of apnoea, bronchospasm and aspiration causing chest infection. In these patients, the symptoms do not appear to be related to prolonged exposure of the lower oesophagus to acid but may occur following relatively short-lived episodes of reflux both during the

day and in association with changes of sleep state. To define the association between respiratory symptoms and reflux, it may be necessary to combine pH studies with recordings of oxygen saturation, dips in oxygen saturation being associated with clinically significant episodes of bronchospasm or apnoea. In those with prolonged episodes of gastro-oesophageal reflux, oesophagitis might be expected to occur and this can be readily detected by endoscopy.

Manometry
Oesophageal manometry can now reliably be carried out in the preterm infant but it is largely a research tool and probably has little part to play in clinical practice. Those interested in this technique should read the recent papers by Omari *et al.*[50, 77]

Stomach and Duodenum

Function of the stomach may be impaired both in terms of integrity of the gastric mucosa (see above) and its ability to process and empty contents into the small intestine. Tolerance of feeds by the very preterm infant is a major problem for many neonatal centres, but despite the very obvious indication for tests of gastric motor function, these are only routinely conducted in a very few research centres. One of the reasons for this is that most tests of gastric motor function and emptying are not readily available or until recently have not been adapted for the premature infant. In addition, they either require a detailed understanding of complex analytical techniques or sophisticated gamma camera and mass spectrometry facilities.

Gastric emptying studies
There are a plethora of methodologies available for measuring gastric emptying including the gold standard gamma scintigraphy. Gamma scintigraphy, however, is inconvenient, expensive and radioisotopes are required which make multiple studies in small children unethical. The alternatives include ultrasound, electrical impedance tomography and stable isotopes.

Ultrasound. This is safe and comfortable for the infant, it can be repeated on multiple occasions and it is possible using milk feeds in small infants. The images, however, are not always very clear and require great skill in both their acquisition and interpretation. Nevertheless, this method has been used by several groups as a useful means of measuring gastric emptying.[78]

Electrical impedance tomography (EIT). This is another non-invasive technique whose results compare favourably with those of scintigraphy. It has the advantage that the equipment is cheap, portable and easy to operate, so that tests can be conducted at the cotside.[79] EIT measures the conductance of gastric contents which can be altered by the ionic composition as well as the volume; therefore, changes in gastric acid secretion that take place during the digestion of a meal may distort gastric-emptying profiles. As a consequence, centres that employ this methodology prefer to block acid secretion with an H_2 blocker. This methodology has the advantage that it is also possible to measure contractile activity of the antral wall and to detect gastro-oesophageal and duodeno-gastric reflux.

Stable isotope breath test. ^{13}C octanoic acid is immediately absorbed in the duodenum and ultimately excreted in the breath. As gastric emptying is the rate-limiting step of the absorption of MCT, the fraction of ^{13}C expired in the breath following a test meal containing the MCT octanoic acid marked with the ^{13}C stable isotope, indicates the rate of gastric emptying. Thus, analysis of the expired ^{13}C fraction in breath samples using isotope ratio mass spectrometry can define a gastric emptying curve and allow emptying parameters to be calculated. This appears to be a safe and non-invasive method of measuring gastric emptying in small infants and allows comparison between various feeding methods.[80]

Gastro-duodenal motor function

Electrogastrography. This is a non-invasive means of measuring electromyographic activity of the stomach by placing ECG electrodes on the infant's abdomen. Analysis of the signals obtained in the frequency domain rather than the time domain has increased understanding of the nature of smooth muscle slow waves and their correlation with contractile activity of the stomach and duodenum.[81] The availability of commercial equipment provides the first means of non-invasively investigating the gastrointestinal neuromusculature and this may have particular application in the preterm infant.

Antro-duodenal manometry. It is possible to measure contractile activity of the stomach and duodenum using manometry but so far this is only available as a research tool in a very few centres; nevertheless Bisset *et al*[51] and Berseth[52] have provided information which should allow logical decisions to be made regarding feeding practices in premature infants.

Neonatal Endoscopy

Both gastroscopy and colonoscopy have become well established procedures in the diagnosis and treatment of gastrointestinal diseases in children. Endoscopic examination can reveal the aetiology for haematemesis and melaena and, sometimes, the reason for feeding difficulties such as oesophagitis. In immunocompromised infants, candida infections are common and can be detected in the oesophagus endoscopically when mouth and throat swab culture is unhelpful. The development of specific neonatal gastroscopes has enabled gastroscopy to be carried out easily in neonates, even in very small preterm infants.

The smallest gastroscope (Olympus GIF N-30) has a diameter of 5.2 mm. It has all the functions of a normal gastroscope: suction, air insufflation, water flushing and a biopsy channel, but these all are carried out through one common channel. The range of tip bending is 180° up and down and 160° to left and right. A specific neonatal colonoscope has not been developed though this could be most useful.

Technical problems

Endoscopy in older children is very safe and reported complications are <1%. They may, however, include transient bacteremia, complications due to sedation, loosened teeth and mucosal haemorrhage. Bowel haematoma or perforations are extremely rare. The few reports in neonates suggest that it is just as safe.[82–84] Endoscopy must, however, always be performed under carefully controlled conditions, so that the infant's blood pressure, oxygen saturation and heart rate are monitored constantly. Most neonates tolerate the procedure well, but during an examination there may be a small increase in the pulse rate while passing the oesophagus, just as there is while inserting a nasogastric tube.[82]

Endoscopy in this age group is only limited by the size of the infant. With the small-diameter gastroscope, it is possible to undertake gastroscopy in neonates weighing as little as 500 g. Due to the narrowness of the oesophagus, nasogastric tubes must be removed from infants weighing <1000 g in order to avoid damage to the thin oesophageal mucosa. Passing the endoscope through the pylorus into the duodenum is usually successful in infants weighing 900 g or more.

Colonoscopy can usually be done in infants >1000 g. There are, however, no special neonatal colonoscopes available and instead either the paediatric colonoscope, preferably the 'floppy' version, or the neonatal gastroscope can be used for colonoscopy. The gastroscope is rather too stiff and the colonoscope too large in diameter for neonates under 2.5 kg; therefore, usually only a left-side colonoscopy can be done and in most cases this is sufficient for diagnosis. However, the colonoscope may fill the whole abdomen and can cause respiratory arrest unless care is taken. Injudicious air insufflation in small infants can quickly fill the colon with air because the endoscope obstructs the rectum and the air cannot be passed out of the rectum. A specific neonatal colonoscope would be a most useful instrument and would enable the whole colon to be assessed. Just as with gastroscopy, it would almost certainly reveal hitherto unsuspected pathology.

Sedation

When carrying out endoscopic examinations in neonates, the endoscopist has to be very careful and light handed. Endoscopies should not cause undue stress or pain to the infant and therefore drugs must be considered carefully on an individual basis. Most neonates on mechanical ventilation receive sedation or analgesia and they can be given additional drugs on the same basis as for any other procedures. The authors have used in addition to phenobarbitol, which infants receive routinely, either morphine 0.1 mg/kg or glycopyrrolate 0.1 mg/kg.[82]

An experienced neonatal nurse, or in the case of the smallest infants, a neonatologist should assist with the procedure. Thus, those who are in charge of the neonate can see the findings with their own eyes and can also be responsible for the welfare of the infant whilst the endoscopist is doing the endoscopy.

Indications

The indications for gastroscopy in neonates include a suspicion of gastrointestinal haemorrhage (symptoms: haematemesis, bloody aspiration of nasogastric tube or melaena),[83] feeding difficulties (severe vomiting, refusal of enteral feeds) and suspicion of infection, e.g. candida infection in neonates who have often received multiple antibiotics.[84] In cases of intractable diarrhoea, the diagnosis can often be achieved by biopsying the small intestinal mucosa through the endoscope.[84]

The indications for colonoscopy are fewer than for gastroscopy. Severe melaena or bloody diarrhoea are the main indications in this age group.

Coagulation studies are mandatory prior to endoscopy. Biopsies should only be taken when there is no evidence of a bleeding diathesis. The biopsies obtained can be subjected not only to histological examination but also to microbiological study and biochemical investigation.

Upper gastrointestinal tract

Gastroscopy has revealed a higher incidence of haemorrhagic disorder than hitherto suspected,[82, 83] oesophagitis, which may be due to excessive aspiration of nasogastric tubes or in older neonates due to gastro-oesophageal reflux, or viral and candida infections. Gastritis or gastric ulcers may be found in infants and are virtually always acute stress phenomena.[83] Microvillous atrophy, duodenitis or autoimmune disease may all be detected in duodenal biopsies[84] in infants with protracted diarrhoea.

Colon

A variety of different forms of colitis may be seen which are usually discontinuous. They vary from mild to severe with patches of variolaform erythema to deep ulceration. Occasionally, the characteristic membranes of pseudomembranous colitis are found, especially when multiple antibiotics have been used. Histologically, lesions vary from resembling necrotizing enterocolitis to ulcerative colitis but are most commonly an eosinophilic colitis usually due to food allergy. In some, an ischaemic or bacterial colitis is found.

The future

Endoscopy is now possible even in the small preterm infants and it is a safe procedure in skilled hands. Endoscopy is revealing a hitherto unsuspected breadth of diseases of the gastrointestinal tract in neonates and specific diagnosis will enable better and more logical treatment in this fragile group. Collaboration between neonatologists and paediatric gastroenterologists is essential for the further development of neonatal gastroenterology.

SUMMARY

In the last decade major advances have been made in understanding the development of the gastrointestinal tract and the ability to investigate both normal events and pathophysiology. Technical advances, particularly in endoscopy, allow hitherto unsuspected pathology to be diagnosed and effectively treated. It seems almost inconceivable that further advances will not be made in the next 10 years and some which are now only available in the research setting should become more generally available.

REFERENCES

1. Lucas A. Programming by early nutrition in man. In: Bock GR and Whelan J (eds) The Childhood Environment in Adult Disease. Chichester: John Wiley & Sons, 1991, pp 38–55.

2. Haffen K, Kedinger M and Semon-Assmann P. Cell contact dependent regulation of enterocytic differentiation. In Lebenthal E (ed) *Human Gastrointestinal Development*. New York: Raven Press, 1989, pp 19–39.
3. Le Douarin NM and Teillet MA. The migration of neural crest cells to the wall of the digestive tract in avian embryo. *J Embryol Exp Morphol* 1973;**30**: 31–48.
4. Moxey PC and Trier S. Specialised cell types in the human fetal small intestine. *Anatomical Rec* 1978;**191**: 269–286.
5. Colony PC and Conforte JC. Morphogenesis in the fetal rat proximal colon: effects of cytocalasin D. *Anatomical Rec* 1993;**235**: 241–252.
6. Winton DJ and Ponder BAJ. Stem cell organisation in mouse small intestine. *Proc R Soc (Lond)* 1990;**23**: 13–18.
7. Suh E and Traber PG. An intestine specific homeobox gene regulates proliferation and differentiation. *Mol Cell Biol* 1996;**16**: 619–625.
8. Louvard D, Kedinger M and Hauri HP. The differentiating intestinal epithelial cells. Establishment and maintenance of functions through interactions between cellular structures. *Ann Rev Cell Biol* 1992;**8**: 157–195.
9. Duluc I, Jost B and Feund JN. Multiple levels of control of the stage and region specific expression of rat intestinal lactase. *J Cell Biol* 1993;**123**: 1577–1586.
10. Henning SJ, Ruben DC and Schulman RJ. Ontogeny of the intestinal mucosa. In: Johnson LR (ed) *Physiology of the Gastrointestinal Tract*. New York, Raven Press, 1994, pp 571–610.
11. Maiuri L, Rai AV, Potter J *et al.* Mosaic pattern of lactase expression by villous enterocytes in human adult type hypolactasia. *Gastroenterology* 1991;**100**: 359–369.
12. Valentich JD and Powell DW. Intestinal sub-epithelial myofibroblast and mucosal immunophysiology current opinions. *Gastroenterology* 1994;**10**: 645–651.
13. Hathen K, Lacroix B and Kedinger M. Inductive properties of fibroblastic cell cultures derived from rat intestinal mucosa on epithelial differentiation. *Differentiation* 1983;**23**: 226–233.
14. Howlett AR and Bissell MJ. The influence of tissue micro environment (stroma and extracellular matrix) on the development and function of memory epithelium. *Epithelial Cell Biol* 1993;**2**: 79–89.
15. Simon-Assmann P, Kedinger M, De Arcangelis A, Russo V and Symo P. Extracellular matrix components in intestinal development. In: Ekblom P (ed) *Extracellular Matrix in Animal Development*. Amsterdam: Experentia, 1985; pp 65–82.
16. Kedinger M, Bouziges F and Simon-Assman P. Influence of cell interactions on intestinal brush border enzyme expression. In: Kotic A, Skoda J, Paces V and Kosca V (ed) *Highlights in Modern Biochemistry*. Zeist: VSP International Science Publishers, 1989, pp 1103–1112.
17. Probstmeier R, Martini R and Schachner M. Expression of J1 tenascin in the crypt villous unit of adult mouse small intestine. Implications for its role in epithelial cell shedding. *Development* 1990;**109**: 313–321.

18. Chawengsaksophak KR, James V, Hammond F, Kontgen F and Beck F. Homeostasis and intestinal tumours in *Cdx2* mutant mice. *Nature* 1997;**385**: 84–87.
19. Lorenz O, Duluc I, De Arcangelis A, Simon-Assmann P, Kedinger M and Froynd JN. Key role of the *Cdx2* homeobox gene in extracellular matrix mediated intestinal cell differentiation. *J Cell Biol* 1997 **139**: 1553–1565.
20. Yntema CL and Hammond WS. The origin of intrinsic ganglia of trunk viscera from vagal neural crest in the chick embryo. *J Comp Neurol* 1954;**101**: 515–541.
21. Peters Van de Sanden MGH, Kirby ML, Gittenberger de Groot AC, Tibboel D, Mulder MP, Meijers C. Oblation of various regions within the avian vagal neural crest has differential effects on ganglion formation in the fore, mid and hind gut. *Dev Din* 1993;**196**: 183–194.
22. Serbedzija GN, Burgan S, Fraser SE and Broner Fraser M. Vital dye labelling demonstrates a sacral neural crest contribution to the enteric nervous system of chick and mouse embryos. *Development* 1991;**111**: 857–866.
23. Pomeranz HD and Gershon MD. Colonisation of the avian hind gut by cells derived from the sacral neural crest. *Dev Biol* 1990;**137**: 378–394.
24. Allan IJ and Newgreen DF. The origin and differentiation of enteric neurons of the intestine of the foul embryo. *Am J Anat* 1980;**157**: 137–154.
25. Tucker GC, Siment G and Thiery JP. Pathways of avian neural crest cell migration in the developing gut. *Dev Biol* 1986;**116**: 430–450.
26. Pham TD, Gershon MD and Rothman TP. Time of origin of neurons in the murine enteric nervous system sequence in relation to phenotype. *J Comp Neurol* 1991;**314**: 789–798.
27. Fujimoto T, Harter J, Yokoyama S and Mitomi T. A study of the extracellular matrix protein as the migration pathway of neural crest cells in the gut: analysis in human embryos with special reference to the pathogenesis of Hirschsprung's disease. *J Pediatr Surg* 1981;**24**: 550–556.
28. Trupp M, Arinas E, Fainzibla M, Nilson AS, Sieber VA and Grigoriou M. Peripheral expression and biological activities of GDNF, a new neurotropic factor for avian and mammalian peripheral neurons. *Nature* 1996;**381**: 789–793.
29. Schuchardt A, D'agati V, Larsson-Blomberg L, Constantini F and Pachnis V. Defects in the kidney and enteric nervous system of mice lacking the tyrosine kinase receptor ret. *Nature* 1994;**367**: 380–383.
30. Kapur RP, Yost C and Palmiter RD. A transgenic model for studying the development of the enteric nervous system in normal and aganglionic mice. *Development* 1992;**116**: 167–175.
31. Hosoda K, Hammer RE, Richardson JA, Baynesh AG, Cheung JC and Giaida A. Targetted and natural pie bald lethal mutations of endothelin B receptor gene produce megacolon associated with spotted coat colour in mice. *Cell* 1994;**79**: 1267–1276.
32. Payette RF, Tennyson VM, Pomeranz HD, Pham TD, Rothman TP and Gershon MD. Accumulation of components of basal laminae: association with the failure of neural crest cells to colonise the presumptive aganglionic bowel of LS/LS mutant mice. *Dev Biol* 1988;**125**: 341–360.

33. Sanchez MP, Selos Santiago I, Frezen J, Bin He, Lira SA and Barbacid M. Renal agenesis and the absence of enteric neurons in mice lacking GDNF. *Nature* 1996;**382**: 70–73.
34. Edery P, Lyonnet S, Mulligan LM, Pelet A, Dow E and Abel L. Mutation of the ret proto oncogene in Hirschsprung's disease. Nature 1994;**367**: 378–380.
35. Lyonnet S, Bellono A, Pelet A *et al.* A gene for Hirschsprung's disease maps to the proximal long arm of chromosome 10. *Nature Genet* 1993;**4**: 346–350.
36. Eng C, Smith DP, Mulligan LM *et al.* Point mutation within the tyrosine kinase domain of the ret proto oncogene in multiple endocrine neoplasia type 2B and related sporadic tumours. *Hum Mol Genet* 1994;**3**: 237–241.
37. Moore MW, Klein RD, Farinas I *et al.* Renal and neuronal abnormalities in mice lacking GDNF. *Nature* 1996;**382**: 76–79.
38. Manak JR and Scott MP. A class act: conservation of homeo domain protein functions. *Development* 1994;**120(Suppl)**: 61–77.
39. McGuinness W and Krumlauf R. Homeobox genes and axial patterning. Cell 1992;**68**: 283–302.
40. Hunt P and Krumlauf R. Hox codes and positional specification invertebrate embryonic axis. *Annu Rev Cell Biol* 1992;**8**: 227–256.
41. Kessel M and Gruss P. Murine development control genes. *Science* 1990;**249**: 374–379.
42. Duboule D and Dollae P. The structural and functional organisation of the murine hox gene family resembles that of Drosphila homeotic genes. *EMBO J* 1989;**8**: 1497–1505.
43. Dolle P, Izpisua-Belmonte JC, Bonchonelli E and Deboule D. The hox 4.8 gene is localised at the '5 prime' extremity of the hox 4 complex and is expressed in the most posterior parts of the body during development. *Mech Dev* 1991;**36**: 3–13.
44. Wilkinson DG, Bhatt S, Cook M, Bonchonelli E and Krumlauf R. Segmental expression of hox 2 homeobox containing genes in the developing mouse hind brain. *Nature* 1989;**341**: 405–409.
45. Hunt P, Gulisano M, Cook M *et al.* A destinct hox code for the branchial region of the vertebrate head. *Nature* 1991;**353**: 861–864.
46. Pitera J, Smith VV and Milla PJ. Normal expression of hox genes in the developing gastrointestinal tract: a basis for understanding abnormalities of enteric neuromusculature. *Gastroenterology* 1997;**112**: A898.
47. Shirasawa S, Yunker AM, Roth KA, Brown GA, Orning S and Korsmeyer S. ENX (hox L11 1) deficient mice develop myenteric neuronal hypoplasia and mega-colon. *Nature Med* 1997;**3**: 646–650.
48. Wolgemuth DJ, Beringer RR, Mostola MP, Brinster RL and Palmiter RD. Transgenic mice overexpressing the mouse homeobox containing gene hox 1.4 exhibit abnormal gut development. *Nature* 1989;**337**: 464–467.
49. Kondo T, Dolle P, Zakany J and Duboule D. Function of posterior hox D genes in the morphogenesis of the anal sphincter. *Development* 1996;**122**: 2651–2659.
50. Omari TI, Miki K, Fraser R et al. Oesophageal body and lower oesophageal sphincter function in healthy premature infants. *Gastroenterology* 1995;**109**: 1757–1764.

51. Bisset WM, Watt JB, Rivers RPA and Milla PJ. Ontogeny of fasting small intestinal motor activity in the human infant. *Gut* 1988;**29**: 453–488.
52. Berseth CL. Gestational evolution of small intestine motility in preterm and term infants. *J Pediatr* 1989;**115**: 646–651.
53. Lichtenberger L. A search for the origin of neonatal hypogastrinaemia. *J Pediatr Gastroenterol Nutr* 1984;**3**: 161–166.
54. Marchini G and Uvnas-Moberg K. Levels and molecular forms of gastrin and somatostatin in plasma and in gastric contents of infants after section delivery. *J Pediatr Gastroenterol Nutr* 1992;**14**: 406–412.
55. Kiviluoto T, Voipio J and Kivilaakso E. Subepithelial tissue pH of rat gastric mucosa exposed to luminal acid, barrier breaking agents and haemorrhagic shock. *Gastroenterology* 1988;**94**: 695–702.
56. Kivilaakso E, Fromm D and Silen W. Relationship between ulceration and intramural pH of gastric mucosa during haemorrhagic shock. *Surgery* 1978;**84**: 70–77.
57. Luen MJM. Cell physiology and pharmacology of gastric acid secretion. *Therapy* 1992;**47**: 93–96.
58. Kelly EJ, Lagopoulous M and Primrose JN. Immunocytochemical localisation of parietal cells and G cells in the developing human stomach. *Gut* 1993;**34**: 1057–1059.
59. Hyman PE, Clark DD and Ucret SL. Gastric acid secretory function in preterm infants. *J Pediatr* 1985;**106**: 467–471.
60. Siegal M, Krantz B and Lebenthal E. The effect of gastric emptying of isocholoric feedings in premature infants. *Pediatr Res* 1984;**18**: 212A.
61. Szabo S. Gastric mucosal injury and protection. *J Clin Gastroenterol* 1991;**13**: S21–34.
62. Hills BA. Gastric surfactant and the hydrophobic mucosal barrier. *Gut* 1996;**39**: 621–627.
63. Dial E and Lichtenberger LM. A role for milk phospholipids in protection against gastric acid. *Gastroenterology* 1984;**87**: 379–385.
64. Dial E and Lichtenberger LM. Development of gastric mucosal protection against acid in the rat. *Gastroenterology* 1986;**91**: 318–325.
65. Maki M, Ruuska T, Kuusela AL, Karikoski R and Ikonen RS. High prevelance of asymptomatic oesophageal and gastric lesions in preterm and term infants in intensive care. *Crit Care Med* 1994;**21**: 1863–1867.
66. Kuusela AL, Ruuska T, Karikoski R *et al.* A randomised controlled study of prophylactic ranitidine in preventing stress induced gastric mucosal lesions in neonatal intensive care unit patients. *Crit Care Med* 1997;**25**: 346–351.
67. Cavell B. Gastric emptying in preterm infants. *Acta Pediatr Scand* 1979;**68**: 725–730.
68. Siegal M, Lebenthal E and Krantz B. Effect of choloric density on gastric emptying in premature infants. *J Pediatr* 1984;**104**: 118–122.
69. Billeaud C, Guillet J and Sandler B. Gastric emptying in infants with or without gastro-oesophageal reflux according to the type of milk. *Eur J Clin Nutr* 1990;**44**: 577–583.

70. Lucas A, Adrian TE, Kristophades N, Bloom SR and Aynsley-Green A. Plasma motilin gastrin and enteroglucagon and enteral feeding in the human newborn. *Arch Dis Child* 1980;55: 673–677.
71. Ruckebusch Y. Development of digestive motor patterns during perinatal life: mechanisms and significance. *J Pediatr Gastroenterol Nutr* 1986;5: 523–536.
72. Wasniak ER, Fenton TR and Milla PJ. The development of fasting small intestinal motor activity in the human neonate. In: Roman CE (ed) *Gastrointestinal Motility*. Lancaster: MTP Press, 1984, pp 265–270.
73. Bisset WM, Watt JB, Rivers RPA and Milla PJ. Postprandial motor response of the small intestine to enteral feeds in preterm infants. *Arch Dis Child* 1989;**64**: 1356–1361.
74. Berseth CL and Nordi CK. Manometry can predict feeding readiness in preterm infants. *Gastroenterology* 1992;**103**: 1523–1528.
75. Baker J and Berseth CL. Postnatal change in inhibitory regulation of intestinal motor activity in human and canine neonates. *Pediatr Res* 1995;**38**: 133–139.
76. Newell SJ, Booth IW, Morgan ME, Durban GM and McNeish AS. Gastro-oesophageal reflux in preterm infants. *Arch Dis Child* 1989;**64**: 780–786.
77. Omari TI, Miki K, Davidson G *et al.* Characterisation of relaxation of the lower oesphageal sphincter in healthy premature infants. *Gut* 1997;**40**: 370–375.
78. Newell SJ, Chapman S and Booth IW. Ultrasonic assessment of gastric emptying in the preterm infant. *Arch Dis Child* 1993;**69**: 32–36.
79. Ruuska TH, Evans DF, Kempsy S and Milla PJ. Foregut motility in the very preterm infant. *J Pediatr Gastroenterol Nutr* 1995;**20**: 460.
80. Van den Driessch E, Peeters K, Ghoos Y, Devlieger H and Veereman-Wauters G. Gastric emptying in formula fed and breast fed infants measured with the 13C octanoic acid breath test. J Pediatr Gastroenterol Nutr 1997;**24**: 480.
81. Devane SP, Ravelli AM, Bisset WM, Smith VV, Lake BD and Milla PJ. Gastric antral dysrhythmias in children with chronic idiopathic intestinal pseudo-obstruction. *Gut* 1992;**33**: 1477–1481.
82. Ruuska T. Gastroscopies in preterms. *Acta Endoscop* 1994;**24**: 151–156.
83. Liebman WM, Thaler MM and Bujanover Y. Endoscopic evaluation of upper gastrointestinal bleeding in the new born. *Am J Gastroenterol* 1978;**69**: 607–608.
84. Ruuska T, Fell JM, Bisset WM and Milla PJ. Neonatal and infantile upper gastrointestinal endoscopy using a new small diameter fibre optic gastroscope. *J Pediatr Gastroenterol Nutr* 1996;**23**: 604–608.

7

Liquid Ventilation: Present and Immediate Future

Thomas H. Shaffer and Marla R. Wolfson

INTRODUCTION

Perfluorochemical (PFC) liquids offer potential for biomedical use and the support of respiration.[1, 2] During fluid breathing, a liquid replaces nitrogen gas as the carrier for oxygen and carbon dioxide. Since the air–liquid interface at the alveolar–capillary surface is eliminated and replaced with a liquid–liquid interface, lung compliance is increased, alveoli are recruited and lung inflation pressures are reduced. Thus, fluid breathing provides a potential form of ventilatory support with reduced risk of barotrauma. While a number of fluids have been explored as breathing media, PFC liquids have shown greatest promise due to the physicochemical properties of low surface tension, high respiratory gas solubility, and the chemically and biologically inert nature of this material. In addition to respiratory applications, PFC liquids have been developed to support other organ systems and are approved for use as synthetic bloods, imaging agents and replacement fluid for the eye.[3–5] As such, a few pure medical-grade PFC liquids exist which meet the physicochemical property requirements as well as purity specifications for respiratory applications. Moreover, new fluorine chemistry methods should enable production of future PFC liquids uniquely designed for the specific biomedical application. There have been several applications and techniques reported for PFC fluids, including both respiratory and non-respiratory support.[1, 2]

The efficiency of the lungs as a gas exchanger is essential for existence in the extrauterine environment at any age. However, premature birth or respiratory insult typically impair the efficiency. Unlike structural abnormalities which cannot be altered acutely, treatment focused at biochemical deficiencies such as exogenous surfactant replacement therapy and antenatal hormone therapy have demonstrated improvement in lung function, decreased ventilatory requirements, and a reduction in mortality. Although significant advances in respiratory care and reduction in mortality of patients with respiratory failure have been demonstrated, morbidity from barotrauma persists and leads to chronic pulmonary sequelae.[6] For these reasons, alternative means to support pulmonary gas exchange while preserving lung structure and function still warrant further investigation.

With this in mind, application of liquid ventilation (LV) technology has the potential to improve the clinical management of neonatal pulmonary pathophysiology, including premature lung disease, aspiration syndromes, pneumonia and pulmonary hypoplasia.[7] Although animal studies have been impressive to date, documentation of efficacy in human disease will be required. To this end and building on more than 30 years of studies in which animals of all ages have been successfully ventilated with PFC fluid and recovered to mechanical gas ventilation with residual PFC in the lung, the first clinical trial of PFC ventilation was performed in neonates in 1989.[8, 9] LV procedures, similar to preclinical animal studies, are currently being tested in neonates, children and adults with a variety of life-threatening lung injuries, including respiratory distress syndrome, congenital diaphragmatic hernia, sepsis, near-drowning, aspiration syndromes and smoke inhalation. To date, about 700 patients across the United States and Canada are being enrolled in LV studies with the PFC fluid known as perflubron (LiquiVent™). Continued research will further define the applications and limitations of this alternative clinical approach to respiratory management. This review presents a summary of the PFC liquids explored and the most recent technical approaches to liquid-assisted ventilation (LAV). The rationale and status of preclinical studies and human experiences are also discussed.

PHYSICAL PROPERTIES OF RESPIRATORY LIQUID MEDIA

PFC liquids are synthetic fluorinated hydrocarbon materials, first produced during World War II as part of the Manhattan Project. These compounds are formulated by replacing all of the carbon-bound hydrogen atoms with fluorine atoms on common organic compounds.[10]

PFC liquids have varying physicochemical properties (Table 7.1) which, in part, are dictated by the arrangement of the carbon–fluorine bonds.[10, 11] Recently, the authors have reported the quantitative structure–activity relationships of 16 perfluorinated hetero-hydrocarbons as potential respiratory media.[12] The physicochemical profile of 16 commercially available PFC liquids were characterized by creating a method for accurate predication of a host of unknown physical properties. The input data were categorized into 3 groups: empiric properties, geometric indices and quantum mechanical descriptors. Algorithms were then developed, one for each independent variable function, including oxygen solubility, partition coefficient (log P), vapor pressure, viscosity and density. This algorithm is expected to assist in the predication of physical properties of PFC liquids, such that PFC production and selection from currently available fluids can be optimized for each liquid-ventilation application.

On the basis that PFC liquids are synthetic materials which are not normally found in the body, PFC uptake, elimination and biodistribution

Table 7.1 Physical properties of typical perfluorochemical fluids used for respiratory applications.

Physical property	Perfluorofuran/pyran	Perfluorodecalin	Perflubron
O_2 solubility @ 25°C (ml gas/100 ml liquid)	52	53	49
CO_2 solubility @ 37°C (ml gas/100 ml liquid)	160	210	140
Surface tension (dynes/cm @ 25°C)	15	18	15
Vapor pressure (torr @ 37°C)	63	11	14
Density @ 25°C (g/ml)	1.78	1.93	1.95
Dynamic viscosity (centipose @ 25°C)	1.46	2.12	5.65
Kinematic viscosity (centistokes @ 25°C)	0.82	1.10	2.90

In general, all of these fluids are inert, odorless and colorless. They have low surface tension (10–19 dyne/cm) and high solubility for oxygen (>40 vol%); and are insoluble in water, sparingly soluble in lipids and in organic solvents, and completely soluble in other fluorinated compounds.
Perfluorofuran/pyran mixture: RM-101, Mercantile Development, Inc; perfluorodecalin: PP-5, BNFL Fluorochemicals Ltd & Air Products & Chemicals; and perflubron, LiquiVent™: Alliance Pharmaceutical Corp & Hoechst-Marion-Roussel.

have been investigated following LV procedures in humans and animals and in mathematical models of LV.[13–18] Since PFC liquids are practically insoluble in water and are soluble to a small degree in lipids, the small quantities of PFC which diffuse across the lung and into the blood dissolve in blood lipid. Despite differences in experimental conditions across studies, very low concentrations (0.25–10 μg PFC/ml blood) of different PFC compounds have been demonstrated in the blood, reaching a plateau by 15–20 min after pulmonary exposure to PFC.[15–18] Blood levels following intratracheal PFC administration are orders of magnitude lower than those following intravascular administration (40–80 mg PFC/ml of blood) of PFC emulsion clinically approved for angioplasty in humans and under investigation as an oxygen carrier or temporary 'blood substitute'.[3, 17] PFC uptake into the blood following intratracheal administration is dependent on PFC vapor pressure, permeability coefficients in the lung, PFC solubility in blood, blood lipid content and ventilation/perfusion matching. Biodistribution of PFC to the various organs is dependent on tissue–blood partition coefficients, tissue blood flow and tissue compartment volume, which is similar to the distribution of drugs in the body. Fat-rich organs have a higher capacity for PFC storage and vessel-rich organs with high blood flow are saturated with PFC more rapidly. The unique chemical structure of PFC liquids means they are not metabolized. PFCs are predominantly eliminated by the lung through volatilization into the expiratory gases; a small amount of PFC may be transpired through the skin. PFC liquids have been shown to be retained in certain tissues for approximately 2 years after LAV (see below) or intravascular injection of emulsions, without any apparent toxic effect.

PFC liquids were first used in 1966 to support normobaric respiration in mammals.[19] Initial liquid breathing investigations of total body immersion or gravity-assisted ventilation demonstrated the ability of PFC to support oxygenation and improve pulmonary compliance;[19, 20] however, this approach failed to maintain physiologic carbon dioxide elimination due to expiratory flow limitations and diffusional gradients.[21] Limitations in gas exchange have been resolved by new liquid ventilator configurations, components and PFC liquids.[22–24]

PHYSIOLOGICAL PRINCIPLES AND PULMONARY APPLICATIONS

Respiratory Support Applications

LAV is defined as augmented pulmonary gas exchange facilitated by tracheal instillation of PFC liquid. The physicochemical properties of the PFC liquid and biophysical effects of the liquid on lung mechanics support favorable physiologic responses in the surfactant-deficient or impaired lung. With PFC instillation in the lung, the gas–liquid interface is replaced with a liquid–liquid interface at the lung surface while supporting an adequate alveolar reservoir for pulmonary gas exchange. At the same time, high surface tension at the gas–liquid interface is eliminated and interfacial tension is reduced.[1,2] Since transmural pressures across the alveolar–capillary membrane are more evenly matched, pulmonary blood flow is more homogenous in the fluid- as compared to gas-filled lung.[1,25,26] At present, LAV techniques for respiratory support consists of tidal liquid ventilation (TLV), and partial liquid ventilation (PLV). The presence of endogenous surfactant or surfactant pretreatment further reduces collapsing pressures in the PFC-treated lung by further decreasing tension at the PFC–lung interface.[27]

Tidal liquid ventilation

Since its origin with saline-[20] and PFC-ventilated animals,[22] TLV (assisted mechanical ventilation) is the transport of respiratory gases solely in dissolved form via tidal volume exchange of liquid to and from the lung. Using this method, all gas–liquid interfacial tension is eliminated and the lung is provided maximal protection from inflation pressures as lung volume is recruited, compliance is increased and inflation pressures and pulmonary barotrauma are reduced.[1,2,28,29] Briefly, TLV is achieved by cycling fluid from a reservoir to and from the lung by a mechanical ventilator which has evolved over the years to include electromechanical bellows pumps,[22] gravity-driven pressure systems[30,31] and modified extracorporeal membrane oxygenation (ECMO) pumps[22–25,31] driven by a variety of pneumatic/fluidic/electronic control systems. Control strategies consisting of constant pressure or flow schemes, manual set time-cycling or demand-controlled timing, pressure (system, airway, or alveolar) and/or volume (lung and tidal volume) limitation have been explored. The most recent approaches are microprocessor based with feedback control.[24] Independent of pumping and control schemes, warmed and oxygenated PFC liquid is pumped from a fluid reservoir into the lung during inspiration. Expiration is accomplished by actively removing liquid from the lung with passive assist of the lung recoil. Fluid is then filtered, returned to a gas exchanger for desired levels of oxygenation and CO_2 scrubbing and returned to the fluid reservoir. PFC fluid is conserved by condensing vapor in the expired gas and non-condensed PFC loss due to evaporation is measured and returned to the system.[32] Along these lines, a recent study compared PFC loss from 2 types of gas exchangers [spray bubbler (SB) and silicone membrane (SM)] as a function of PFC liquid vapor pressure, gas flow, PFC liquid flow and liquid temperature.[33] It was found that PFC loss from both exchangers increased as a function of gas flow, vapor pressure and temperature. In addition to these factors, PFC loss from the SM was increased with increasing PFC flow, thus suggesting that the type of gas exchanger should be matched to a specific PFC ventilation fluid.

The TLV process is initiated by instilling PFC fluid (25–35 ml/kg) into the gas-filled lung while gently manipulating the thorax to assist removal of resident gas volumes. TLV algorithms which address optimum frequency (3–8 breaths/ min), tidal volume (15–20 ml/kg) and inspiratory:expiratory timing ratio (1:2 or 1:3) have been developed to maintain adequate CO_2 elimination (up to 4-fold steady-state values), minimize resistive pressures, overcome expiratory flow limitations associated with liquids, and overcome diffusional dead space associated with CO_2 diffusivity in a liquid respiratory media.[21] Proximal airway pressures are rapidly dissipated along the tracheo-bronchial tree during TLV, such that alveolar pressures are markedly lower than proximal airway pressures.[1, 18]

Over 20 years, basic studies have shown that TLV can effectively improve lung mechanics and ventilation/perfusion matching, and decrease intrapulmonary shunt, thereby supporting pulmonary gas exchange and cardiovascular stability in experimental animal preparations. In this regard, TLV has been explored in adult, neonatal, and preterm animal preparations with respiratory distress of various etiologies.[1, 2, 18, 22, 23, 29–31, 34–37] Because TLV maintains a liquid–liquid alveolar interface in the immature lung, this ventilatory approach provides a useful tool in creating an animal preparation to study developmental processes beginning as early as 102 days' gestation in the lamb (65% gestation; correlating to human development of 18–20 weeks).[23] Unlike the use of exogenous surfactant therapy in the very early stages of development or extracorporeal gas exchange, there is no known physiological limitation to the duration of TLV. Most recent studies have shown safe and effective ventilation with TLV in premature lambs up to 72 hours postnatally.[37] Morphological studies of animals of various ages, with and without lung injury, suggest that TLV actually minimizes damage typically incurred as a result of gas ventilation.[28, 35–37] After TLV, gas exchange spaces are clear, the air–blood interface is thin walled, the capillaries are intact and thin walled, the epithelial cell membranes remain intact, and abundant surfactant is noted in lamellar bodies indicating maintenance of lung ultrastructure.[28, 38] Differences between the gas-ventilated and TLV lung are profound: there is a substantial reduction in pulmonary consolidation, atelectasis, hemorrhage, disruption of alveolar–capillary membrane and an absence of inflammatory infiltrates in the latter.[28]

Partial liquid ventilation

Initial TLV studies with respiratory distress in lambs demonstrated not only an improvement in gas exchange and lung function during ventilation with PFC but also residual improvements in pulmonary function upon return to gas ventilation (GV).[1, 25, 29, 34] Originally, it was suggested that the administration of PFC liquid to the lungs may work as an artificial surfactant for respiratory distress syndrome (RDS) or a lavage media for certain other types of pulmonary dysfunction;[8, 9, 29, 34, 39, 40] however, these studies with high vapor pressure liquids, such as FC-75 and Rimar 101, proved to be short lived or ineffective in improving or sustaining lung function. More recently, several researchers have studied the utility of tracheal instillation of newer PFC liquids such as perflubron (LiquiVent™) in combination with GV in newborn piglets,[41] neonatal lambs,[35, 36, 42, 43] rabbits,[44] the congenital diaphragmatic hernia (CDH) lamb model,[45] premature human infants and adults with respiratory failure.[46–52] This combined ventilation scheme with PFC liquids and GV has been described as PLV and is characterized by filling and maintaining the lung with a functional residual capacity of PFC liquid while conventional GV is performed. It has been proposed that residual PFC is oxygenated and carbon dioxide is exchanged in the lungs by means of the tidal gas movement provided by GV.

Despite differences in the magnitude of the responses, it has been shown that PLV provides adequate or improved gas exchange at reduced airway pressures compared to conventional GV in a wide range of animal preparations with respiratory failure induced by various mechanisms. The histological picture of lungs treated with PLV has been reported to be greatly improved compared to other forms of respiratory support or untreated control groups, and PLV-treated lungs from healthy full-term animals reflect preserved architecture. However, closer inspection has demonstrated marked regional differences in pulmonary histology in the lungs of preterm and neonatal lambs with RDS following PLV.[35, 42–45] These changes were associated with stratification of the PFC and gas to the dependent and independent regions of the lung, respectively, which was corroborated by radiologic evaluation and gross inspection of the lung.[42–45] The dependent region of the lungs appeared to be preserved while little improvement in the non-dependent regions was noted. The studies indicate that for a number of pulmonary abnormalities, it is possible to achieve some degree of pulmonary improvement with PLV;

however, further refinement in this technique is necessary to offer maximum protection of the lung.

A number of techniques have been explored for PLV. Thus far, investigators have considered brief periods of LV (3–5 min),[8, 9, 40, 53] rapid instillation of a bolus (30 ml/kg) of oxygenated PFC,[39–41] as well as a slow infusion of non-preoxygenated PFC in doses up to 30 ml/kg over 15 min.[42–45,47–52] The technical aspect of instilling PFC liquid and adjustment of the gas ventilator are familiar to the clinician; however, effective ventilation of a lung which is partly filled with liquid and partly with gas is more challenging since there are many unknowns with respect to the distribution of PFC fluid in the lung, oxygen and carbon dioxide saturation of resident PFC, continually changing lung mechanics, evaporative loss of PFC, and changing volumes of gas and PFC lung volumes. Maintenance of a therapeutic PFC liquid volume following initial instillation in the lungs is dependent upon a number of factors. Studies employing an analyzer system designed to quantify expired PFC vapor have shown that PFC liquid volume loss and evaporation rate from the lungs is influenced by time, PFC physical properties, gas–liquid contact, ventilation strategy, lung pathophysiology, repositioning of the subject, and the administration of supplemental PFC doses to the lungs.[32] The optimum PFC filling strategy, initial and subsequent dosing schedule, and subsequent GV scheme is still under extensive investigation.

Non-Respiratory Support Applications

Lavage

Several initial studies with PFC liquids were directed at lavaging the lungs of alveolar debris.[25, 39] The rationale for this procedure was that PFC liquid would provide a means for bilateral lavage of the lungs with a reduction in the risk of hypoxemia and hypercapnia typically associated with saline lavage procedures. In an early study of meconium aspiration, PFC liquid was used to ventilate lambs delivered by cesarean section with evidence of meconium aspiration.[25] At birth, poor oxygenation, acidosis and low pulmonary compliance were present during GV in all lambs; however, during subsequent TLV, improvements were noted in PaO_2, alveolar–arterial oxygen gradient and pulmonary compliance. In addition, $PaCO_2$ was lower during TLV and pulmonary blood flow was more uniform. Based on these findings, it was concluded that TLV improved pulmonary perfusion, and ventilation/perfusion matching. Furthermore, it was suggested that these changes in pulmonary function were associated with the removal of meconium which was observed in the expired liquid. The effectiveness of this procedure for lung lavage has also been shown in a number of other acute animal studies with injured lungs.[35, 40]

Drug delivery

Delivery of biologically active agents to the neonatal lung is often part of the management regime of pulmonary dysfunction. Theoretically, if gas exchange could be maintained during the process, insufflation of an agent directly to the lung surface and tissue presents advantages for distribution and uptake of pulmonary-targeted agents. This technique is particularly attractive in the liquid-filled lung since pulmonary blood flow is more homogeneously distributed and ventilation/perfusion is more evenly matched.[54] Finally, because gas exchange can be supported by inert PFC liquid, potential side effects due to the interaction between the biological agent and the vehicle (PFC) can be ameliorated. Several studies have demonstrated the utility of PFC LV techniques to deliver aqueous-based pharmacological agents (i.e. vasopressors, antibiotics, adenovirus for gene transfer) directly to the lung parenchyma when administered intratracheally during LAV in preterm lambs with RDS, normal or lung injured full-term lambs, and normal rabbits.[54–56] It is also noteworthy that, despite the lack of miscibility of the aqueous agents in PFC liquid, the physiological responses, serum uptake and intrapulmonary distribution of agents demonstrate that TLV provides an effective method to deliver a number of agents to the pulmonary and systemic circulation.

In addition to aqueous agents, other studies have demonstrated physiologic responses to inspired nitric oxide (NO) during PLV with PFC liquid.[57] The ability to deliver NO during PLV is probably related to the PFC-facilitated recruitment of lung volume, distribution of NO in the gas and liquid regions of the lung, and the solubility and diffusion of NO in the PFC liquid.

Taken together, these studies indicate that PFC liquid may be useful in delivering other agents (i.e. bronchodilators, exogenous surfactant, antibiotics, steroids, chemotherapeutics, mucolytics, antioxidants and gene therapy products) directly to the lung surface, while protecting non-targeted organs from iatrogenic pharmacological effects. It appears that this approach has a promising therapeutic role in the management of variety of neonatal problems, such as surfactant deficiency, exudative processes, gene therapy, persistent or acquired pulmonary hypertension, chronic lung disease, pneumonia and airway reactivity.

Pulmonary imaging

PFC liquids, in general, are useful contrast media when instilled into anatomical structures such as the lungs. Because these fluids are inert, radiopaque, support gas exchange and are vaporized from the lung, they provide a useful diagnostic imaging tool to evaluate pulmonary structure–function without intrinsic problems related to existing contrast agents.[13, 58]

Multimodal imaging techniques of conventional X-ray and high-resolution computed tomography (HRCT) of the PFC-filled lung may be used to evaluate lung structures, PFC distribution and sequential elimination.[58] The addition of bromine atoms to PFC compounds provides greater radiopacity. Anterior–posterior (A–P) views combined with cross-table lateral (L) views are required qualitatively to evaluate the distribution pattern of the PFC during gas ventilation (PLV). During the elimination phase of breathing, plain film X-rays indicate a predominant central clearance pattern, whereas sequential HRCT images identified central as well as peripheral clearance with a calculated 45% decrease in overall density related to PFC clearance by 30 min.[58]

Conventionally, the ability to evaluate small airway pathology with bronchographic agents has been limited by poor resolution of the bronchioles at the secondary lobule level. Because of its density, low surface tension and intense radiopacity, perflubron has been used as a bronchographic contrast agent for HRCT. This PFC liquid has allowed direct visualization of the airways through the centrilobar bronchioles and their first-order branches with definition within a millimeter of the lung surface.[59]

The advent of helical CT has allowed for volumetric data acquisition with markedly improved multiplanar reconstruction, 3D rendering and, with post-processing software, has permitted direct visualization of the inside of large airways (so-called 'virtual bronchoscopy'). A recent study showed that the instillation of a dose of liquid perflubron increased airway contrast and therefore increased airway resolution.[60] Bronchoscopic CT without perflubron only allowed visualization of the first 2 generations with poor resolution of third-order branches. In contrast, images with perflubron permitted improved resolution of the tracheobronchial tree to the fifth-order branches. These preliminary studies demonstrate that perflubron liquid in the lungs can enhance bronchoscopic CT images of the tracheobronchial tree by improving contrast and resolution of more distal generations of airways.

Anti-inflammatory activity

In several *in vivo* animal models of acute lung injury, it has been shown that ventilation with perflubron reduces alveolar hemorrhage, pulmonary permeability, edema and neutrophil infiltration. It has been suggested that ventilation with perflubron may attenuate the inflammatory response in acute lung injury in these models.[35, 36] In a cobra venom factor (CVF) lung injury model, it was shown that pulmonary neutrophil infiltration in rat lungs was significantly reduced during PLV when compared to conventional GV support.[61] Along the same lines, exposure of alveolar macrophages from rabbit lungs demonstrated that perflubron liquid *in vitro* decreased the responsiveness of macrophages to potent stimuli.[62] The mechanism of perflubron as a non-specific anti-inflammatory agent is still under extensive investigation.

Lung expansion

Recent studies have shown the potential of LV as an alternative treatment in supporting gas exchange and lung mechanics in the presence of pulmonary hypoplasia. The basis of this application is related to low pressure alveolar recruitment and respiratory support to facilitate improved ventilation to perfusion matching. PLV studies of CDH in a lamb preparation, supported either prophylactically at birth or rescued after a period of GV, showed improved gas exchange and compliance as compared to conventional GV support.[45, 57] Based on lung histology and morphometry in the rescue CDH study, PFC tracheal instillation did not seem to be any less traumatic as compared to GV-treated controls.[45] This may in part be explained by the severity of the CDH and the delayed initiation of liquid treatment. The CDH lamb preparation prophylactically treated with PFC at delivery demonstrated improved function and histology as compared with rescue treatment.[57]

Clinical Experiences

A number of case reports and small population patient trials have been presented (Table 7.2). In 1989, the first human trial with PFC liquid was initiated in near-death infants with severe respiratory failure.[8, 9] LV was given in two 3–5-min cycles separated by 15 min of GV. Although all infants in these studies ultimately died from their underlying respiratory disease, it was shown that LV was able to support gas exchange and that residual improvement in pulmonary function was observed following return to GV. Further clinical trials were limited by the need for a medical-grade breathing fluid and a medically approved liquid ventilator.

Based on the encouraging results of this first infant trial and the continued success of neonatal and adult animal trials with liquid-assisted gas ventilation, a multicenter trial was designed to evaluate the safety and efficacy of PLV with sterile perflubron (LiquiVent™; Alliance Pharmaceutical Corp.) in the treatment of premature infants with severe respiratory failure who had declined on conventional therapy.[49] Thirteen patients with a gestational age of 24–34 weeks and weight of

Table 7.2 Reported clinical case reports and studies.

Date	Patients	Reference
1989	Preterm – RDS	8
1991	Preterm – RDS	9
1995	Infants – ARDS	48
1996	Infants, children and adults – ARDS, ECMO	47
1996	Adults – ECMO	50
1996	Infants – CDH, ECMO	52
1996	Adult – ARDS, ECMO	46
1996	Preterm – RDS	49
1996	Infants – ARDS, ECMO	51

600–2000 g met study criteria and were enrolled. Ten received treatment for 24–76 hours. PLV was discontinued in 3 infants in favor of high-frequency ventilation. During the first hour of PLV, oxygen tension and lung compliance increased 138% and 61%, respectively. There were no serious adverse events related to PLV and 8 patients survived to 36 weeks' corrected gestational age. It was reported that PLV could be achieved for up to several days in critically ill infants without serious adverse events. Furthermore, PLV-associated clinical improvements were clearly demonstrated.

Based on previously successful animal trials combining intratracheal PFC instillation and ECMO,[36] several studies recently evaluated the safety and efficacy of PLV with sterile perflubron in a series of adults, children and neonates who were in respiratory failure and on ECMO support.[47, 50–52] It was shown that during PLV, the A-a O_2 difference decreased and static pulmonary compliance increased: 11 of 19 patients survived. In another small case study, clinical and radiographic findings were reported in 2 infants in whom ECMO support was supplemented with the tracheal instillation of perflubron.[48] Although clinical response and outcome were inconclusive, radiographically it was shown that perflubron was an effective contrast agent for evaluation of neonatal pulmonary abnormalities.[46, 48, 51]

CONCLUSION

To date, numerous animal studies and a few clinical reports have shown that insufflation of preterm lungs and acutely injured adult lungs with a PFC liquid reduces elevated interfacial surface tension. In contrast to conventional GV alone, more effective oxygenation, ventilation, and acid–base balance can be achieved during LAV at lower and safer alveolar inflation pressures. Initial findings from safety and efficacy clinical studies are encouraging in that all patients tolerated LAV without serious adverse effects and demonstrated some residual improvement in pulmonary function. Although many patients ultimately died of their underlying respiratory disease, clinical improvements were clearly demonstrated. These clinical trials demonstrate that LAV can support gas exchange, even in preterm infants, newborn infants and adults with severe and prolonged lung disease.

The application of non-respiratory support techniques with PFC liquids, such as lung lavage, pulmonary administration of drugs, pulmonary imaging enhancement, anti-inflammatory action and lung expansion, provides unique clinical advantages for the treatment and diagnosis of several types of pulmonary disease.

Finally, LAV techniques have the potential to treat lung disease with less risk of barotrauma and may provide the means for complementing other forms of respiratory management, such as ECMO, high-frequency ventilation and NO administration. For LV to assume a role in clinical medicine, it must be shown to be safe and effective with respect to other therapies or in combination with current treatments. Controlled multicenter trials are warranted and in progress.

Acknowledgments

The authors gratefully acknowledge the National Institutes of Health, American Heart Association, Alliance Pharmaceutical Corp, Hoechst-Marion-Roussel Corp., Miteni, s.r.l., BNFL, and 3M Corporation, and the expanding team of clinical and basic scientists affiliated with Temple University School of Medicine for their active involvement, encouragement and foresight.

REFERENCES

1. Shaffer TH, Wolfson MR and Clark LC. State-of-the-art: Liquid ventilation. *Pediatr Pulmonol* 1992;**14**: 102–109.
2. Wolfson MR and Shaffer TH. Liquid ventilation during early development: theory, physiologic processes and application. *J Dev Physiol* 1990;**13**: 1–12.
3. Riess JG. Overview of progress in the fluorocarbon approach to *in vivo* oxygen delivery. [Review]. *Art Cells Blood Subs Immob Biotech* 1992;**20**: 20–24.
4. Haidt SJ, Clark LC and Ginsbery J. Liquid perfluorocarbon replacement of eye tissue. *Invest Ophthamol* 1982;**22**: 233–238.

5. Mattrey RF. Perfluorooctylbromide: a new contrast agent for CT, sonography and MR Imaging. *Am J Radiol* 1989;**152**: 247–252.
6. Hack M, Horbar JD, Mallory MH, Tyson JE, Wright E and Wright L. Very low birthweight outcomes of the National Institute of Child Health and Human Development Neonatal Network. *Pediatrics* 1991;**87**: 587–597.
7. Shaffer TH and Wolfson MR. Liquid ventilation: An alternative ventilation strategy for management of neonatal respiratory distress. *Eur J Pediatr* 1996;**155 (Suppl 2)**: 530–534.
8. Greenspan JS, Wolfson MR, Rubenstein SD and Shaffer TH. Liquid ventilation of preterm baby [letter]. *Lancet* 1989;**2**: Nov: 1095.
9. Greenspan JS, Wolfson MR, Rubenstein SD and Shaffer TH. Liquid ventilation of human preterm neonates. *J Pediatr* 1990;**117**: 106–111.
10. Sargent JW and Seffl RJ. Properties of perfluoronated liquid. *Fed Proc* 1970;**29**: 1699–1703.
11. Moore RE and Clark LC Jr. Chemistry of fluorocarbons in biomedical use. *Int Anesthesiol Clin* 1985;**23**: 11–24.
12. Gabriel JL, Miller TF, Wolfson MR and Shaffer TH. Quantitative structure–activity relationships of perfluorinated hetro-hydrocarbons as potential respiratory media: Application to oxygen solubility, logP, viscosity, vapor pressure, and density. *ASAIO* 1996;**42**: 968–973.
13. Long DM, Liu MS, Szanto PS *et al.* Efficacy and toxicity studies with radiopaque perfluorocarbon. *Radiology* 1972;**105**: 323–332.
14. Tuazon AS, Cox C, Stavis RL, Wolfson MR and Shaffer TH. Tissue uptake of perfluorochemical (PFC) during liquid ventilation (LV): A peripheral exchange. *Faseb J* 1994;**8**: 413A.
15. Shaffer TH, Wolfson MR, Greenspan JS, Hoffman RE, Davis SL and Clark LC Jr. Liquid ventilation in premature lambs: uptake, biodistribution and elimination of perfluorodecalin liquid. *Repro Fertil Dev* 1996;**8**: 409–416.
16. Calderwood HW, Ruiz BC, Tham MK, Modell JH, Saga S and Hood CI. Residual levels and biochemical changes after ventilation with perfluorinated liquid. *J Appl Physiol* 1975;**39**: 603–607.
17. Keipert PE, Otto S, Flaim SF *et al.* Influence of perflubron emulsion particle size on blood half-life and febrile response in rats. *Art Cells Blood Subs Immob Biotech* 1994;**22**: 1169–1174.
18. Shaffer TH, Greenspan JS and Wolfson MR. Liquid ventilation. In: Boynton BR, Carlo WA and Jobe AH (eds) *New Therapies for Neonatal Respiratory Failure: A Physiological Approach.* New York: Cambridge University Press, 1994, pp 279–301.
19. Clark LC Jr and Gollan F. Survival of mammals breathing organic liquids equilibrated with oxygen at atmospheric pressure. *Science* 1966;**152**: 1755–1756.
20. Kylstra JA, Paganelli CV and Lanphier EH. Pulmonary gas exchange in dogs ventilated with hyperbarically oxygenated liquid. *J Appl Physiol* 1966;**21**: 177–184.
21. Koen PA, Wolfson MR and Shaffer TH. Fluorocarbon ventilation: maximal expiratory flows and CO_2 elimination. *Pediatr Res* 1988;**24**: 291–296.

22. Shaffer TH and Moskowitz GD. Demand-controlled liquid ventilation of the lungs. *J Appl Physiol* 1974;**36**: 208–213.
23. Wolfson MR, Tran N, Bhutani VK and Shaffer TH. A new experimental approach for the study of cardiopulmonary physiology during early development. *J Appl Physiol* 1988;**65**: 1436–1443.
24. Wolfson MR, Heckman J, Cox C and Shaffer TH. Liquid ventilation equipment and methodology: A historical perspective. *11th Annual CNMC ECMO Symposium Keystone Co*, 1995.
25. Shaffer TH, Lowe CA, Bhutani VK and Douglas PR. Liquid ventilation: effects on pulmonary function in distressed meconium-stained lambs. *Pediatr Res* 1984;**18**: 47–52.
26. Lowe CA and Shaffer TH. Pulmonary vascular resistance in the fluorocarbon-filled lung. *J Appl Physiol* 1986;**60**: 154–159.
27. Tarczy-Hornoch P, Hildebrandt J, Mates EA, Standaert TA, Lamm WJE and Jackson JC. Effects of exogenous surfactant on lung pressure–volume characteristics during liquid ventilation. *J Appl Physiol* 1996;**80**: 1764–1771.
28. Wolfson MR, Greenspan JS, Deoras KS, Rubenstein SD and Shaffer TH. Comparison of gas and liquid ventilation: clinical, physiological, and histological correlates. *J Appl Physiol* 1992;**72**: 1024–1031.
29. Shaffer TH, Rubenstein D, Moskowitz D and Delivoria-Papadopoulos M. Gaseous exchange and acid–base balance in premature lambs during liquid ventilation since birth. *Pediatr Res* 1976;**10**: 227–231.
30. Jackson JC, Standaert TA, Truog WE and Hodson WA. Full-tidal liquid ventilation with perfluorocarbon for prevention of lung injury in newborn non-human primates. *Art Cells Blood Subs Immob Biotech* 1994;**22**: 1121–1132.
31. Hirschl RB, Merz SI, Montoya JP *et al.* Development and application of a simplified liquid ventilator. *Crit Care Med* 1995;**23**: 157–163.
32. Shaffer TH, Foust R, Wolfson MR, Miller TF. Analysis of perfluorochemical elimination from the respiratory system. *J Appl Physiol* 1997;**83(3)**: 1033–40.
33. Miller TF, Wolfson MR, Peck GA and Shaffer TH. Multifactorial analysis of perfluorochemical (PFC) liquid conservation during liquid ventilation (LV). *Faseb J* 1996;**10**: 807A.
34. Shaffer TH, Douglas PR, Lowe CA and Bhutani VK. The effects of liquid ventilation on cardiopulmonary function in preterm lambs. *Pediatr Res* 1983;**17**: 303–306.
35. Foust R, Tran NN, Cox C *et al.* Liquid assisted ventilation: An alternative strategy for acute meconium aspiration injury. *Pediatr Pulmonol* 1996;**21**: 316–322.
36. Hirschl RB, Parent A, Tooley R *et al.* Liquid ventilation improves pulmonary function, gas exchange, and lung injury in a model of respiratory failure. *Ann Surg* 1995;**221**: 79–88.
37. Stavis RL, Wolfson MR, Cox CA *et al.* Prolonged total liquid ventilation in premature lambs. *Pediatr Res* 1997;**4**: 108A.
38. Forman DL, Bhutani VK, Hilfer SR and Shaffer TH. A fine structure study of the liquid-ventilated rabbit. *Fed Proc* 1984;**43**: 647.

39. Shaffer TH, Ferguson JD, Koen PA, Moskowitz GD and Delivoria-Papadopoulos M. Pulmonary lavage in preterm lambs. *Pediatr Res* 1978;**12**: 695–698.
40. Richman PS, Wolfson MR and Shaffer TH. Lung lavage with oxygenated perfluorochemical liquid in acute lung injury. *Crit Care Med* 1993;**21**: 768–774.
41. Fuhrman BP, Paczan PR and DeFrancisis M. Perfluorocarbon-associated gas exchange. *Crit Care Med* 1991;**19**: 712–722.
42. Wolfson MR, Kechner NE, Friss H, Rubenstein SD and Shaffer TH. Improved gas exchange during and following slow tracheal instillation of perfluorochemical liquid in neonatal respiratory distress. *Am J Resp Crit Care Med* 1994;**149**: A545.
43. Wolfson MR, Kechner NE, Miller TF, Friss HE, Roache R, Dechaderavian JP, Shaffer TH. Perfluorochemical rescue after surfactant treatment: effect of perfluoron dose and ventilatory frequency. *J Appl Physiol* 1998; **84(2)**: 624–640.
44. Tutuncu AS, Faithfull NS and Lachmann B. Comparison of ventilatory support with intratracheal perfluorocarbon administration and conventional mechanical ventilation in animals with acute respiratory failure. *Am Rev Resp Dis* 1993;**148**: 785–792.
45. Major D, Cadenas M, Cloutier R, Fourier L, Shaffer TH and Wolfson MR. Combined ventilation and perfluorochemical (PFC) tracheal instillation as an alternative treatment for near-death congenital diaphragmatic hernia. *J Pediatr Surg* 1995;**30**: 1178–1182.
46. Jamadar DA, Kazerooni EA and Hirschl RB. Pneumomediastinum: elucidation of the anatomic pathway by liquid ventilation. *J Comput Assist Tomography* 1996;**20**: 309–311.
47. Hirschl RB, Pranikoff T, Gauger P, Schreiner RJ, Dechert R and Bartlett RH. Liquid ventilation in adults, children, and full-term neonates. *Lancet* 1995;**346**: 1201–1202.
48. Gross GW, Greeenspan JS, Fox WW, Rubenstein SD, Wolfson MR and Shaffer TH. Use of liquid ventilation with Perflubron during extracorporeal membrane oxygenation: Chest radiographic appearances. *Radiology* 1995;**194**: 717–720.
49. Leach CL, Greenspan JS, Rubenstein SD *et al* and for the LiquiVent Study Group. Partial liquid ventilation with perflubron in premature infants with severe respiratory distress syndrome. *N Engl J Med* 1996;**335**: 761–767.
50. Hirschl RB, Pranikoff T, Wise C *et al.* Initial experience with partial liquid ventilation in adult patients with acute respiratory distress syndrome. *JAMA* 1996;**275**: 383–389.
51. Greenspan JS, Fox WW, Rubenstein SD, Wolfson MR, Spinner SS, Shaffer TH and The Philadelphia Liquid Ventilation Consortium. Partial liquid ventilation in critically ill infants receiving extracorporeal life support. *Pediatrics* 1997;**99**: 1–5.
52. Gauger PG, Pranikoff T, Schreiner RJ, Moier FW and Hirschl RB. Initial experience with partial liquid ventilation in pediatric patients with acute respiratory distress syndrome. *Crit Care Med* 1996;**24**: 16–22.

53. Valls-i-Soler A, Wolfson MR, Kechner N, Foust R and Shaffer TH. Comparison of natural surfactant and brief liquid ventilation rescue treatment in very immature lambs. *Biol Neonate* 1996;**69**: 275–283.
54. Wolfson MR, Greenspan JS and Shaffer TH. Pulmonary administration of vasoactive drugs (PAD) by perfluorocarbon liquid ventilation. *Pediatrics* 1996;**97**: 449–455.
55. Zelinka MA, Wolfson MR, Calligaro S, Rubenstein SD, Greenspan JS and Shaffer TH. A comparison of intratracheal and intravenous administration of gentamicin during liquid ventilation. *Eur J Pediatr* 1997;**156**: 401–404.
56. Lisby D, Gonzales LW, Fox WW, Wolfson MR, Shaffer TH and Ballard PL. Liquid ventilation facilitates pulmonary distribution of adenovirus-mediated gene transfer. *Pediatr Res* 1996;**39**: 389A.
57. Wilcox DT, Glick PL, Karamanoukian HL, Morin FC, Fuhrman BP and Leach CL. Perfluorocarbon associated gas exchange (PAGE) and nitric oxide in the lamb with congenital diaphragmatic hernia model. *Pediatr Res* 1994;**35**: A260.
58. Wolfson MR, Stern RG, Kechner N, Sekins KM and Shaffer TH. Utility of a perfluorochemical liquid for pulmonary diagnostic imaging. *Art Cells Blood Subs Immob Biotech* 1994;**22**: 1409–1420.
59. Stern RG, Wolfson MR, McGuckin JF, Forge JA and Shaffer TH. High-resolution computed tomographic bronchiolography using perfluoroctylbromide (PFOB): An experimental model. *J Thoracic Imag* 1993;**8**: 300–304.
60. Milestone B, Miller TF, Wolfson MR, Stern RG and Shaffer TH. Virtual bronchoscopy with perfluoronated hydrocarbon (PFC) enhancement. *Acad Radiol* 1997;**4(8)**: 583–586.
61. Colton DM, Hirschl RB, Johnson KJ, Til GO, Deab SB and Bartlett RB. Neutrophil infiltration is reduced during partial liquid ventilation in the setting of lung injury. *Surg Forum* 1994;**45**: 668–670.
62. Smith TM, Steinhorn DM, Thusu K, Fuhrman BP and Dandona P. Liquid perfluorochemical decreases the *in vitro* production of reactive oxygen species by alveolar macrophages. *Crit Care Med* 1995;**23**: 1533–1539.

8

Bronchopulmonary Dysplasia: A Team Approach

Mary E. Wearden and James M. Adams

INTRODUCTION

Bronchopulmonary dysplasia (BPD) has emerged as the dominant pulmonary disease of the newborn as surfactant replacement therapy has promoted a striking reduction in low birth weight mortality. Occurrence of BPD is inversely related to birth weight and may exceed 75% among babies < 750 g. Outcome varies among tertiary care centers, with mortality ranging from 25–40% but risk of death is closely related to duration of mechanical ventilation. Death rates of 21–57% are reported for infants requiring > 1 month on intermittent positive pressure ventilation (IPPV) and may reach 90% when ventilation exceeds 4 months.[1, 2]

Management of the ventilator-dependent infant during a prolonged course of hospitalization presents a unique challenge. Increased risk of growth failure, hearing loss, retinopathy of prematurity (ROP) and neurodevelopmental handicaps have been reported among these infants and many have oral motor dysfunction and associated feeding problems. No small part of their care involves attempts to minimize the adverse impact of the intensive care environment. In attempting to meet this challenge, the authors have developed a comprehensive, team approach to the chronic ventilator patient using a critical care pathway as a guideline for multidisciplinary management over time.

The team care approach, using multidisciplinary members, represents a co-ordinated approach to patient care.[3–6] This is particularly important in optimizing the care of the chronically-ill patient who requires complex care and integrated decision making. The goal of this approach is to simplify and stabilize the infant's clinical course to optimize the infant's development and achieve hospital discharge in a timely fashion. This model has been used successfully in the care of many chronically ill patients, including those with cleft lip and palate, cerebral palsy, cancer, and diabetes.[7–10] This chapter will first present a composite picture of the medical care of the BPD patient. These interventions were compiled from the literature, outcome studies, and expert local opinion. The final section details the role of the multidisciplinary team in the care of infants with BPD.

CARDIOPULMONARY PHYSIOLOGY

In advanced BPD there is increased airway resistance, decreased dynamic compliance, reduction in tidal volume and severe pulmonary clearance delay. Uneven airway obstruction promotes gas trapping with hyperinflation; bronchomalacia is often present. Little improvement in pulmonary function occurs before 6 months of age but by 3 years of age compliance is near normal and airway resistance only about 30% higher than controls.[11] Most deaths are related to infection or cardio-pulmonary failure associated with persistent pulmonary hypertension and cor pulmonale.

Heart–lung interaction is extremely fragile part of the pulmonary vascular bed has been obliterated, reducing cross-sectional area. Uneven airway obstruction, with alveolar hypoxia and hypoxic vasoconstriction in underventilated lung units, promotes a further increase in pulmonary vascular resistance. Well-ventilated lung units, with intact vasculature, must accept a disproportionate amount of pulmonary blood flow at the expense of high microvascular pressures and increased fluid filtration. High right-sided cardiac pressures inhibit pulmonary lymphatic drainage and add further to the formation of pulmonary edema. Any ventilatory variation that further decreases alveolar PO_2 induces additional hypoxic vasoconstriction in underventilated lung units and forces yet more blood through well-ventilated ones, resulting in even more pulmonary hypertension and pulmonary edema. Understanding this fragile interaction is the essence of management of severe BPD.

MANAGEMENT STRATEGIES

Since improvement in pulmonary function can occur only slowly as a result of lung growth and remodeling, interim pulmonary care is largely supportive. The primary goals of care are:

1. Provision of complete, balanced nutrition together with time to allow growth of new lung and remodeling of the pulmonary vascular bed;
2. Avoidance of cor pulmonale, a major cause of death, by comprehensive care and monitoring to lower pulmonary vascular resistance.

Supportive Care and Nutrition

Adequate growth requires provision of all essential nutrients, often in conjunction with significant fluid restriction. Long-term dietary intake should meet American Academy of Pediatrics guidelines for term and preterm infants.[12, 13] Modest fluid restriction of 150 ml/kg/day can be achieved using a commercial 24 cal/oz, mineral-enhanced premature formula, a standard 24 cal/oz formula (term babies) or human milk with added commercial fortifier (Mead Johnson & Company, Evansville, Indiana) containing supplemental protein, minerals and vitamins. Additional calories may be added as corn oil. If severe fluid restriction (as low as 110 ml/kg/day) is required, caloric supplements alone will not provide adequate protein and trace nutrients. A commercial 27 cal/oz formula may be fortified with protein (Casec to achieve protein intake of 3–3.5 g/kg/day) as well as corn oil and glucose polymers to increase caloric density to 30–32 cal/oz, but osmolarity will exceed 410 mOsmol/l. In babies 5–6 months of age, adequate weight gain has been achieved using Pediasure with fiber (PF, Ross Labs, Columbus, Ohio) with BPD and requiring severe fluid restriction.[14] Infants receiving a special formula in restricted amounts require iron and vitamin supplements, as well as close monitoring of protein and mineral status. Mineral wasting associated with diuretics and catabolic effects of corticosteroids are significant problems.

Cardiopulmonary Care

A comprehensive program is used to enhance pulmonary function and minimize pulmonary vascular resistance. Certain techniques are well described for this purpose. These are temporaryizing measures, however, which avoid cor pulmonale while allowing sufficient time for lung growth. They do nothing to enhance the repair process itself.

Oxygen

Persistent pulmonary hypertension is a predictor of mortality in BPD[15, 16] and oxygen is the primary tool to minimize pulmonary vascular resistance and avoid death from cor pulmonale.

Diuretics

Diuretics enhance the effects of fluid restriction in promoting stability of oxygenation. Several dosage schedules are reported to minimize metabolic side effects.[17, 18] It is particularly important to avoid hypochloremic metabolic alkalosis and most patients require chloride supplementation, part of which should be provided as KCl.

Bronchodilators

Increased resting airway tone has been demonstrated in infants with BPD and numerous studies have reported improved lung mechanics following administration of β_2 agonists and other agents to ventilator-dependent infants.[19–21] Three agents have potential use in BPD and may be administered during IPPV by metered dose inhaler (MDI) using a commercial spacer device.

1. *Albuterol*: Dose–response relationships and strategies for administration of this agent have been described.[22, 23] In the absence of sensitive bedside pulmonary function tests, its empiric use during the period of ventilator dependency appears to be indicated. High-dose therapy may be necessary if acute episodes of bronchospasm occur.[24, 25]
2. *Ipratropium bromide*: A definitive role for cholinergic blockade in BPD has not been established but limited data suggest this agent lowers respiratory system resistance in some infants with BPD in a manner similar to albuterol.[21] A dose-dependent effect has been demonstrated in infants and young children with asthma.[26, 27]
3. *Inhaled corticosteroids*: LaForce and Brudno reported improved airway resistance and lung compliance in a group of ventilator-dependent preterm infants following nebulization of beclomethasone for > 2 weeks.[28]

Systemic Corticosteroids

Three distinct strategies for systemic steroid use in BPD have been suggested, all using dexamethasone.

1. Reduction in duration of assisted ventilation among infants with established BPD.[29] Short-term lung mechanics are improved in part by brisk diuresis and reduced lung water.[30] Adrenal suppression can be avoided if treatment does not exceed 1 week.[31] Some infants who initially respond require chronic steroid therapy, however.
2. Early treatment during the first 2 weeks of life to interrupt the lung injury cycle.[32, 33] Many of these infants also require a prolonged course of daily treatment.
3. A preventive role, using dexamethasone initiated during the first 12 hours of postnatal life.[34, 35]

Duration of treatment in these reports varied between 1 and 12 days. Chronic steroid therapy adds significantly to difficulties of nutritional management.

PATHOGENESIS AND CLINICAL COURSE

BPD is an evolving injury sequence initiated by the interaction of mechanical ventilation and the lung of a predisposed host. The surfactant-deficient or structurally-immature lung is particularly vulnerable to bronchiolar lesions induced by IPPV[36] and airway injury occurs very early in the course.[37, 38] Activation of an intense inflammatory response by this stimulus is associated with further lung damage and progressive clinical symptomatology. A disordered process of regeneration and repair follows, which either progresses to death or becomes quiescent and allows recovery after 1–3 years of lung growth. The clinical course of BPD is more insidious now than that originally described by Northway et al.[39] Most patients have a history of surfactant treatment, birth weight < 1250 g and no hyaline membrane disease but required mechanical ventilation during the first week of life for apnea or anatomic immaturity of the lungs. Three distinct phases in the hospital course form the basis for a comprehensive clinical pathway to guide multidisciplinary management (Figure 8.1). Key points in management using the clinical pathway are discussed below.

Phase I: Acute Course and Diagnosis

This evolves during the first month of life and most closely corresponds to Northway stages 1–2. A relatively benign course during the first 2 weeks gives way to continued ventilator dependency with deteriorating pulmonary function, rising oxygen requirements and opacification of previously clear lung fields radiographically. Wide

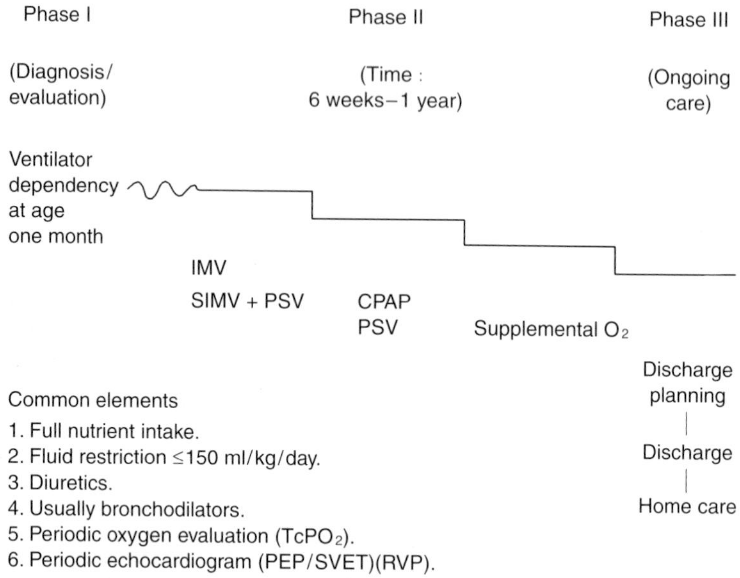

Figure 8.1. Clinical pathway for the patient with bronchopulmonary dysplasia (BPD). This graph represents the 3 phases of BPD. In Phase I, the undulating line represents both the high acuity of care and the unstable nature of the illness at this point. Infants in Phase II are generally much more stable but still require complex therapies. By Phase III, the infant's care has been simplified and the course is very stable. CPAP = continuous positive airway pressure; SIMV = synchronized intermittent mandatory ventilation; PSV = pressure support ventilation; PEP = pre-ejection period; RVET = right ventricular ejection time; IMV = intermittent mandatory ventilation; RVP = right ventricular pressure estimation.

swings in PaO_2 and oxygen saturation values are characteristic.[40] Despite treatment of patent ductus arteriosus (PDA), control of apnea and lack of evidence of infection, the infant remains ventilator dependent. Widespread necrosis of bronchial mucosa is accompanied by the presence of numerous inflammatory markers in tracheal fluid[41] and microvascular permeability is increased markedly. Airway obstruction with necrotic debris produces atelectasis alternating with early cyst formation. Once the diagnosis is made, most patients begin a regimen of fluid restriction, diuretics, and inhaled bronchodilators. Strategies using systemic steroids to limit lung injury or facilitate weaning from mechanical ventilation are employed during this phase. A decision to initiate steroids must consider risks of infection and impairment of growth, as well as estimate whether any short-term improvement in pulmonary function can be sustained safely over the long period necessary for lung growth and repair.

Phase II: Course of Chronic Ventilator Dependency

This phase includes features of Northway stages 3 and 4 as bronchiolar metaplasia, hypertrophy of smooth muscle and interstitial edema produce uneven airway obstruction with worsening hyperinflation of the lung. Obliteration and abnormal muscularization of the pulmonary vascular bed progresses. Active inflammation is slowly replaced by a disordered process of structural repair. The early weeks of this phase remain quite unstable with frequent changes in oxygen requirement and characteristic episodes of acute deterioration. After 4–6 weeks, the clinical course becomes more static as fibrosis, hyperinflation and pulmonary edema come to dominate the clinical picture. Increased airway smooth muscle is present and resting airway tone is increased. Tracheobronchomalacia is common.[42, 43] Elevated pulmonary vascular resistance and high right ventricular afterload leave the infant vulnerable to episodes of acute cor pulmonale. This phase evolves over 3–9 months. During this time, growth and remodeling of lung parenchyma and the pulmonary vascular bed is associated with gradual improvement in pulmonary function. Oxygen requirements fall to 40% or less and the patient can be weaned from IPPV to breathe spontaneously on CPAP or a Pressure Support mode of ventilation. Subsequently, extubation and supplemental oxygen alone become possible.

Management during this period is constantly focused on the 2 primary goals. A nutritional plan is developed to achieve long-term growth within the fluid tolerance of the individual patient. Diuretics and bronchodilator therapy are combined with liberal oxygen supplementation to optimize lung mechanics and minimize pulmonary venous resistance (PVR). Critical environmental modifications include age-appropriate activity scheduling, play therapy, uninterrupted sleep time and avoidance of stimuli triggering episodes of hypoxemia.

Certain monitoring parameters, periodically obtained, aid in assuring a consistent plan of care and achievement of the goals of care.

Nutritional monitoring

Patients should be weighed every 1–3 days with length and frontal occipital circumference (FOC) measurements obtained weekly. Nutritional monitoring includes periodic determination of blood urea nitrogen (BUN), serum albumin, prealbumin, calcium, phosphorus and alkaline phosphatase. The nutritionist specialist should evaluate dietary profile and growth parameters every 1–2 weeks.

Oxygen monitoring

Long-term maintenance of adequate oxygenation is the key to preventing death from cor pulmonale. FiO_2 should be adjusted to maintain

PaO_2 above 55 mmHg.[44, 45] Insidious hypoxemia is common during feedings and sleep and additional oxygen supplements may be necessary during these periods.[46] Status can be evaluated by a 6–8-hour strip recording of transcutaneous oxygen tension ($TcPO_2$) or pulse oximetry (SpO_2) every 1–2 weeks. Attempts should be made to keep $TcPO_2$ above 55 mmHg and SpO_2 above 94% in term and older infants (90–95% range in small prematures). Arterial blood gas samples must be obtained periodically. The impact of oxygen on outcome cannot be overemphasized. The need for supplemental O_2 extends well beyond the period of positive pressure support and overzealous attempts to wean supplemental O_2 may precipitate acute cardiopulmonary failure and even death.

Echocardiograms

The value of echocardiography in screening for pulmonary hypertension and assessing response of the pulmonary vascular bed to oxygen has been described in several studies.[16, 44, 47] Tricuspid regurgitation is commonly present and flow velocity can be determined by Doppler. A modified Bernoulli equation can be used to calculate the pressure gradient across this valve:

$$\text{Pressure gradient} = 4(V_{max})^2$$

This value plus assumed right atrial pressure provides an estimate of right ventricular systolic pressure. Increased mortality risk has been associated with pre-ejection period/right ventricular ejection time (PEP/RVET) ratios > 0.30[16] and it is recommended that sufficient oxygen be given to avoid ratios > 0.34.[44] These two echocardiographic parameters can be measured every 4–6 weeks to estimate right ventricular afterload and assess adequacy of pulmonary care. If either is abnormal, an increase in supplemental oxygen, as well as other components of pulmonary care, should be considered.

Preventive care

Immunizations should be given as recommended by the 1998 guidelines of the American Academy of Pediatrics.[48] Inactivated polio vaccine is indicated for these hospitalized infants.

Phase III: Discharge Planning and Transition to Home Care

This phase encompasses the transition from IPPV to the home care environment. Active, inflammatory lung damage has ceased and the process of repair has become more orderly. Lung growth and remodeling has progressed sufficiently to allow more stable pulmonary function without the need for positive pressure support. Lung mechanics remain quite abnormal, however, and hyperinflation, fibrosis and cysts often remain visible radiographically. Many more months of lung growth will be required to overcome these derangements.

The most important aspect of this phase is the recognition that, although the lungs have improved, both structure and function remain quite abnormal. Close monitoring of adequacy of oxygenation is essential for several weeks following extubation to be sure a subtle rise in PVR will not lead to insidious development of cor pulmonale.

Developmental screening

Hearing screening should be done prior to discharge or before 6 months of age to allow early intervention by an audiologist, if needed. Developmental assessment may begin during the hospital stay as part of comprehensive long-term follow-up after discharge. Specific attention to oral motor function and feeding disorders may be necessary.

During this period, discharge planning can begin. Hearing and developmental needs should receive special attention with increased emphasis on play therapy and any physical therapy required. Effects of feeding on oxygenation must be evaluated closely. Special home care needs should be identified and a home dietary plan chosen and implemented. Infants with oral motor dysfunction may require special techniques of feeding. Most infants will be discharged with low flow O_2 by nasal cannula, an oral diuretic and modest fluid restriction (150 ml/kg/day) using a standard 24 cal/oz formula that is readily available commercially. Continuation of nebulized bronchodilators by mask is often necessary. As long as the infant requires oxygen, fluid restriction and diuretics will make lung function more efficient and help minimize PVR.

Preventive care

Infection is a significant cause of post-discharge hospitalization and death in BPD. Immunizations should be up to date prior to discharge. Infants with BPD who are receiving oxygen or have received it within the past 6 months prior to the respiratory syncytial virus season should be considered for immunoprophylaxis with a respiratory syncitial virus antibody preparation during the active RSV season.[49, 50]

CO-ORDINATION OF CARE

The primary goals of care can best be achieved by a multidisciplinary care team directed by an experienced neonatologist or pediatric pulmonologist complimented by other physicians skilled in developmental assessment and nutrition. In addition to these physicians, team members include NICU nurses, social workers, respiratory therapists, child life specialists, physical and occupational therapists, a dietitian, unit-specific pharmacist (if available), and audiologist. The team should have regularly scheduled meetings and rounds to foster communication among the team members and to evaluate progress of each patient with regards to goals of care. Such a team can maintain consistent, goal-directed care for each patient with a long-term view toward optimizing the infant's overall development while his/her lung function and clinical condition are improving.

In our NICU, team meetings are held twice a month. One meeting is devoted to representation and presentation by all of the patient-care disciplines. The infant's history is briefly presented by the pediatric resident caring for the patient that month. The issues that are emphasized are current ventilator/oxygen support, medications, nutrition, growth parameters, developmental progress, and family issues (see Figure 8.2). Each team member contributes their knowledge of the particular issue in open discussion and then the plan and goals for that particular issue are summarized by the team leader and recorded into the patient's care plan by the nursing staff. The care plan is kept in a central location as a reference for the health-care staff. The second team meeting of the month consists of bedside rounds led by the team leader. This meeting serves to address any intercurrent issues and reconfirm the overall goals for the infant.

C. Everett Koop in the 1987 Surgeon General's report on *Children with Special Health Care Needs* has emphasized the importance of family-centered care.[51] The team approach by its very design fosters the concept of family-centered care. The infant's parents and extended family (if they are involved) are invited to the multidisciplinary meetings to participate in the discussion and decision-making process. Realistically, this usually occurs for infants whose course has been very complex in order to review their course to date and emphasize the achievements necessary before discharge can occur. Near the time of hospital discharge, the family is invited to participate in the team rounds to get a clear picture of what the patient's home care will be and what training they will need to complete before discharge.

Since the infant with BPD may be hospitalized for a prolonged period, it is important to address the environmental issues to which the infant is exposed. The team is particularly adept at establishing a social environment that minimizes adverse aspects of chronic ventilator care and the ICU environment. Early in the course of ventilator dependency, prematures benefit from environmental modifications that reduce noise and discomfort and minimize the stress response. As infants

CHRONIC PULMONARY CARE TEAM

Name: ____________________ Date: ____________________
DOB: ____________________ DOL:# ____________________
Birth Wt: ____________________ Born at: ____________________
Gest Age: ____________________

History

____
____
____
____
____
____

Current Information

Wt: ________
Vent: ______ IMV: ________ Ti: ______ Pressure Support: ______
PIP: ________ CPAP: ________________
Peep: ________ Nasal Cannula ________
FiO_2: ________
Feeds: _____ cc Kg/day.
Type ___________ Method: ______________
Additives: ____
Medications:

____
____
____
____

HUS: ____
Eye Exams: ____
Audiology: ____
____
Lab: ____
____
Other: ____
____

Figure 8.2. This form is used as a guide for presentation of the infants with BPD at the multidisciplinary care meeting. HUS = head ultrasound.

become older, parents and caregivers must work together to provide a friendly, play-oriented environment. Some infants with BPD have associated neurological dysfunction or hearing deficits and feeding disorders are common. Resources to manage such disorders must be assembled and integrated into a regular schedule of play therapy against a backdrop of ongoing medical care. Maintenance of an appropriate social environment for these chronically hospitalized infants presents a considerable challenge and has significant positive impact on the medical course.

In addition to modifying the NICU environment in terms of light and noise, the multidisciplinary team, particularly the child life specialist and bedside nurses, works in concert to develop a consistent daily schedule for the chronically ventilated infants. The number of different caregivers is limited by assignment of primary nurses, respiratory and occupational therapists. The caregivers are encouraged to learn the infant's stress responses and to respond to these cues promptly to prevent escalation. This has been invaluable in decreasing the number of desaturation episodes by intervening early in the agitation/hypoxia cycle. One of the most valuable aspects of consistency in caregivers is that they are able to learn each individual infant's cues and comfort measures. Noxious interventions such as blood draws and suctioning are clustered during the day and interventions are minimized as much as possible. The infant's daily schedule is posted at the bedside so all caregivers will adhere to it (Figure 8.3). Sleep–wake cycles are also promoted with the eventual goal (when it is age appropriate) of sleep 6–8 hours at night.

The multidisciplinary team also functions to educate the health- care workers in the NICU. In addition to bedside teaching rounds and team meetings, inservices are held to encourage the philosophy surrounding the care of and goals for the infants with BPD. This has been well received by the staff and has aided in extending the team objectives to rotating house staff and faculty as well as the NICU staff.

Since prognosis for long-term recovery in BPD is good, the psychology of BPD care is particularly important. It is essential that caregivers maintain an involved, optimistic attitude toward these infants. The team has worked to encourage this positive attitude among caregivers and to foster support for the bedside caregivers who are proficient in the care of the infant with chronic lung disease.

CONCLUSIONS

Despite surfactant therapy, BPD remains a significant source of chronic lung disease in the neonate. Care of the infant with BPD is largely

Dear Hospital People:

I am getting to know my surroundings better. Please try to follow my routine as closely as possible. Encourage me to be awake during the day and to consistently sleep through the night. Once I go home my Momma and Daddy are going to need all the sleep they can get at night. My sister and I will keep them very busy.

7am–1pm
- Assessment
- 8am Eat
- 8am Respiratory treatment
- Up in swing
- 11am Eat
- 10am–12noon Nap time
- PT

1pm–7pm
- 2pm Eat
- 1pm–3pm Nap time
- Child Life
- 2pm Respiratory treatment
- 5pm Eat
- Resting and/or play time in bed

7pm–7am
- Up in swing
- Assessment
- 8pm Eat
- Bath
- 8pm Respiratory treatment
- 10pm–8am Sleeping/Cluster care
- 11pm Eat

<u>These are some things I like to do:</u>
- Listen to you talk or read to me.
- Look at faces, especially my Momma's and Daddy's.
- Listen to music or to you singing to me.
- Look at bright colors and different shapes.
- Be held and cuddled.
- Be rocked.
- Sit up in my chair (Kaylin's glider chair.)

Thanks for taking such great care of me.

Figure 8.3. Sample daily schedule used in the authors' NICU for infants with bronchopulmonary dysplasia.

supportive until improvement occurs as a function of lung growth, which is a slow process. Acknowledging this fact, the authors have adapted a multidisciplinary team care approach to provide consistent medical care for these infants. They have found that consistency of care at all levels allows recovery to progress with minimal setbacks. This concept has been enormously successful and well accepted in their unit. Using the techniques outlined in this chapter, the team care approach for the patient with BPD can be adapted to any ICU setting.

REFERENCES

1. Wheater M and Rennie JM. Poor prognosis after prolonged ventilation for bronchopulmonary dysplasia. *Arch Dis Child* 1994;**71**: F210–F211.
2. Overstreet DW, Jackson JC, van Belle G and Truog WE. Estimation of mortality risk in chronically ventilated infants with bronchopulmonary dysplasia. *Pediatrics* 1991;**88**: 1153–1160.
3. Brita-Rossi P *et al.* Improving the process of care: The cost-quality value of interdisciplinary collaboration. *J Nursing Care Qual* 1996;**10**: 10–16.
4. Crepeau E. Three images of interdisciplinary team meetings. *Am J of Occup Ther* 1994;**48**: 717–722.
5. Vinicor F. Interdisciplinary and intersectoral approach: a challenge for integrated care. *Patient Educ and Counseling* 1995;**26**: 267–272.
6. McHugh M, West P, Assathly C *et al.* Establishing an interdisciplinary patient care team. *JONA* 1996; **26**: 21–27.
7. Elmendorf EN, D'Antonio LL and Hardesty RA. Assessment of the patient with cleft lip and palate. *Clin Plastic Surg* 1993;**20**: 607–621.
8. DeLuca PA. The musculoskeletal management of children with cerebral palsy. Pediatr Clin of North America 1996;**43**: 1135–1150.
9. Packer RJ. An overview of pediatric oncology as a model for interdisciplinary care. *Child's Nervous System* 1995;**11**: 13–16.
10. Van Buskirk MC and Vanderbilt D. Evaluating patient care by the use of a diabetic ketoacidosis CareMap in an intensive care unit setting. *J Nursing Care Qual* 1995;**9**: 59–68.
11. Bancalari E *et al.* Bronchopulmonary dysplasia. *Pediatr Clin North Am* 1996;**33**: 1.
12. Committee on Nutrition, American Academy of Pediatrics. Introduction of solid foods. In: *Pediatric Nutrition Handbook*, 3rd edn. Elk Grove, IL: American Academy of Pediatrics, 1993.
13. Committee on Nutrition, American Academy of Pediatrics. Guidelines for nutrient intake. In: *Pediatric Nutrition Handbook*, 3rd edn. Elk Grove, IL: American Academy of Pediatrics, 1993, pp 64–164.
14. Valentine C, Schanler R, and Abrams S. Appropriate growth of infants 4–12 months of age with bronchopulmonary dysplasia (BPD) using a specialized pediatric formula. *19th Clinical Congress Nutrition Practice*, 1995, Poster A177, p 599.

15. Goodman G, Perkin RM, Anas NG *et al.* Pulmonary hypertension in infants with bronchopulmonary dysplasia. *J Pediatr* 1988;**112**: 67–72.
16. Fouron J, Le Guennec J, Villrmant D *et al.* Value of echocardiography in assessing the outcome of bronchopulmonary dysplasia in the newborn. *Pediatrics* 1980;**65**: 529–535.
17. Rush MG, Englehardt B, Parker RA *et al.* Double-blind, placebo-controlled trial of alternate day furosemide therapy in infants with chronic bronchopulmonary dysplasia. *J Pediatr* 1990;**117**: 112–118.
18. Kao LC, Warburton D, and Cheng MH. Effect of oral diuretics on pulmonary mechanics in infants with chronic bronchopulmonary dysplasia: Results of a double blind crossover sequential trail. *Pediatrics* 1984;**74**: 37–44.
19. Kao LC, Warburton D, Platzker ACG and Keens TG. Effect of isoproterenol inhalation on airway resistance in chronic bronchopulmonary dysplasia. *Pediatrics* 1984;**73**: 509–513.
20. Soslulski R, Abbasi S and, Fox WW. Therapeutic value of terbutaline in bronchopulmonary dysplasia. *Pediatr Res* 1982;**16**: 309A.
21. Wilkie RA and Bryan MH. Effect of bronchodilators on airway resistance in ventilator dependent neonates with chronic lung disease. *J Pediatr* 1987;**111**: 278–282
22. Denjean A, Guimaraes H, Migdal M *et al.* Dose related bronchodilator response to aerosolized salbutamol (albuterol) in ventilator dependent premature infants. *J Pediatr* 1992;**120**: 974–979.
23. Kramer R, Birrer P, Modelska K *et al.* A new baby spacer device for aerosolized bronchodilator administration in infants with bronchopulmonary disease. *Eur J Pediatr* 1992;**151**: 57–60.
24. Schuh S, Parkin P, Rajan A *et al.* High versus low dose, frequently administered, nebulized albuterol in children with severe, acute asthma. *Pediatrics* 1989;**83**: 513–518.
25. US Department of Health and Human Services. *Guidelines for Diagnosis and Management of Asthma.* National Asthma Education Report, Publication No. 91, 3042. US Government Printing Office, 1991.
26. Henry RL, Hiller EJ, Mulner AD *et al.* Nebulized ipratropium bromide and sodium cromoglycate in the first two years of life. *Arch Dis Child* 1984;**59**: 54–57.
27. Davis A, Vickerson F, Worsley G *et al.* Determination of dose response relationship for nebulized ipratropium in asthmatic children. *J Pediatr* 1984;**105**: 1002–1005.
28. LaForce WR and Brudno S. Controlled trial of beclomethasone dipropionate by nebulization in oxygen and ventilator dependent infants. *J Pediatr* 1993;**122**: 285–288.
29. Avery GB, Fletcher AB, Kaplan M and Brudno DS. Controlled trial of dexamethasone in respirator dependent infants with bronchopulmonary dysplasia. *Pediatrics* 1985;**7**: 106–111.
30. Gladstone IM, Jacobs HC and Ehrenkranz RA. Pulmonary function tests (PFT) and fluid balance (FB) in neonates with chronic lung disease (CLD) during dexamethasone (DEX) treatment (RX). *Pediatr Res* 1989;**25**: Abstract 1277.

31. Stephure DK, Singhal N and McMillian DD. Safety of dexamethasone (DXM) for bronchopulmonary dysplasia (BPD). *Pediatr Res* 1989;**25**: Abstract 546.
32. Brozanski BS, Jones JG, Gilmour CH *et al.* Effect of pulse dexamethasone therapy on the incidence and severity of chronic lung disease in the very low birth weight infant. *J Pediatr* 1995;**126**: 769–776.
33. Durand M, Sardesai S and McEvoy C. Effects of early dexamethasone therapy on pulmonary mechanics and chronic lung disease in very low birth weight infants: a randomized, controlled trial. *Pediatrics* 1995;**95**: 584–590.
34. Yeh TF, Torre JA, Rastogi A *et al.* Early postnatal dexamethasone therapy in premature infants with severe respiratory distress syndrome: a double-blind, controlled study. *J Pediatr* 1990;**117**: 273–282.
35. Rastogi A, Akintorin SM, Betz ML *et al.* A controlled trial of dexamethasone to prevent bronchopulmonary dysplasia in surfactant treated infants. *Pediatrics* 1996;**98**: 204–210.
36. Nilsson R, Grossmann G and Robertson B. Lung surfactant and the pathogenesis of neonatal bronchiolar lesions induced by artificial ventilation. *Pediatr Res* 1978;**12**: 249–255.
37. Robertson B. The evolution of neonatal respiratory distress syndrome into chronic lung disease. *Eur Respir J* 1989;**2(Suppl 3)**: 33s–37s.
38. Goldman SL, Gerhardt T, Sonni S *et al.* Early prediction of chronic lung disease by pulmonary function testing. *J Pediatr* 1983;**102**: 613–616.
39. Northway WH, Rosan RC and Porter DY. Pulmonary disease following respirator therapy of hyaline membrane disease. *N Engl J Med* 1967;**276**: 357–368.
40. Bolivar JM, Gerhardt T, Gonzalez A *et al.* Mechanisms for episodes of hypoxemia in preterm infants undergoing mechanical ventilation. *J Pediatr* 1995;**127**: 767–773.
41. Groneck P, Gotze-Speer B, Oppermann M *et al.* Association of pulmonary inflammation and increased microvascular permeability during the development of bronchopulmonary dysplasia: A sequential analysis of inflammatory mediators in respiratory fluids of high risk preterm neonates. *Pediatrics* 1994;**93**: 712–718.
42. McCubbin M, Frey EE, Wagener JS *et al.* Large airway collapse in bronchopulmonary dysplasia. *J Pediatr* 1989;**114**: 304–307.
43. Miller RW, Woo P, Kellman RK and Slagle TS. Tracheobronchial abnormalities in infants with bronchopulmonary dysplasia. *J Pediatr* 1987;**111**: 779–782.
44. Halliday HL, Dumpit Fe M and Brady JP. Effects of inspired oxygen on echocardiographic assessments of pulmonary vascular resistance and myocardial contractility in bronchopulmonary dysplasia. *Pediatrics* 1980;**65**: 536–540.
45. Abman SH, Wolfe RR, Accurso FJ *et al.* Pulmonary vascular response to oxygen in infants with severe bronchopulmonary dysplasia. *Pediatrics* 1985;**75**: 80–84.
46. Garg M, Kruzner SI, Bautista DB and Keens TG. Clinically unsuspected hypoxia during sleep and feeding in infants with bronchopulmonary dysplasia. *Pediatrics* 1988;**81**: 635–642.

47. Benatar A, Clarke J and Silverman M. Pulmonary hypertension in infants with chronic lung disease: non-invasive evaluation and short term effect of oxygen treatment. *Arch Dis Child* 1995;**72**: F14–F19.
48. *Recommended Childhood Immunization Schedule – United States, January–December 1997*. *Pediatrics* 1998;**101**: 154.
49. American Academy of Pediatrics, Committee on Infectious Diseases, Committee on Fetus and Newborn. Respiratory syncitial virus immune globulin: intravenous indications for use. *Pediatrics* 1997;**99**: 645–650.
50 The IMpact-RSV Study Group. Palivizumab, a humanized respiratory syncitial virus monoclonal antibody, reduces hospitalization from respiratory syncitial virus infection in high-risk infants. *Pediatrics* 1998;**102**: 531.
51. Koop CE. *Surgeon General's Report: Children with Special Health Care Needs*. US Government Printing Office, 1987, pp 184–200.

9

Using New Information in Retinopathy of Prematurity

Dale L. Phelps

INTRODUCTION

Understanding of retinopathy of prematurity (ROP) has expanded biphasically since the disorder was first described by Terry in 1942.[1] The flurry of publications surrounding its original description and the research leading to the causal link with prolonged, unnecessary oxygen use[2] were followed by quiet years. Retrolental fibroplasia (RLF) as it was called then, was nearly forgotten in the 1960s. However, with the increasing survival of ever smaller infants, and their greater susceptibility to ROP, the disorder and active research returned together (Figure 9.1). This chapter focuses on the more recent information and application of this knowledge in practice and covers the changing picture of ROP, concepts in pathophysiology, prevention and treatment, and the elements of an effective screening, tracking and follow-up program.

CHANGING PICTURE AND CLASSIFICATION

ROP was called retrolental fibroplasia (RLF) from the 1940s until the early 1980s when the primary role of prematurity in its etiology was acknowledged, and the name reverted to that originally proposed by Terry.[3, 4] A great deal more than the name has changed in medicine's ability to describe and treat the disease.

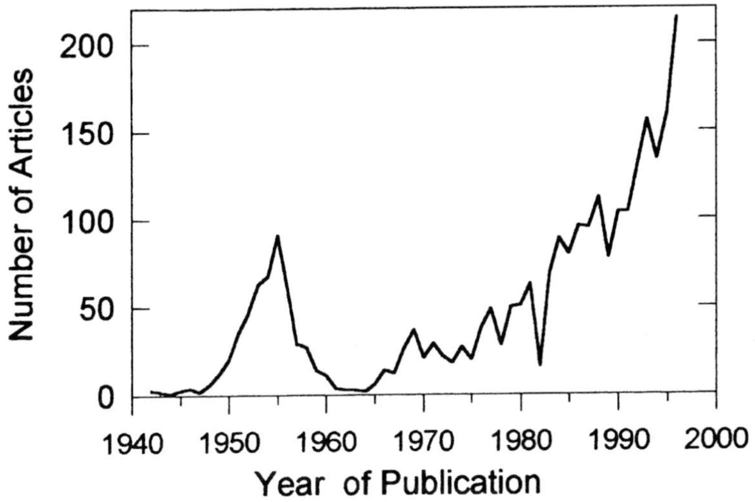

Figure 9.1 Annual number of publications identified relating to ROP, using data searches from Medline, EMBASE, *Current Contents*, and bibliographic backwards searching. Updated from Silverman, WA, *Retrolental Fibroplasia: a Modern Parable*. Grune & Stratton 1980, p. 54 with permission.

The estimated annual numbers of infants who have lost vision to ROP in the USA has varied over the years (Fig. 9.2), reaching its first peak in the late 1940s when prolonged administration of routine oxygen injured the growing retinal vessels and led to many cases of vision loss among premature infants who grew up with few other morbidities.[5] Restricting the use of oxygen to just that required to avoid cyanosis dropped the incidence of vision loss after 1953, but ROP began to resurface in the 1970s when the survival of extremely premature infants started to rise.[6, 7] This increase in the projected absolute number of cases continued until the effectiveness of cryotherapy in treating ROP was announced,[8–10] allowing the projected number of cases of blindness due to ROP to fall, despite the continued increase in survival of ever more premature infants. Co-morbidities such as cerebral palsy and learning impairments are more common among the children with severe ROP in this second wave,[11–13] as compared to individuals from the 1940s and 50s. While some have argued this may reflect over-restriction of oxygen use,[14, 15] it is more likely related to the extreme fragility of ever lower birth weight infants. As understanding, skills and research continue to improve the care of these smallest infants, the incidence of major mor-

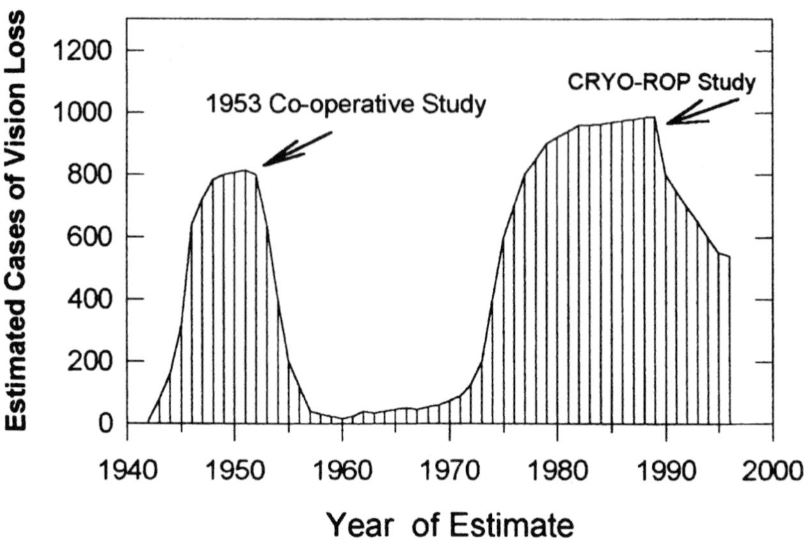

Figure 9.2 Estimated number of individuals experiencing vision loss from ROP annually in the USA. Both the 'Cooperative Study of RLF and the Use of Oxygen', whose results were announced in 1953,[2] and the 'Cryotherapy for ROP Study', whose preliminary results were announced in 1988,[8] had profound effects on these estimates. Estimates are projected from birth rates and combined estimates of ROP incidence rates and the effectiveness of cryotherapy.[5, 7] No official records of the incidence or etiology of vision loss among infants are required in the USA, thus these are estimates only.

bidities continues to fall,[16, 17] and some recent case series suggest that the birth weight-specific incidence of ROP may be falling, even if it is not understood precisely why.[18] The fascinating early history of ROP is well portrayed by Silverman.[5]

The International Classification of ROP (ICROP) was developed and published in 1984–87 to enable investigators and clinicians consistently and accurately to describe and communicate their findings in active ROP as it evolves.[19, 20] The ICROP emphasized the location in the eye (zone), extent (number of clock hours), stage (degree of neovascularization), and presence of 'plus disease' as the characteristics most affecting prognosis. Figure 9.3 illustrates the location of the 3 zones as described in ICROP superimposed on an artist's rendition of the immature retina of a premature infant's eye.

Staging describes the degree of neovascularization at the vascular–avascular border of the anteriorly growing vessels; the extent of neo-

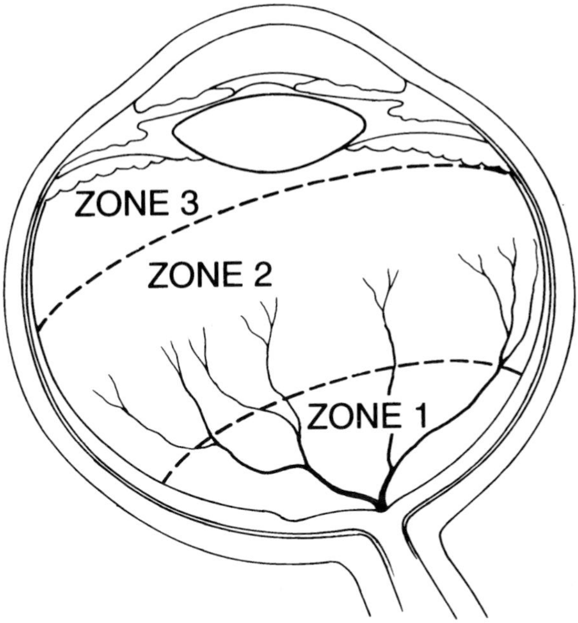

Figure 9.3 Viewed from above, horizontal section through a premature infant's eye, showing the nasal retina to the right and the temporal retina to the left. The zones of the ICROP are indicated by the dashed lines. Modified from *Pediatrics Rev* 1995; **16**, 50–56 with permission.

vascularization is described in clock hours (maximum of 12). When the posterior pole vessels become engorged and tortuous, this incremental increase in the severity of ROP is recognized with the descriptor 'plus disease'. The CRYO-ROP Multicenter Cooperative Group followed 4099 surviving infants of <1251 g birth weight, born in 1986–87, defining the natural history of ROP using the then new ICROP terminology. Beyond the gestation and birth weight, the strongest predictors of a poor outcome were zone 1 ROP at presentation, plus disease and greater extent (more clock hours) of ROP.[21–23] For the individual infant, these data have been combined with other baseline characteristics using multiple regression, and the results published both as a report, and made available as a software program that predicts ROP risk for individual patients.[23] Changes in neonatal practice, such as surfactant, prenatal steroids and prophylactic indomethacin may alter these risks as compared to infants born in 1986–87, but the clinician is still likely to find the information useful.

PATHOPHYSIOLOGY

The scarring and traction on the retina that leads to vision loss from ROP is the result of disordered healing after injury to the growing retinal capillaries. Most of the observations in both humans and mammalian models of ROP are consistent with the *theory* of ROP proposed below.

Normal Growth

The retinal vessels that provide circulation to the inner retina are almost fully developed and well established in the term infant, but have only just started to make progress from the disk where they arise in the fetus at 15–16 weeks' gestation. Michaelson proposed that the retina produced a growth factor to induce retinal vascularization as needed,[24] and recent research points to vascular endothelial growth factor (VEGF) as at least one of the important growth factors that participates in both the normal vascularization of the retina and in ROP.[25–29] Increasingly sophisticated studies of the human retina during development improve the understanding of how maturation of the retina expands from zone 1 near the disk towards the ora serrata in orderly sequential ripples of development. As the primitive neuroretina differentiates and develops photoreceptors, cells supportive of the vasculature invade the inner retina from the region of the disc, followed by vascular precursor cells which then form a primitive capillary network. Remodeling of this network develops the mature pattern of retinal arterioles and venules.[27, 30–33] In a very young premature infant, all of these stages can be observed histologically at the same point in time along the distance from the disk to the ora serrata. Once the vessels have completed remodeling and develop a basement membrane, pericytes and glia limitans, they become highly resistant to subsequent injury.

Injury

The delicate capillary bed of the immature retina is easily injured. Animal models for this disorder most often use high blood oxygen levels (50–100% inspired oxygen in neonatal animals with normal lungs, resulting in arterial oxygen levels of 200–600 torr) to injure the growing capillaries of the retina. Studies in the rat,[34] mouse,[35, 36] cat,[37–39] and dog[40, 41] have all contributed to the understanding of how the developing retina responds to such an injury. In the human infant today, such hyperoxemia is vigorously avoided, yet ROP still occurs.

Examination of the clinical correlates with ROP among infants matched for degree of retinal maturation (i.e. gestation and birth weight adjusted) provide some clues. Compared to infants of similar gestation or birth weights who do not have ROP, those infants who develop severe ROP have more often experienced major physiologic instability requiring prolonged periods of oxygen administration and ventilation,[42–46] intraventricular hemorrhage, septic or hemorrhage shock, etc.[42–45, 47, 48] Each year, as techniques for providing a more stable and less eventful neonatal course improve, ROP is increasingly being restricted to the smaller, less mature infants.[18, 49]

Repair/Healing

Once injury has occurred, the continued differentiation of the neuroretina and increasing metabolic demands requires an increased vascular supply.[50] The tissue response is to make and release a cascade of vasogenic factors that act in concert to promote new vessel formation, the healing process which can be seen as the ROP neovascularization. The majority of the time this process is orderly and the new vessels grow and supply the retina, reducing the stimulus for new vessel growth. Growth factors are then presumably down regulated, and excessive amounts of new vessel growth fade. While the vessels always remain mildly abnormal in appearance,[51, 52] the danger of traction on the macula or retinal detachment mostly resolves with this regression. There may therefore be only a small degree of difference in the pathophysiology between the majority of infants whose ROP regresses (heals), and the much smaller number of infants whose ROP progresses to macular traction/fold or detachment leading to visual impairment.

An important timing feature of the healing process has emerged from natural history studies of ROP. The onset of visible neovascularization and timing of the progression of the disease is developmentally regulated rather than postnatally regulated.[21, 53] Counting from the last menstrual period prior to pregnancy, where a term gestation is 40 weeks, most infants who develop ROP are <32 weeks at birth. When examinations are performed starting at 4–6 weeks after birth and repeated biweekly, ROP reaches the CRYO-ROP prethreshold stage at a median age of 36 weeks' and not before 31 weeks' postmenstrual age (PMA). Threshold ROP, when it occurs, has an onset about 1 week later at a median age of 37 weeks and is not observed prior to 32 weeks' PMA.[21] These findings support the hypothesis that basic metabolic changes related to retinal maturation drive the timing of retinal neovascularization, and are consistent with the release of growth factors in relation to retinal vascularization.[24, 27, 35, 50] They also provide practical guidance for the institution of screening policies for ROP.

Genetics

A final point in the discussion of pathophysiology relates to 2 similar developmental retinopathies. Familial exudative vitreoretinopathy (FEVR) and Norrie's disease both cause a neovascular retinal disorder that can lead to traction and retinal detachments, and are unrelated to premature delivery.[54–56] Such cases account for the sporadic reports of 'ROP' in full-term infants. However, the link is becoming even more interesting; recently, premature infants with ROP unexpectedly severe for their gestation were studied and found to have missense mutations in the gene for Norrie's disease.[57] This is an area to watch for future developments and may explain some of the outlier cases of ROP.

PREVENTION

The relationship between gestation and the incidence of ROP makes clear that reducing premature birth is the most effective means of preventing vision loss from ROP. This point was thoughtfully made in 2 evaluations of morbidities associated with assisted conception.[58, 59] Premature births, however, are rarely under the control of the neonatologist, who can nonetheless still affect the incidence of ROP among them.

In a randomized controlled trial, limiting the use of oxygen to just what is necessary to avoid cyanosis has been clearly demonstrated to reduce the incidence of ROP as compared to routine administration of over 50% oxygen to all infants to reduce apnea of prematurity.[2] Today, this is accomplished through the judicious use of arterial blood gases, transcutaneous oxygen monitoring and pulse oximetry; however, there are as yet no clearly established safe values for oxygen administration.[60] Several guidelines have been used over the years based on the best rationale that a group of reasonable physicians could agree on, and arterial PaO_2 values of 50–80 torr are currently recommended for premature infants.[61] Similarly, no standards for pulse oximetry ranges have been established, but a survey of practices in the United States in 1986 showed that over half of units were using target ranges of 90–95% saturation.[62]

Several case–control studies have identified medical conditions independently associated with ROP after controlling for the dominant effects of gestation and/or birth weight. Duration of oxygen administration consistently is the strongest association, followed by duration of ventilation and then multiple indicators of an unstable neonatal course such as intraventricular hemorrhage, pneumothorax, symptomatic patent ductus arteriosis, small for gestational age status, sepsis, shock, etc. With the widespread use of prenatal steroids in preterm labor, surfactant therapy for respiratory distress, indomethacin prophylaxis for intraventricular hemorrhage, early intravenous nutrition, and multiple other interventions, the overall homeostasis of the premature newborn is continuously being enhanced. In aggregate, these efforts are likely to continue to reduce retinal capillary injuries, and therefore consequent ROP.

Pharmacologic prophylaxis for ROP has been the subject of considerable investigation, based on the hypothesis that oxygen injury to the retinal capillaries is oxidative in origin. Unfortunately, none of the studies to date has provided clear evidence of a benefit. Reducing environmental light was expected to reduce capillary oxidant injury from the expected interaction of light energy and oxygen, producing oxygen free radicals. However, a recent meta-analysis of the well controlled trials published through to August 1998 does not support this hypothesis for reducing the incidence of any ROP, although the number of infants studied to date is insufficient to rule out a moderate effect on the incidence of severe ROP.[63–66] The 1998 publication of a randomized controlled trial of light reduction through the wearing of dark goggles from the day of birth through to 31 weeks in 409 infants <1251 grams birth weight provides additional strong supporting data. No difference was found in the incidence of any ROP (54% goggle wearers vs 68% controls), nor in the incidence of threshold ROP (5% in both groups).[66]

Vitamin E prophylaxis has similarly been intensively studied in multiple centers, and again the systematic evaluation of published randomized controlled clinical trials fails to demonstrate a benefit, although again the numbers studied may be insufficient to demonstrate a small, but important, effect.[67–69]

D-Penicillamine is a chelator of heavy metals and as such can reduce the oxidant potential of an infant's serum. When administration of D-penicillamine to reduce hyperbilirubinemia was followed by an unexpected reduction in ROP,[70] the investigators instigated a randomized controlled trial that similarly showed a reduction in stage 2 or greater ROP among premature infants treated from birth. No adverse effects were observed.[71] This finding from a single institution in a study of 141 survivors requires replication, but may be promising.

Inositol supplementation of intravenous feedings is another intervention that was serendipitously noted to reduce the incidence of ROP.[72, 73] It also requires replication in other settings to determine if inositol has a true effect in reducing ROP, its magnitude and safety limitations.

TREATMENT

Neonatal

Peripheral ablation for acute ROP

Treatment of active acute ROP has become a reality since first reported by Nagata in 1968.[74] The concept now involves ablation of the peripheral avascular retina which is the putative source of angiogenic growth factors driving the neovascularization. This drastic measure to destroy part of the organ to be rescued was met with initial scepticism. Early pilot studies gave mixed results,[75–77] but these were sufficiently promising to lead Palmer *et al* to organize a multicenter randomized controlled trial of cryotherapy ablation of the avascular peripheral retina in infants with ROP sufficiently severe to have a predicted 50% risk of retinal detachment. The study demonstrated a nearly 50% reduction in unfavorable retinal outcomes for infants with zone 1 or 2 ROP and at least 5 contiguous or 8 composite clock hours of stage 3 with plus disease.[8, 10, 78]

Laser photocoagulation of the avascular peripheral retina has become a popular alternative to cryotherapy in recent years, accomplishing the same peripheral ablation of avascular retina. A limited number of randomized comparisons have demonstrated that laser therapy is at least as effective as cryotherapy, and infants experience less postoperative instability and local reaction following laser treatment.[79–81] However, discussion continues as to whether the argon laser, which makes relatively large spots leading to a shorter procedure, or a diode laser is preferred. There have been reports of cataracts following laser treatment and, although these are not common, they are particularly troublesome since their necessary removal results in an aphakic eye.[82, 83]

Irrespective of the mode of treatment selected by the ophthalmic surgeon, neonatologists have an important role in providing medical support for the infant during and following surgery. Both cryotherapy and laser photocoagulation are painful procedures and local and/or general anesthesia is needed. Pressure on the globe during the procedure increases the frequency of bradycardia and can be countered with atropine.[84] In the 1–2 days following the procedure, apnea and increased oxygen requirements are common and may be related to serosanguinous nasal discharge which is more common with cryotherapy.

Infants require careful monitoring in the postoperative period, making this a procedure that usually requires continued hospitalization.

The criteria for selecting ROP for treatment deserve special mention. While a 50% reduction in vision loss from ablative treatment is of clear benefit, physicians have quickly become dissatisfied with even this tremendous improvement; it still leaves about a quarter of treated infants with unfavorable outcomes. The impulse to treat ROP before it reaches the severe stages meeting CRYO-ROP criteria for 'threshold' is strong and understandable. However, doing so means many infants who would never reach threshold are treated, and increases the number of eyes exposed to potential and as yet not fully understood long-term consequences of extensive peripheral retinal ablation. For example, if infants were to be treated at the point where they developed prethreshold ROP, 3 infants would have to be treated for each that would progress to threshold. Since 4 threshold infants have to be treated to prevent 1 case of vision loss, the number of prethreshold infants that would have to be treated to prevent 1 case of vision loss would be 12. At this ratio, the incidence and long-term consequences of treatment become very important. It is known that the visual fields may be only mildly affected by treatment,[85–87] and that color vision is not impaired.[88] The 10-year follow-up of survivors from the original cohort of 291 infants in the CRYO-ROP study currently being conducted will increase understanding of the longer term consequences of this intervention. Efforts to select those infants most likely to progress to poor outcomes,[23] for early or alternative treatments, are being evaluated, particularly for zone 1 disease.

Retinal detachment rescue

Efforts to rescue the retina once detachment has begun are often disappointing. Some ophthalmic surgeons attempt early application of a buckle around the globe of the eye to bring the sclera closer to the retina, combined with laser or cryotherapy to hold the retina in place. This may keep the retina attached in up to half of eyes, particularly where the macula remains attached at the time of surgery.[89–91] In some cases, formed vision has been retained, and in more cases at least light/dark perception. If total retinal detachment (stage 5) occurs, vitrectomy with or without lens sparing is even less successful. Even when the retina is reattached, visual results are disappointing, but in some children light perception or the ability to distinguish moving objects may still be considered worth the effort.[92–96] It is important that parents have realistic expectations about such surgery, and that the infant's total overall health status be considered so that the potential benefits can be balanced against the risks of major, long duration ophthalmic surgery.

Investigational areas

Considering the discussions above, there is still much to be learned about ROP. Two of the interesting treatment questions that are being asked at this time are whether treatment should be considered of ROP stages of less than the CRYO-ROP threshold severity, and also whether supplemental use of oxygen can downregulate the growth factors and control neovascularization in prethreshold ROP. The latter question is being investigated in a multicenter randomized controlled trial.[97] The study is based on laboratory findings of harmful effects of marginal hypoxia during the healing phase in an animal model of ROP,[98] the beneficial effects of oxygen supplementation in the same model,[37] and some clinical data suggesting that a similar benefit may occur in human ROP.[99, 100]

Follow-Up Eye Care for Premature Infants

Early care for the infant with sight

Myopia is a serious problem for premature infants and occurs more commonly than in full-term infants. This is true even if the premature infant never had ROP (13–16% for any myopia, 1.7% for high myopia at 2 years).[101, 102] With ROP, the risk more than doubles; 25% of infants who had ROP have myopia of –0.25 diopters or worse at 1–2 years, and 6% have high myopia, defined as >–5 diopters.[101] Just as ROP can be asymmetrical, so can the myopia (anisometropia), and an infant will suppress the use of a myopic eye in favor of using the one with more normal focus. Left untreated, this 'lazy eye' or amblyopia result following premature birth can lead to a functionally blind eye that still has a well attached retina with good potential. This is particularly tragic if the other eye later experiences vision loss.

Retinoscopy performed by an ophthalmologist by about 3 months following discharge from the NICU is a straightforward procedure and permits an estimate of the degree of myopia. Glasses, contact lens, patching and other interventions by a trained ophthalmologist will permit the optimal salvage of useful vision. Initial cryotherapy and preservation of retinal attachment alone is not enough. It is particularly rewarding for parents to observe the gains in visual attention and interaction with the environment when an infant with severe nearsightedness becomes able to see further than a few inches in front of his/her face. The child with bilateral refractive error usually responds in this way. The child requiring correction in only one eye is behaviorly far more difficult because no immediate benefit is perceived and he/she is being forced to use a less preferred eye.

Cataracts may arise in conjunction with severe ROP, and may become more common now that laser treatment is increasingly used. If there is a total retinal detachment, cataract treatment is not emergent. However, if a cataract develops in a child with attached retina, it should be evaluated, and usually treated immediately. Without a focused image falling on the retina, development of the interaction between visual cortex and retina efferents will fail and the eye will be functionally blind.

Early treatment of low vision

During the initial years following birth, it is difficult to assess the learning capacity and function of children who are blind. One of the important senses used in learning about the world has been lost. All such families need early intervention to teach alternative communication and learning skills to these children. Their tactile, auditory and kinesthetic skills need to be emphasized and developed, and families and teachers make critical differences in their ability to learn to function as they grow up. This should start within weeks of the time vision loss is suspected. While some children will have multiple handicaps and limited ability to benefit from such interventions, there is no way to be certain of this during the initial months when intervention must begin.[103]

Infants who experience total retinal detachments may also have medical ophthalmic complications that require treatment. Glaucoma can be subtle in onset and cause pain. Children who show a change in behavior, tears or excessive eye rubbing should be suspected of glaucoma and promptly referred to the ophthalmologist. Fortunately, this complication can often be successfully treated with topical steroids,[104] but sometimes enucleation of the blind eye offers the only relief.

Total retinal detachment can also lead to phthisis, lack of growth of the eye and orbit and consequently a cosmetically, as well as functionally, unsatisfactory result. For appropriate children, enucleation and use of gradually enlarging prostheses will encourage normal growth of the orbit. Or if there is satisfactory growth but still a poor cosmetic look because of leukocoria, a scleral shell can be inserted over the globe to gain a more normal appearance.[105]

Late complications

Having navigated the rigors of treatment for acute ROP in infancy and glasses and amblyopia treatment in childhood, the teen and adult former-ROP patient unfortunately remains at risk from their disorder, but to an unknown degree. There are no data based on a large inception cohort to determine the frequency of late traction and detachments or cataracts. However, case series and individual patients all too clearly attest to this reality.[106–108] Retinal detachments proceeding from progressive retinal thinning and finally tears during the teenage years can often be successfully treated with cryotherapy, laser and/or scleral buckling procedures. Individuals with retinal scarring, or following cryo or laser treatment for ROP, should remain in active follow-up with an ophthalmologist familiar with ROP, effectively for life. Sadly, it is the individual with vision loss already in one eye who is most likely to progress to later problems in the fellow eye because of the severity of the original process.

IMPLEMENTATION OF A SCREENING/TRACKING PROGRAM FOR ROP

Each neonatal service caring for premature infants must have in place an effective ROP program for screening and follow-up to ensure timely treatment if ROP progresses. The program must be jointly planned with neonatologists, ophthalmologists and support personnel, and will differ in its final format at each center. The elements to be included, however, must be:

1. identification of appropriate infants for examination;
2. tracking for follow-up examinations according to the findings in hospital or following discharge or transfer;
3. treatment plans for threshold infants; and
4. longer-term follow-up for refraction in year 1.

At all stages, communication with families is an essential ingredient.

Who?

The natural history arm of the CRYO-ROP study has provided some of the best systematic data on the incidence of ROP,[21,22] and is largely in agreement with various guidelines from the National Pediatric and Ophthalmic Societies.[109–111] In recent years, severe ROP requiring treatment appears to be increasingly less common among infants of >32 weeks', or even 28 weeks', gestation at birth, and therefore the USA guidelines were revised in 1997 to recommend routine examinations only in those infants of 28 weeks' gestation or less or 1500 g birth weight or less. In addition, the individual premature infant (over 28 weeks' gestation at birth) who is suspected of being at high risk should be examined at the request of the neonatologist. Those factors which place an infant at particularly high risk, however, are not delineated. Based on case reports[42, 43, 45, 48, 112–114] and the analyses of risk factors discussed above, the author's personal, and still growing, list of high-risk factors are listed in Table 9.1.

When?

Traditional recommendations were for the first examination to be performed at 4–6 weeks following delivery, but not later than discharge home from the nursery. However, analysis of the onset of ROP and of threshold ROP has increasingly supported a change in practice to perform the first examination at 30–32 weeks PMA. Thus, the 24-week infant would not have a first examination until 6–8 weeks after birth, while the 28-week infant would be examined 2–4 weeks following birth.[111] The recommendations are mute for the infant born at 32 weeks with sufficient risk factors to have an examination; however, it would appear wise to complete this within 2–3 weeks of birth.[21, 115] The onset of threshold ROP was not observed before 31 weeks PMA in 291 infants with threshold ROP in the CRYO-ROP study, and therefore this approach should be safe in terms of detecting threshold ROP in time for treatment. As premature infants improve in their overall progress through the NICU, dates of discharge home now sometimes precede these dates (see below), and pose a serious tracking problem.

Table 9.1 High-risk events as indicators for ROP screening in infants of 29–36 weeks' gestation.

Significant acidosis
Overt necrotizing enterocolitis
Grade II or worse intraventricular hemorrhage
Cerebral infarct
Seizures
Prolonged period of arterial oxygen >90 torr
Shock or hypotension (hypovolemic, septic, cardiogenic, other)
Period of profound anemia
Hydrops fetalis (immune or non-immune)
Other significant alteration in homeostasis during the perinatal period
Small for gestational age status at birth
Surgery requiring general anesthesia in the neonatal period
Other serious medical events affecting circulatory or metabolic integrity

Medical Aspects

The ROP screening examinations require a dilated pupil and scleral depression in order to visualize the ora serrata. Concentrated eye drops can cause hypertension and some gastrointestinal dysmotility, and therefore are used at lower concentrations for premature infants.[116, 117] The most commonly used is Cyclomydril® (cyclopentolate 0.2% and phenylephrine 1.0%).[116] Infants with heavily pigmented irises may sometimes require 2.5% phenylephrine (or 1% tropicamide) to achieve a dilated pupil, and this is also true when ROP has advanced to very active stages. During the examination infants are likely to have bradycardic episodes associated with the well recognized occulo-cardiac reflex, in addition to their own predisposition to apnea of prematurity.[9, 118] The neonatal team must monitor the infant carefully during the examination, and the ophthalmologist performing follow-up examinations of recently discharged infants in the outpatient setting should have assistance in observing such infants for apnea, although this is far less likely as they age beyond 42 weeks' PMA.

Tracking Repeat Examinations

When newborn centers first began scheduling and tracking the initial early ROP examination for all infants, logistic difficulties were encountered.[119] However, these pale in comparison to the complexities of ensuring appropriate follow-up examinations in the era of early discharges and back transfers to referring hospitals.[120] The median age for threshold ROP to appear is 37 weeks' PMA, approximately the time that many of these infants are being discharged home. It is possible for ROP to progress from prethreshold to threshold soon after discharge home, and this is a time when parents are particularly stressed and often fail to keep follow-up appointments. While the practice in many centers has been to keep premature infants at high risk of progression to threshold ROP in hospital, there is increasing recent pressure from families and from managed care plans to have these infants cared for at home. It is essential to remember the 'danger zone' of onset of threshold ROP shown in Figure 9.4. It falls unhappily at one of the otherwise most optimistic times for these tiny brave survivors and their families.

Each center's ROP tracking system must be organized to cut through the barriers of back transfer to regional hospitals or discharge home. The family is one of the greatest potential risks in such a program, but they can also be its greatest strength.

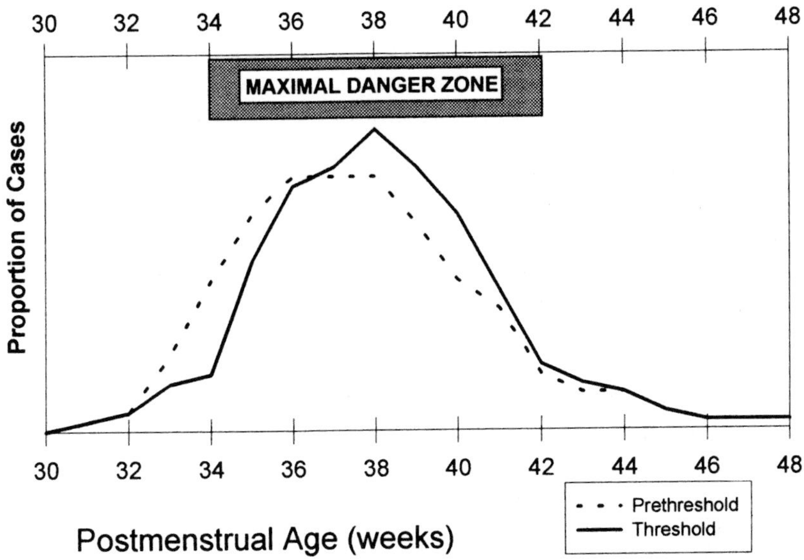

Figure 9.4 Postmenstrual age (PMA) and the onset of prethreshold and threshold ROP. The curves show all data for those infants who developed prethreshold ROP (dashed lines) and threshold ROP (solid lines) according to the PMA at the time of diagnosis. The median age for first diagnosis of prethreshold ROP was 36 weeks and for threshold ROP was 37 weeks. Graph developed by smoothing the data published by the CRYO-ROP study and reproduced with permission from Palmer EA, Flynn JT, Hardy RJ *et al.* Incidence and early course of retinopathy of prematurity. The Cryotherapy for Retinopathy of Prematurity Cooperative Group. *Ophthalmology* 1991;**98**: 1628–1640

Informing and Involving the Family

While bad news is traumatic for families, repeatedly in retrospect they state that the hardest thing of all is not knowing what is going to happen. Published information enables the neonatal team to provide families with valuable prognostic information,[23, 121, 122] and at the same time enlist their help in ensuring appropriate follow-up.

Predelivery

When time permits, in depth discussion about the risks of extremely preterm delivery, including vision impairment, are discussed.

Immediate days following birth

Even if discussed prior to delivery, once the infant is likely to survive, common complications among infants of <28 weeks' gestation are discussed in the context of what is to be expected in the coming weeks.

2–6 weeks following birth

During this period, parents are alerted to the timing of the first eye examination and provided written material about ROP in general. The low likelihood of serious disease is emphasized for the more mature and less ill infants, but is not minimized for those that are extremely immature or unstable. The need for follow-up examinations to determine a final outcome, and a visit during the first months following discharge, is introduced. Informational material for parents is available from a number of sources, and the material used by the CRYO-ROP study can be accessed without charge via the internet.[121]

After the first examination

Based on the initial examination findings (zone and stage of vessels/ROP) and PMA, data from the CRYO-ROP study are used to determine the probability of progression to threshold ROP.[22, 23] Some of these published aggregate data are reproduced in Table 9.2 and have provided a useful 'pocket-guide' in the intensive care nursery.

Explicit percentages mean a great deal to some families while others wish only generalities. Physicians can better support families and ensure follow-up when they know the statistical probabilities and can interpret them for the family. Fortunately, in many screened cases, mature or nearly mature vessels in zone 3 allow great reassurance. It is important to remember, however, that the finding of 'no ROP' is not reassuring in an eye with incompletely developed vessels – such a finding nearly always precedes ROP and is especially common at <32 weeks' PMA.

Follow-up examinations

Using the data from CRYO-ROP at each follow-up examination allows further refinement of the probabilities specific for that infant.[122, 23] Parents will always seek the time when they are 'home free', but this rarely occurs much before 36 weeks' PMA in those with no ROP or mild ROP, and usually not until after 44 weeks in those that have more severe stages of ROP acutely. By the time families take their infant home, or threshold ROP develops, they are usually prepared for and proactive in the follow-up process. If surgical intervention is needed, they are better prepared to discuss the options with the surgeon, and continue in follow-up postoperatively.

Examination at 3–6 months

Families who have learned that prematurity can cause nearsightedness or crossed or lazy eyes during the earlier counseling will be more likely to complete the 3–6 month follow-up needed for detection and treat-

Table 9.2 Probability (%) of reaching cryotherapy criteria. Modified with permission from Ref. 22.

	Post-menstrual age (weeks)					
	≤32	33–34	35–36	37–38	39–40	41–42
Zone 1						
Incomplete Z1	33	37	7	36	°	°
Stage 1–	18	33	°	°	°	°
All others	°	°	°	°	°	°
Zone 2						
Incomplete Z2	9	6	3	1	2	0.0
Stage 1–†	8	6	4	2	1	1.0
Stage 2–	4	6	4	2	1	1.3
Stage 3–	°	16	13	8	2	0.0
Stage 1+†	°	83	42	°	°	°
Stage 2+	°	44	34	25	17	0.0
Stage 3+	°	77	61	34	31	14.3

° = too few infants to calculate risk.
†'+' means with plus disease ROP, '–' means without plus disease.

ment of important myopia, or anisometropia in these children. When they do not understand the importance of these examinations, other priorities surrounding child rearing will take precedence.

SUMMARY

New treatments and ongoing research show that ROP remains a serious problem despite all efforts to prevent it. Screening examinations for ROP can be adjusted for PMA, and can be limited to somewhat younger infants than previously, but it remains critically important to detect and treat infants with threshold ROP in a timely fashion to ensure the best possible visual outcome for this disorder. Early discharge programs pose a serious threat to the success of these plans, but family education can help to overcome this, and also prepare those individuals who have retinal scars for a lifetime of ophthalmic follow-up.

Acknowledgments

The author was supported in part by an Unrestricted Grant from Research to Prevent Blindness, Inc. and the National Eye Institute, EY09962 and EY09959.

REFERENCES

1. Terry T. Extreme prematurity and fibroblastic overgrowth of persistent vascular sheath behind each crystalline lens. *Am J Ophthalmol* 1942;**25**: 203–204.
2. Kinsey V, Jacobus J and Hemphill F. Retrolental fibroplasia: Cooperative study of retrolental fibroplasia and the use of oxygen. *Arch Ophthalmol* 1956;**56**: 481–547.
3. Retinopathy of prematurity/idiopathic fibroplasia. *Pediatrics* 1981;**67**: 751–752.
4. Ashton N. Retrolental fibroplasia now retinopathy of prematurity. *Br J Ophthalmol* 1984;**68**: 689.
5. Silverman WA. *Retrolental Fibroplasia: A Modern Parable*. New York: Grune & Stratton, 1980.
6. Gibson DL, Sheps SB, Uh SH, Schechter MT and McCormick AQ. Retinopathy of prematurity-induced blindness: birth weight-specific survival and the new epidemic. *Pediatrics* 1990;**86**: 405–412.
7. Phelps DL. Retinopathy of prematurity: an estimate of vision loss in the United States – 1979. *Pediatrics* 1981;**67**: 924–925.
8. Cryotherapy for Retinopathy of Prematurity Cooperative Group. Multicenter trial of cryotherapy for retinopathy of prematurity. Preliminary results. *Arch Ophthalmol* 1988;**106**: 471–479.
9. Cryotherapy for Retinopathy of Prematurity Cooperative Group. Multicenter trial of cryotherapy for retinopathy of prematurity. Three-month outcome. *Arch Ophthalmol* 1990;**108**: 195–204.
10. Cryotherapy for Retinopathy of Prematurity Cooperative Group. Multicenter trial of cryotherapy for retinopathy of prematurity. One-year outcome – structure and function. *Arch Ophthalmol* 1990;**108**: 1408–1416.
11. Fledelius HC. Central nervous system damage and retinopathy of prematurity – an ophthalmic follow-up of prematures born in 1982–84. *Acta Paediatr* 1996;**85**: 1186–1191.
12. Takahashi A, Majima A, Suzuki C *et al.* The association between retinopathy of prematurity and chronic general complications. *Jpn J Clin Ophthalmol* 1995;**49**: 935–938.
13. Msall ME, Buck GM, Rogers BT, Duffy LC, Mallen SR and Catanzaro NL. Predictors of mortality, morbidity, and disability in a cohort of infants ≤28 weeks' gestation. *Clin Pediatr* 1993;**32**: 521–527.
14. Cross KW. Cost of preventing retrolental fibroplasia? *Lancet* 1973;**2**: 954–956.
15. Bolton DP and Cross KW. Further observations on cost of preventing retrolental fibroplasia. *Lancet* 1974;**1**: 445–448.
16. Pennefather PM, Tin W, Clarke MP, Fritz S and Strong NP. Retinopathy of prematurity in a controlled trial of prophylactic surfactant treatment. *Br J Ophthalmol* 1996;**80**: 420–424.
17. Fowlie PW. *Prophylactic Intravenous Indomethacin in Very Low Birth Weight Infants*. The Cochrane Library, Neonatal Module 1997. Cochrane Collaboration Update Software Ltd., Oxford, UK.
18. Gehrs KM, Barnes CH, Rosenthal WN and Lee S. The infant with threshold retinopathy of prematurity in the 1990s. *Invest Ophthalmol Vis Sci* 1997;**38**: S746.

19. International Committee for Classification of ROP. An international classification of retinopathy of prematurity. *Arch Ophthalmol* 1984;**102**: 1130–1134.
20. The International Committee for the Classification of the Late Stages of Retinopathy of Prematurity. An international classification of retinopathy of prematurity. II. The classification of retinal detachment. *Arch Ophthalmol* 1987;**105**: 906–912 [published erratum appears in *Arch Ophthalmol* 1987;**105**: 1498].
21. Palmer EA, Flynn JT, Hardy RJ *et al.* Incidence and early course of retinopathy of prematurity. The Cryotherapy for Retinopathy of Prematurity Cooperative Group. *Ophthalmology* 1991;**98**: 1628–1640.
22. Schaffer DB, Palmer EA, Plotsky DF *et al.* Prognostic factors in the natural course of retinopathy of prematurity. The Cryotherapy for Retinopathy of Prematurity Cooperative Group. *Ophthalmology* 1993;**100**: 230–237.
23. Hardy RJ, Palmer EA, Schaffer DB *et al.* Outcome-based management of retinopathy of prematurity. *J Am Assoc Pediatr Ophthalmol Strabis* 1997;**1**: 46–54. To download the 'Freeware' for Outcome-Based Management of Retinopathy of Prematurity (An application of Microsoft Access®), log into: http: //www.sph.uth.tmc.edu/rmrop/.
24. Michaelson I. The mode of development of the vascular system of the retina, with some observation on its significance for certain retinal diseases. *Trans Ophthalmol Soc UK* 1948;**68**: 137–180.
25. Donahue ML, Phelps DL, Watkins RH, Lomonaco MB and Horowitz S. Retinal vascular endothelial growth factor (VEGF) mRNA expression is altered in relation to neovascularization in oxygen induced retinopathy. *Curr Eye Res* 1996;**15**: 175–184.
26. Aiello LP, Avery RL, Arrigg PG *et al.* Vascular endothelial growth factor in ocular fluid of patients with diabetic retinopathy and other retinal disorders. *N Engl J Med* 1994;**331**: 1480–1487.
27. Stone J, Chan-Ling T, Pe'er J, Itin A, Gnessin H and Keshet E. Roles of vascular endothelial growth factor and astrocyte degeneration in the genesis of retinopathy of prematurity. *Invest Ophthalmol Vis Sci* 1996;**37**: 290–299.
28. Pierce EA, Foley ED and Smith LEH. Vascular endothelial growth factor: A critical factor in the vaso obliterative phase of retinopathy of prematurity. *Invest Ophthalmol Vis Sci* 1996;**37**: 608.
29. Young TL, Smith LEH, Foley E, Pierce EA and Anthony DC. Histopathological results and vascular endothelial growth factor messenger RNA: Expression in the retina of an infant with asymmetric retinopathy of prematurity. *Invest Ophthalmol Vis Sci* 1995;**36**: S67.
30. Chan-Ling T, Gock B and Stone J. The effect of oxygen on vasoformative cell division. Evidence that 'physiological hypoxia' is the stimulus for normal retinal vasculogenesis. *Invest Ophthalmol Vis Sci* 1995;**36**: 1201–1214.
31. Diaz-Araya CM, Provis JM, Penfold PL and Billson FA. Development of microglial topography in human retina. *J Compar Neurol* 1995;**363**: 53–68.
32. Penfold PL, Provis JM, Madigan MC, van Driel D and Billson FA. Angiogenesis in normal human retinal development: the involvement of

astrocytes and macrophages. *Graefes Arch Clin Exp Ophthalmol* 1990;**228**: 255–263.

33. Kretzer FL and Hittner HM. Spindle cells and retinopathy of prematurity: interpretations and predictions. *Birth Defects Original Article Series* 1988;**24**: 147–168.
34. Penn JS, Henry MM, Wall PT and Tolman BL. The range of PaO_2 variation determines the severity of oxygen-induced retinopathy in newborn rats. *Invest Ophthalmol Vis Sci* 1995;**36**: 2063–2070.
35. Pierce EA, Foley ED and Smith LEH. Regulation of vascular endothelial growth factor by oxygen in a model of retinopathy of prematurity. *Arch Ophthalmol* 1996;**114**: 1219–1228 [correction of errata in *Arch Ophthalmol* 1997;**115**: 427].
36. Gyllenstein L, Hellstrom BE. Experimental approach to the pathogenesis of retrolental fibroplasia II. The influence of the developmental maturity on oxygen-induced changes in the mouse eye. *Am J Ophthalmol* 1955;**39**: 475–488.
37. Phelps DL. Reduced severity of oxygen-induced retinopathy in kittens recovered in 28% oxygen. *Pediatr Res* 1988;**24**: 106–109.
38. Ashton N. Animal experiments in retrolental fibroplasia. *Am Acad Ophthalmol Otolaryngol Soc Trans* 1954;**58**: 51–54.
39. Patz A. The role of oxygen in retrolental fibroplasia. *Trans Am Ophthalmol Soc* 1968;**66**: 940–985.
40. McLeod DS, Crone SN and Lutty GA. Vasoproliferation in the neonatal dog model of oxygen-induced retinopathy. *Invest Ophthalmol Vis Sci* 1996;**37**: 1322–1333.
41. McLeod DS, Brownstein R and Lutty GA. Vaso-obliteration in the canine model of oxygen-induced retinopathy. *Invest Ophthalmol Vis Sci* 1996;**37**: 300–311.
42. Gunn TR, Easdown J, Outerbridge EW and Aranda JV. Risk factors in retrolental fibroplasia. *Pediatrics* 1980;**65**: 1096–1100.
43. Keith CG, Smith ST and Lansdell BJ. Retrolental fibroplasia: a study of the incidence and aetiological factors, 1977–1979. *Med J Aust* 1981;**2**: 589–592.
44. Wolbarsht ML, George GS, Kylstra J and Landers MB. Does carbon dioxide play a role in retrolental fibroplasia? *Pediatrics* 1982;**70**: 500–501.
45. Yu VY, Hookham DM and Nave JR. Retrolental fibroplasia – controlled study of 4 years' experience in a neonatal intensive care unit. *Arch Dis Child* 1982;**57**: 247–252.
46. Maheshwari R, Kumar H, Paul VK, Singh M, Deorari AK and Tiwari HK. Incidence and risk factors of retinopathy of prematurity in a tertiary care newborn unit in New Delhi. *Natl Med J Ind* 1996;**9**: 211–214.
47. Bassiouny MR. Risk factors associated with retinopathy of prematurity: a study from Oman. *J Trop Pediatr* 1996;**42**: 355–358.
48. Jandeck C, Kellner U, Kossel H, Bartsch M, Versmold HT and Foerster MH. Retinopathy of prematurity in infants of birth weight greater-than-2000 g after haemorrhagic shock at birth. *Br J Ophthalmol* 1996;**80**: 728–731.
49. Nodgaard H, Andreasen H, Hansen H and Sorensen HT. Risk factors associated with retinopathy of prematurity (ROP) in Northern Jutland, Denmark 1990–1993. *Acta Ophthalmol Scand* 1996;**74**: 306–310.

50. Weiter JJ, Zuckerman R and Schepens CL. A model for the pathogenesis of retrolental fibroplasia based on the metabolic control of blood vessel development. *Ophthal Surg* 1982;**13**: 1013–1017.
51. Baum JD. Retinal artery tortuosity in ex-premature infants. 18-year follow-up on eyes of premature infants. *Arch Dis Child* 1971;**46**: 247–252.
52. Hellstrom A, Hard A, Chen Y, Niklasson A and Albertsson-Wikland K. Ocular fundus morphology in preterm children. *Invest Ophthalmol Vis Sci* 1997;**38**: 1184–1192.
53. Quinn GE, Johnson L and Abbasi S. Onset of retinopathy of prematurity as related to postnatal and postconceptional age. *Br J Ophthalmol* 1992;**76**: 284–288.
54. Benson WE. Familial exudative vitreoretinopathy. *Trans Am Ophthalmol Soc* 1995;**93**: 473–521.
55. Bergen RL and Glassman R. Familial exudative vitreoretinopathy. *Ann Ophthalmol* 1983;**15**: 275–276.
56. Mintz-Hittner HA, Ferrell RE, Sims KB *et al.* Peripheral retinopathy in offspring of carriers of Norrie disease gene mutations – possible transplacental effect of abnormal norrin. *Ophthalmology* 1996;**103**: 2128–2134.
57. Shastry BS, Pendergast SD, Hartzer MK, Liu X, Trese MT. Identification of missense mutations in the Norrie disease gene associated with advanced retinopathy of prematurity. *Arch Ophthalmol* 1997;**115**: 651–655.
58. Mckibbin M and Dabbs TR. Assisted conception and retinopathy of prematurity. *Eye* 1996;**10**: 476–478.
59. Choyce DP. Selective abortion. Fifth of babies born after assisted conception have retinopathy of prematurity. *Br Med J* 1996;**313**: 1005
60. Bancalari E, Flynn J, Goldberg RN *et al.* Influence of transcutaneous oxygen monitoring on the incidence of retinopathy of prematurity. *Pediatrics* 1987;**79**: 663–669.
61. Fetus and Newborn Committee of the AAP. Clinical considerations in the use of oxygen. In: *Guidelines for Perinatal Care*, 4th ed. Elk Grove, IL: AAP, ACOG, 1997, pp 188–192.
62. Phelps DL and Colf NE. Home oxygen administration and retinopathy of prematurity: survey of 1988 practices. *Am J Dis Child* 1990;**144**: 141–142.
63. Phelps DL and Watts JL. *Early Light Reduction to Prevent ROP*. The Cochrane Library, Neonatal Module 1997; Issue 3 and Updates. Cochrane Collaboration Update Software Ltd., Oxford, UK.
64. Locke JC and Reese AB. Retrolental fibroplasia. The negative role of light, mydriatrics, and the ophthalmoscopic examination in its etiology. *Arch Ophthalmol* 1952;**48**: 44–47.
65. Seiberth V, Linderkamp O, Poepel B, Knorz MC and Liesenhoff H. Light and acute retinopathy of prematurity: A controlled clinical trial. *Invest Ophthalmol Vis Sci* 1992;**33**: 1085.
66. Reynolds JD, Hardy RJ, Kennedy KA *et al.* Lack of efficacy of light reduction in preventing retinopathy of prematurity. Light Reduction in Retinopathy of Prematurity (LIGHT-ROP). Cooperative Group. *New Engl J Med* 1998;**338**;1572–1576.

67. Phelps DL. Vitamin E and retinopathy of prematurity: the clinical investigator's perspective on antioxidant therapy: side effects and balancing risks and benefits. *Birth Defects Original Article Series* 1988;**24**: 209–218.
68. *Vitamin E and Retinopathy of Prematurity: Report of a Study by a Committee of the Institute of Medicine, Division of Health Sciences Policy*. Washington, DC: National Academic Press, 1986.
69. Watts JL. Retinopathy of prematurity. In: Sinclair JC and Bracken MB (eds) *Effective Care of the Newborn Infant*. Oxford: Oxford University Press, 1992, pp 617–639.
70. Lakatos L, Hatvani I, Karmazsin L and Oroszlan G. Prevention of retrolental fibroplasia in very low birth weight infants by D-penicillamine. *Eur J Pediatr* 1982;**138**: 199–200.
71. Lakatos L, Hatvani I, Oroszlan G *et al.* Controlled trial of D-penicillamine to prevent retinopathy of prematurity. *Acta Paediatr Hung* 1986;**27**: 47–56.
72. Hallman M, Pohjavuori M and Bry K. Inositol supplementation in respiratory distress syndrome. *Lung* 1990;**168**: 877–882.
73. Hallman M, Bry K, Hoppu K, Lappi M and Pohjavuori M. Inositol supplementation in premature infants with respiratory distress syndrome. *N Engl J Med* 1992;**326**: 1233–1239.
74. Nagata M. Therapeutic possibility in retrolental fibroplasia in the premature infant with light coagulation. *Ganka Ophthalmol* 1968;**10**: 719–727.
75. Kingham JD. Acute retrolental fibroplasia. II. Treatment by cryosurgery. *Arch Ophthalmol* 1978;**96**: 2049–2053.
76. Hindle NW and Leyton J. Prevention of cicatricial retrolental fibroplasia by cryotherapy. *Can J Ophthalmol* 1978;**13**: 277–282.
77. Ben-Sira I, Nissenkorn I, Grunwald E and Yassur Y. Treatment of acute retrolental fibroplasia by cryopexy. *Br J Ophthalmol* 1980;**64**: 758–762.
78. Cryotherapy for Retinopathy of Prematurity Cooperative Group. Multicenter trial of cryotherapy for retinopathy of prematurity. Snellen visual acuity and structural outcome at 5½ years after randomization. *Arch Ophthalmol* 1996;**114**: 417–424.
79. Clarkson JG, Capone JA, Sternberg JP *et al.* Laser therapy for retinopathy of prematurity. *Arch Ophthalmol* 1994;**112**: 154–156.
80. Iverson DA, Trese MT, Orgel IK and Williams GA. Laser photocoagulation for threshold retinopathy of prematurity. *Arch Ophthalmol* 1991;**109**: 1342–1343.
81. Hunter DG and Repka MX. Diode laser photocoagulation for threshold retinopathy of prematurity. A randomized study. *Ophthalmology* 1993;**100**: 238–244.
82. Pogrebniak AE, Bolling JP and Stewart MW. Argon laser-induced cataract in an infant with retinopathy of prematurity. *Am J Ophthalmol* 1994;**117**: 261–262.
83. Christiansen SP and Bradford JD. Cataract following diode laser photoablation for retinopathy of prematurity. *Arch Ophthalmol* 1997;**115**: 275–276.
84. Brown GC, Tasman WS, Naidoff M, Schaffer DB, Quinn GE and Bhutani VK. Systemic complications associated with retinal cryoablation for retinopathy of prematurity. *Ophthalmology* 1990;**97**: 855–858.

85. Quinn GE, Dobson V, Hardy RJ, Tung B, Phelps DL and Palmer EA. Visual fields measured with double-arc perimetry in eyes with threshold retinopathy of prematurity from the cryotherapy for retinopathy of prematurity trial. *Ophthalmology* 1996;**103**: 1432–1437.
86. Kremer I, Nissenkorn I, Lusky M and Yassur Y. Late visual field changes following cryotherapy for retinopathy of prematurity stage 3. *Br J Ophthalmol* 1995;**79**: 267–269.
87. Nissenkorn I, Ben-Sira I, Kremer I *et al.* Eleven years' experience with retinopathy of prematurity: visual results and contribution of cryoablation. *Br J Ophthalmol* 1991;**75**: 158–159.
88. Dobson V, Quinn GE, Abramov I *et al.* Color vision measured with pseudoisochromatic plates at five-and-a-half years in eyes of children from the CRYO-ROP study. *Invest Ophthalmol Vis Sci* 1996;**37**: 2467–2474.
89. Ricci B, Santo A, Ricci F, Minicucci G and Molle F. Scleral buckling in stage 4 retinopathy of prematurity. *Graefes Arch Clin Exp Ophthalmol* 1996;**234**: S38–S41.
90. Gobel W and Richard G. Retinopathy of prematurity – current diagnosis and management. *Eur J Pediatr* 1993;**152**: 286–290.
91. Noorily SW, Small K, de Juan EJ and Machemer R. Scleral buckling surgery for stage 4B retinopathy of prematurity. *Ophthalmology* 1992;**99**: 263–268.
92. Wicharz A, Paulmann H and Stojanov D. Results of surgical therapy of advanced stages of retinopathy of prematurity. *Fortschritte Ophthalmol* 1991;**88**: 477–481.
93. Quinn GE, Dobson V, Barr CC *et al.* Visual acuity in infants after vitrectomy for severe retinopathy of prematurity. *Ophthalmology* 1991;**98**: 5–13 [published erratum apppears in *Ophthalmology* 1991;**98**: 1005].
94. Hirose T, Katsumi O, Mehta MC and Schepens CL. Vision in stage 5 retinopathy of prematurity after retinal reattachment by open-sky vitrectomy. *Arch Ophthalmol* 1993;**111**: 345–349.
95. Mintz-Hittner HA, O'Malley RE and Kretzer FL. Long-term form identification vision after early, closed, lensectomy-vitrectomy for stage 5 retinopathy of prematurity. *Ophthalmology* 1997;**104**: 454–459.
96. Quinn GE, Dobson V, Barr CC *et al.* Visual acuity of eyes after vitrectomy for retinopathy of prematurity: follow-up at 5½ years. The Cryotherapy for Retinopathy of Prematurity Cooperative Group. *Ophthalmology* 1996;**103**: 595–600.
97. Phelps DL, Palmer EA and Wood NE. Supplemental oxygen for prethreshold retinopathy of prematurity. In: Shapiro MJ, Biglan AW and Miller MM (eds) *Retinopathy of Prematurity*. Amsterdam: Kugler Publications, 1995, pp 139–141.
98. Phelps DL and Rosenbaum AL. Effects of marginal hypoxemia on recovery from oxygen-induced retinopathy in the kitten model. *Pediatrics* 1984;**73**: 1–6.
99. Szewczyk T. Retrolental fibroplasia and related ocular diseases: Classification, etiology, and prophylaxis. *Am J Ophthalmol* 1953;**36**: 1333–1361.
100. Gaynon MW, Stevenson DK, Sunshine P, Fleischer BE and Landers MB. Supplemental oxygen may decrease progression of prethreshold disease to threshold retinopathy of prematurity. *J Perinatol* 1997;**17**: 434–438.

101. Quinn GE, Dobson V, Repka MX *et al.* Development of myopia in infants with birth weights less than 1251 grams. The Cryotherapy for Retinopathy of Prematurity Cooperative Group. *Ophthalmology* 1992;**99**: 329–340.
102. Nissenkorn I, Yassur Y, Mashkowski D, Sherf I and Ben-Sira I. Myopia in premature babies with and without retinopathy of prematurity. *Br J Ophthalmol* 1983;**67**: 170–173.
103. Teplin SW. Development of blind infants and children with retrolental fibroplasia: implications for physicians. *Pediatrics* 1983;**71**: 6–12.
104. Kushner BJ and Sondheimer S. Medical treatment of glaucoma associated with cicatricial retinopathy of prematurity. *Am J Ophthalmol* 1982;**94**: 313–317.
105. Summers G, Phelps DL, Tung B and Palmer EA. Ocular cosmesis in retinopathy of prematurity. The Cryotherapy for Retinopathy of Prematurity Cooperative Group. *Arch Ophthalmol* 1992;**110**: 1092–1097.
106. Tasman W and Brown GC. Progressive visual loss in adults with retinopathy of prematurity (ROP). *Trans Am Ophthalmol Soc* 1988;**86**: 367–379.
107. Brown MM, Brown GC, Duker JS, Tasman WS and Augsburger JJ. Exudative retinopathy of adults: a late sequela of retinopathy of prematurity. *Int Ophthalmol* 1994;**18**: 281–285.
108. Krolicki TJ and Tasman W. Cataract extraction in adults with retinopathy of prematurity. *Arch Ophthalmol* 1995;**113**: 173–177.
109. Wilkinson AR, Clark D, Fielder A, Marlow N, Schulenburg WE and Weindling AM. Retinopathy of prematurity: Guidelines for screening and treatment. The report of a joint working party of the Royal College of Opthalmologists and the British Association of Perinatal Medicine. *Early Hum Dev* 1996;**46**: 239–258.
110. Fleck BW, Wright E, Dhillon B, Millar GT and Laing IA. An audit of the 1995 Royal College of Ophthalmologists guidelines for screening for retinopathy of prematurity applied retrospectively in one regional neonatal intensive care unit. *Eye* 1995;**9**: 31–35.
111. Screening examination of premature infants for retinopathy of prematurity – a joint statement of the American Academy of Pediatrics, the American Association for Pediatric Ophthalmology and Strabismus, and the American Academy of Ophthalmology. *Ophthalmology* 1997;**104**: 888–889.
112. Shohat M, Reisner SH, Krikler R, Nissenkorn I, Yassur Y and Ben-Sira I. Retinopathy of prematurity: incidence and risk factors. *Pediatrics* 1983;**72**: 159–163.
113. Kellner U, Jandeck C, Helbig H *et al.* Evaluation of published recommendations for screening studies of retinopathy of prematurity. *Ophthalmologie* 1995;**92**: 681–684.
114. Pallas ACR, Tejada PP, Medina LMC, Martin PMJ, Orbea GC and Barrio AMC. Premature retinopathy: Our experience. *Anales Espanoles Pediatr* 1995;**42**: 52–56.
115. Nissenkorn I, Kremer I, Gilad E, Cohen S and Ben-Sira I. 'Rush' type retinopathy of prematurity: report of three cases. *Br J Ophthalmol* 1987;**71**: 559–562.

116. Isenberg S, Everett S, Parelhoff E. A comparison of mydriatic eyedrops in low-weight infants. *Ophthalmology* 1984; 91: 278–279.
117. Merritt JC and Kraybill EN. Effect of mydriatics on blood pressure in premature infants. *J Pediatr Ophthalmol Strabis* 1981;**18**: 42–46.
118. Frishberg Y, Amir J, Nissenkorn I, Ben-Sira I and Davidson S. Severe bradycardia and nodal rhythm complicating cryopexy for retinopathy of prematurity. *J Pediatr Ophthalmol Strabis* 1986;**23**: 258–260.
119. Trainor S, White GLJ, Trunnell E and Kivlin JD. Compliance with a standard of care for retinopathy of prematurity in one neonatal intensive care unit. *J Pediatr Ophthalmol Strabis* 1988;**25**: 237–239.
120. Demorest BH. Retinopathy of prematurity requires diligent follow-up care. *Surv Ophthalmol* 1996;**41**: 175–178.
121. Patient materials may be downloaded from the CRYO-ROP linked site on the American Academy of Pediatric Ophthalmology and Strabismus Homepage: http: //med-aapos.bu.edu/
122. Phelps DL. Retinopathy of prematurity. *Pediatr Rev* 1995;**16**: 50–56.

10

Infections in Newborn Infants and the Potential for New Prevention and Treatment Strategies

Paola Papoff and Robert D. Christensen

INTRODUCTION

Recent successful efforts to prevent hyaline membrane disease have resulted in the rescue of a new population of preterm neonates. Unfortunately, these extremely low birth weight (ELBW) infants, who are now surviving to populate neonatal intensive care units (NICUs), have an extraordinarily high risk of developing nosocomial infections. Such infections, proven by blood culture, occur in >50% of infants delivered at <750 g birth weight, and 30% of these develop more than one episode of infection prior to hospital discharge. Indeed, up to 40% of ELBW infants who die *after* their first week of life, do so as a result of an infection. ELBW infants who survive a nosocomial infection incur the costs of a prolonged hospitalization and an increased likelihood of a chronic condition.[1]

Several underlying mechanisms account for the high susceptibility of ELBW neonates to infections. Immaturity of their respiratory and digestive systems can necessitate prolonged endotracheal intubation and intravascular catheterization. These measures can constitute ports of entry for micro-organisms. Also, incomplete development of certain aspects of the immune system can enhance susceptibility to infections, and can delay the killing and clearance of organism once an infection has begun. The aim of this chapter is to review the common infections observed in NICUs and to outline some of the promising new approaches to the prevention and treatment of these infections.

EARLY-ONSET NEONATAL INFECTIONS

Early-onset infections are those that arise within the first 72 hours of life. Incidence rates for early-onset neonatal sepsis range from 1 to 8 cases per 1000 live births, with the highest rates in the infants of the lowest birth weight.[2] A recent report from the National Institute of Child Health and Human Development Neonatal Research Network revealed that among infants of ≤1500 g birth weight, the majority of early-onset infections are caused by Gram-positive bacteria, such as Group B streptococcus (GBS), *Streptococcus viridans* and coagulase-negative staphylococci (CONS) (Figure 10.1). Among Gram-negative organisms, *Escherichia coli* remains one of the most frequently isolated organism followed by *Enterobacter*, *Klebsiella*, and *Pseudomonas*. Although *Candida* species rarely are responsible for early-onset infection, they account for a significant number of late-onset cases.

Intrauterine Infection

During the past 15 years, numerous reports have emphasized the association of intrauterine infections (IUI), preterm delivery and early-onset neonatal infections.[3–5] IUI can be classified according to the location of the micro-organisms, e.g. if the organisms are found in the chorioamnion and/or amnion, the amniotic fluid, or the decidua. The specific micro-organisms involved in IUI are not always identified; however, *Ureaplasma urealyticum* is the agent most commonly associated with histologic chorioamnionitis.[6, 7] Bacteria, such as GBS and *Fusobacterium* species, and *Candida albicans* can also be responsible.[8]

The commonest pathway of development of IUI is the ascending route. Rupture of the amnion and chorion is not a prerequisite because micro-organisms can cross intact membranes.[9] Once in the amniotic cavity, the bacteria may directly gain access to the fetal lung, ear, eye and/or umbilical cord. Another pathway of IUI development is the spread of an infection from the decidua parietalis to the decidua basalis and from there directly to the fetal villous circulation.

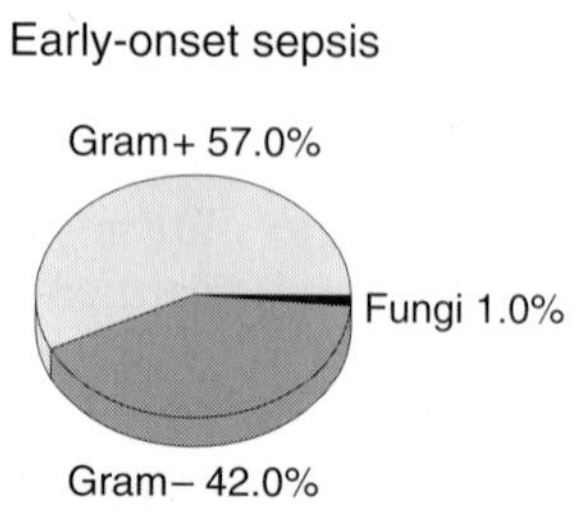

Gram+	%	Gram−	%	Fungi	%
GBS	31	*E. coli*	16	Candida spp.	1
Strep. viridans	9	*H. influenzae*	11		
Other streptococci	7	Klebsiella	5		
CONS	7	Other	10		
Staph. aureus	3				

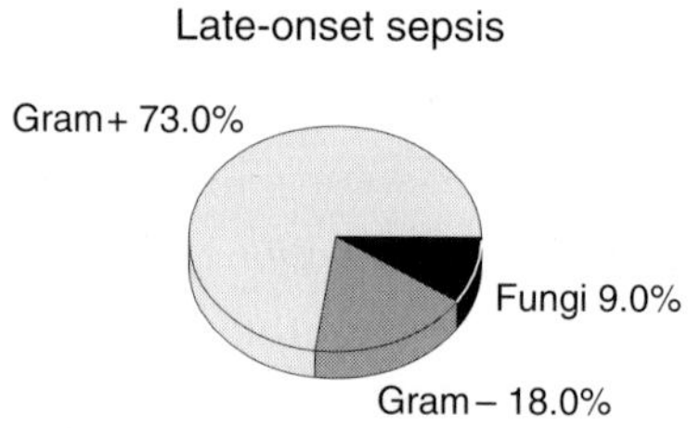

Gram+	%	Gram−	%	Fungi	%
CONS	55	Enterobacter	4	*C. albicans*	5
Staph. aureus	9	*E. coli*	4	*C. parapsilosis*	2
Enterococcus	5	Klebsiella	4	Other	2
GBS	2	Pseudomonas	2		
Other	2	Other	4		

Figure 10.1 Distribution of pathogens associated with sepsis in preterm neonates (birth weight <1501 g). Reproduced with permission from Ref 2.

Prophylactic Antepartum Antibiotics

The association between prolonged preterm rupture of membranes (PPROM), chorioamnionitis and GBS colonization, and the development of early-onset sepsis, has prompted the consideration of prophylactic antepartum antibiotic administration to pregnant women as an approach to decrease the incidence of neonatal infections. Various criteria for the institution of prophylactic antibiotics have been tested. A meta-analysis of 7 somewhat similar clinical trials, encompassing 795 women with preterm delivery, indicated that antepartum antibiotics produce a small reduction in the risk of neonatal pneumonia and necrotizing enterocolitis, but have no effect on other neonatal or maternal outcomes.[10] More positive results were obtained from using antepartum antibiotics following PPROM. Specifically, 2 meta-analyses of studies that employed antimicrobial therapy in PPROM showed improved maternal and fetal outcomes:

- the number of women delivering within 1 week of treatment was decreased;
- maternal morbidity, including chorioamnionitis and postpartum infection, were reduced; and
- fetal morbidity from sepsis and intraventricular hemorrhage was reduced, but no effect was observed on respiratory distress syndrome, necrotizing enterocolitis, or overall neonatal mortality.[11, 12]

The Lancefield Group B *Streptococcus agalactiae* has been a leading cause of perinatal infections for many years in the United States. In neonates, these infections include congenital pneumonia, sepsis and meningitis. Although the incidence varies by geographic region, 12 000 infants in the United States are estimated to develop GBS-associated morbidity or mortality annually. The overall mortality rate for early-onset GBS disease is 2–8% in term infants, but 25–30% in preterm infants. Several preventative regimens have been suggested. One approach is to identify women who are colonized with GBS, and to then eradicate the GBS colonization. GBS are generally harbored in the genitourinary and lower gastrointestinal tracts of adults. When both lower vaginal and anorectal sites are sampled, GBS are found in 15–40% of pregnant women. Colonization rates do not appear to vary significantly by trimester. Carriage may be chronic, transient or intermittent. Vertical transmission of GBS to neonates occurs in 40–73% of culture-positive women, but only 1–2% of their infants develop early-onset disease. Factors associated with GBS sepsis include gestation <37 weeks, rupture of membranes for >18 hours, fever during labor and GBS bacteriuria. Multiple studies employing oral antibiotics to eradicate GBS colonization showed high rates of recurrences of colonization by the time of delivery.

In 1975, Steigman *et al* reported that there had been no cases of GBS infections for 22 years at Mount Sinai Medical Center in New York, and hypothesized that this was due to administration of penicillin G within 30 min of delivery for prophylaxis against ophthalmia neonatorum.[13] This observation was followed by several prospective studies which suggested that intrapartum chemoprophylaxis of GBS carriers is an effective method of preventing neonatal GBS disease.[14] On the basis of these studies, in 1992, the Committee on Infectious Diseases and Committee on Fetus and Newborn of the American Academy of Pediatrics provided guidelines for prevention of early-onset GBS disease through intrapartum prophylaxis of selected maternal GBS carriers.[14] Since 1992, additional data have become available, and more experience with the guidelines has been gained. Recently, consensus guidelines were developed by obstetricians, pediatricians, family practitioners, and public health authorities, and published by the Center for Disease Control and Prevention.[15] These recommendations are based on a choice of two strategies: one based on screening cultures and risk factors (Figure 10.2); the other on identifiable risk factors without screening cultures (Figure 10.3). Figure 10.4 is the algorithm suggested for management of infants born to women receiving intrapartum chemoprophylaxis to prevent GBS disease. Whether or not intrapartum chemoprophylaxis is given, neonates with signs of sepsis should have a complete diagnostic evaluation, including a complete blood count and differential cell count, a blood culture and a chest X-ray if respiratory symptoms are present, and initiation of empiric therapy (ampicillin and gentamicin) pending culture results. In neonates without signs of sepsis, initial clinical evaluation depends on gestational age. In fact, compared to term infants, premature neonates have a 10–15-fold increased risk for early-onset GBS sepsis. Asymptomatic infants <35 weeks' gestation should be evaluated and observed for at least 48 hours without antibiotic therapy. If systemic infection is suspected, complete diagnostic evaluation and empiric therapy are indicated. The management of infants of 35 weeks' gestation or longer is dictated by the duration of maternal intrapartum prophylaxis. Two or more doses of intrapartum antibiotics should prevent early-onset GBS sepsis. Thus, evaluation and observation is recommended only for infants whose mothers have received <2 doses of intrapartum antibiotics.

Perinatal Infections with *Ureaplasma urealyticum*

One of the earliest reports of *U. urealyticum* causing human perinatal disease was by Tafari *et al* in 1976.[16] They described the isolation of this organism from the lungs of 42 of 290 stillborn infants who had histologic evidence of pneumonitis. Many cases of congenital infection with mycoplasma have been reported subsequently, with the identification of both *U. urealyticum* and *Mycoplasma hominis* from fetal lung, blood, and cerebrospinal fluid.[17–21]

U. urealyticum is a common inhabitant of the urogenital tract of pregnant women. Transmission to the fetus can occur *in utero* by transplacental passage from the mother's blood, *in utero* by organisms ascending from the colonized maternal urogenital tract, or at delivery by passage of the fetus through a colonized birth canal. The rate of vertical transmission among colonized women ranges from 18 to 55% for full-term infants, and from 29 to 55% for preterm infants.[22–24] The transmission rate does not appear to be affected by the mode of delivery, but it is significantly increased when clinical chorioamnionitis is present.[24] Colonization of an infant with *U. urealyticum* has been reported despite delivery by cesarean section with intact membranes.

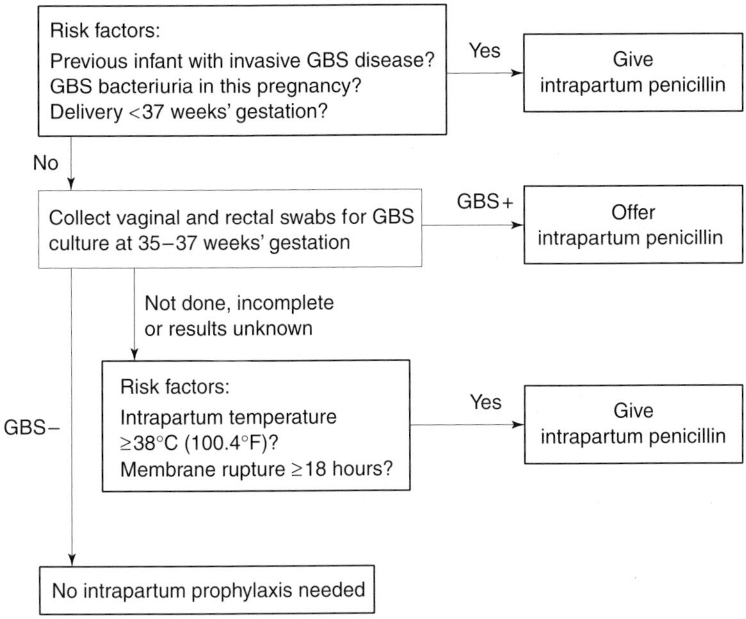

Figure 10.2 Prevention strategy for early-onset Group B streptococcus (GBS) disease using prenatal culture screening at 35–37 weeks. Reproduced with permission from Ref 15.

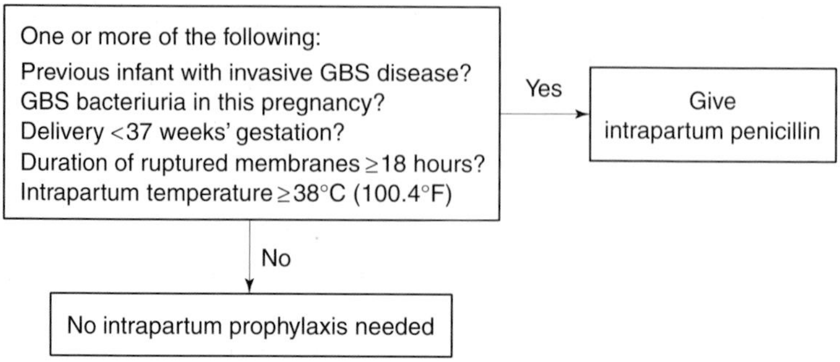

Figure 10.3 Prevention strategy for early-onset Group B streptococcus (GBS) disease using risk factors without prenatal culture screening.

The rate of neonatal colonization appears to be higher in very low birth weight (VLBW) infants. Given this finding, as well as the potential for serious disease from *U. urealyticum*, investigators postulated that prenatal eradication of the organism would improve neonatal outcome. Indeed, in several studies, treating women with antibiotics that were active against *U. urealyticum* appeared to reduce prematurity and increase birth weight.[25] In a recent multicenter, randomized, double-blind trial, pregnant women who were colonized with *U. urealyticum* were treated with erythromycin or placebo, 3 times a day, starting between 26 and 30 weeks' gestation and continuing through 35 com-

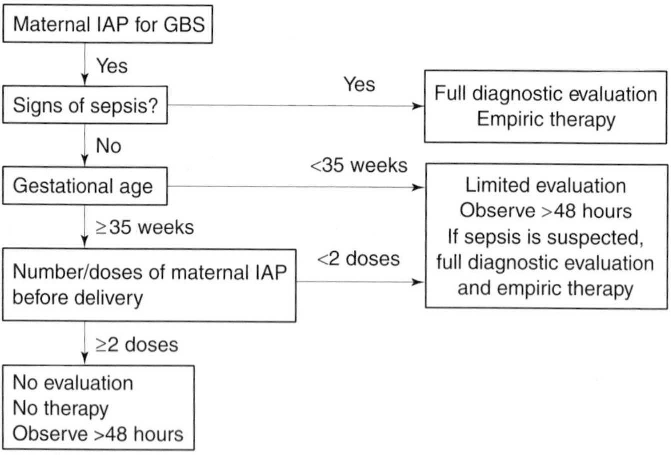

Figure 10.4 Empiric management of a neonate born to a mother who received intrapartum antimicrobial prophylaxis (IAP) for early-onset Group B streptococcus (GBS) disease.

pleted weeks. Unfortunately, erythromycin administration did not eliminate *U. urealyticum* from the women's lower genital tract.[26] Furthermore, there were no significant differences, between erythromycin and placebo recipients in terms of birth weight or gestational age at delivery, frequency of PROM or neonatal outcome.

Another putative approach for decreasing neonatal morbidity from *U. urealyticum* infection is identification, and antibiotic treatment, of colonized neonates. There is limited experience in the treatment of neonates found to have *U. urealyticum* in the lower respiratory tract or other sites from which microbiologic follow-up was performed. Walsh *et al* treated 3 infants with chronic lung disease who had proven infection with *U. urealyticum*, based on open lung biopsy;[27] 2 remained positive despite treatment. Waites *et al* randomized 14 preterm neonates (<1500 g) to receive either 25 or 40 mg/kg/day of erythromycin lactobionate in divided doses at 6-hour intervals. Post-treatment cultures of tracheal aspirates were obtained in 10 of these neonates, 9 of whom were negative. In this study no phlebitis, ototoxicity, cardiac arrhythmias, hematic dysfunction or evidence of other toxicity thought to be associated with administration of erythromycin were observed.[28] Hentschel *et al* treated 1 premature infant with *U. urealyticum*-positive cerebrospinal fluid culture first with erythromycin and then with chloramphenicol, obtaining sterilization of the spinal fluid after 20 days of treatment with chloramphenicol.[29]

Therefore, currently there are no precise recommendations for the treatment of *U. urealyticum* infection in neonates. However, it is suggested that no treatment is needed for colonized infants who display minimal or no disease, while antimicrobials should be initiated in colonized infants with symptoms not otherwise explained. *U. urealyticum* is generally susceptible to all tetracyclines, although reports of resistance have occurred.[30–32] Erythromycin is the drug of choice for neonatal infections due to *U. urealyticum*; however, *M. hominis* is uniformly resistant and usually require treatment with clindamycin, lincomycin, chloramphenicol or tetracyclines. Hazards and relative contraindications of tetracyclines and chloramphenicol in infants are recognized; yet, for cases of meningitis and especially those due to *M. hominis*, currently there may be no alternative.

NEONATAL NOSOCOMIAL INFECTIONS

The risk of systemic nosocomial infections in neonates increases with:

- decreasing birth weight and gestational age;
- intrauterine infection;

- traumatic delivery;
- fetal hypoxia; and
- prolonged intravascular catheterization.

Nosocomial infections are substantially different in neonates from adults. For example, among adult patients, urinary tract infections are the most frequent type of nosocomial infections, followed by surgical-site infections, pneumonia and sepsis.[33] In adults, nosocomial pneumonia is often due to Gram-negative bacilli, and nosocomial sepsis is generally caused by staphylococci. In neonates, sepsis is the most frequently diagnosed variety of nosocomial infection, and most cases occur in patients with central intravenous catheters. Nosocomial pneumonia is the second commonest infection and eye, ear, nose and throat infections are less commonly reported.[34]

The most common nosocomial pathogens among neonates of all weights are CONS, *Staphylococcus aureus*, enterococci, *Enterobacter* species, *Escherichia coli*, and *Candida* species.[4] Most of the CONS relevant to humans are commonly isolated from normal skin and mucous membranes. In virtually all infants these organisms are acquired early in life, either during passage through a colonized birth canal or as a result of exposure to nursery personnel. Leyden found that by 48 hours of age, 100% of normal infants carried CONS on the scalp, axilla and groin.[35] D'Angio *et al* studied surface colonization of premature infants admitted to an intensive care nursery by culturing the nasopharynx, rectum, axilla and behind the ear; by 4 days of age, all infants were colonized by CONS at every site studied.[36]

In most cases, nosocomial infections develop when colonizing organisms overcome the integrity of the skin or mucous membranes. A somewhat speculative potential route involves bloodstream entry from the intestinal tract after injury to the epithelium. Another potential portal for entry of bacteria into the bloodstream is through the respiratory tract. Evidence for this route is provided by Davies *et al* who noted that 12 of 14 premature infants in whom CONS bacteremia was diagnosed had a preceding increase in requirement for mechanical ventilation.[37] In a number of reports, mechanical ventilation was initiated just before the recognition of bacteremia.

The species of CONS most frequently associated with infection is *Staph. epidermidis*. This is likely to be due to the overwhelming preponderance of *Staph. epidermidis* on the skin. However, *Staph. haemolyticus* also frequently colonizes the skin and mucous membranes of hospitalized patients, including neonates, and can cause infection.[38, 39]

Resistance of *Staph. epidermidis* to penicillin, oxacillin, and gentamicin is very common, but resistance to vancomycin is rare. Therefore, vancomycin is a recommended initial empiric therapy for infants at risk for CONS disease. The treatment regimen can subsequently be modified when the antimicrobial susceptibility testing has been accomplished. Occasionally, a CONS infection persists despite treatment with an antimicrobial agent with good *in vitro* activity. In this circumstance, synergistic antibiotic therapy may be necessary. Vancomycin plus rifampin is one such combination. However, if the persistence of CONS despite treatment occurs in a neonate with an indwelling catheter, removal of that catheter may be necessary. This is particularly recommended if the CONS isolate is slime-producing. The same is true for meningitis resulting from an infected cerebrospinal fluid shunt. In this case, intraventricular administration of vancomycin may be necessary in order to eradicate the infection, because of the poor penetration of vancomycin through the blood–brain barrier. No consensus has been developed on the proper duration of systemic antimicrobial treatment for neonates septic with CONS. Based on information with other organisms, antibiotics are generally continued 10–14 days for septicemia and for at least 14 days for meningitis.

The glycopeptide teicoplanin has been suggested as an alternative to vancomycin for the treatment of nosocomial infections with Gram-positive bacteria.[40–42] Teicoplanin is a complex of 5 closely-related glycopeptide antibiotics similar to vancomycin in chemical structure and mechanism of action (inhibition of cell wall biosynthesis by binding to the terminal acyl-D-alanyl-D-alanine residue of cell wall peptidoglycan). Like vancomycin, the antibacterial activity of teicoplanin is restricted to Gram-positive micro-organisms. Susceptible micro-organisms include *Staph. aureus*, CONS, and clostridia; the antibacterial activity is not affected by methicillin resistance or β-lactamase production. However, while resistance of Gram-positive bacteria to vancomycin is rare, reduced susceptibility to teicoplanin has been regularly reported in Europe and the USA.[43] Resistance to teicoplanin is encountered among CONS, particularly *Staph. haemolyticus. Staph. epidermidis* can also be resistant to vancomycin. The mechanisms accounting for resistance of CONS to teicoplanin have not been completely characterized, but possibly involve enzymatic destruction or modification of the molecule; an increase in the amount of peptidoglycan might increase the number of high-affinity teicoplanin-binding sites involved in non-target binding of the antibiotic, with the result that the number of molecules available to bind the specific target would be reduced. O'Hare and Reynolds analyzed the membrane proteins of clinical isolates of *Staph. epidermidis* and *Staph. haemolyticus* resistant to teicoplanin but sensitive to vancomycin and found an increased production of a major membrane protein (39 kDa) in the resistant strains.[44]

Prophylactic administration of antimicrobials has been suggested for the prevention of CONS colonization and disease. In 3 randomized controlled trials,[45–47] vancomycin or teicoplanin added to parenteral nutrition solution virtually eliminated Gram-positive bacteremia in VLBW neonates. The routine prophylactic administration of these glycopeptides is not recommended, however, because of the high likelihood of developing glycopeptide-resistant organisms.

Fungal infections, previously considered rare in neonates, are now frequently diagnosed.[48–50] *Candida albicans* is implicated in 80–90% of human fungal infections. In neonates, fungal infections secondary to non-albicans species are generally due to *C. parapsilosis, C. lusitaniae* or *C. glabrata*. Non-candidal fungal infections among neonates do not appear to have increased in recent years, with the exception of *Malassezia furfur*,[51, 52] which tends to occur in epidemics. *Candida* is part of the normal flora of the gastrointestinal tract,[53] and antibiotic suppression of bacterial flora can permit *Candida* proliferation and overgrowth. This overgrowth can be associated with tissue invasion and subsequent dissemination. A second factor predisposing neonates to fungal infections is the use of indwelling catheters,[54] which provide a port of entry through an otherwise intact cutaneous barrier. The material delivered to the neonates through such catheters can also predispose to candidal disease. Specifically, fungi may contaminate hypertonic glucose solution or fat emulsions.[55, 56] Prolonged endotracheal intubation and the use of tracheostomies also predispose to fungal sepsis.

Attempts at prophylaxis against fungal infection, using oral nystatin, have had limited success. Sims *et al* administered oral nystatin (100 000 units every 8 hours until 1 week after extubation) to VLBW infants who were at risk for developing systemic candidiasis.[57] The incidence of fungal colonization and infection was significantly lower in the nystatin-treated infants than in controls. The drug of choice for systemic antifungal therapy is amphotericin B, a polyene macrolide antibiotic. The concurrent use of 5-fluorocytosine is frequently, but not consistently, recommended. Both drugs cross the blood–brain barrier.

PUTATIVE NEW AGENTS FOR PREVENTION OR TREATMENT OF INFECTIONS

Despite advances in the potency and spectrum of activity of antibiotics over recent decades, a major impact on mortality has yet to be demonstrated in the treatment of neonates with sepsis. In the last few years, however, advances in investigative immunobiology have allowed a better definition and characterization of the biology of septic syndrome, and have therefore increased the potential for new strategies of treatment, aiming either at correcting developmental immune deficiencies or modulating the inflammatory response.

Intravenous Immunoglobulin

Immunotherapy was a common method of treating infectious diseases in the pre-antibiotic era. 'Serotherapy' and administration of immunoglobulin harvested from various large animals were popular approaches to serious infections but were associated with a significant risk of anaphylaxis and serum sickness. Once antibiotics became available, immunotherapy was limited to specific situations such as rabies, tetanus and hepatitis.

In human neonates, antibody-mediated immunity is derived primarily from maternal immunoglobulin G (IgG) transferred transplacentally. Such transfer begins at 8–10 weeks' gestation, but accelerates during the second half of the last trimester. Significant synthesis of IgG by the neonate generally does not begin until several months after birth. Because of the timing of maternal to fetal transfer of IgG, infants delivered prematurely have a lower endowment of IgG, and this decreases further over their first weeks of life. Their subsequent deficiency in humoral immunity may contribute to their high rate of nosocomial infections.

Opsonic antibody, which enhances phagocytosis and killing of bacteria by neutrophils, is an important component of immunity against encapsulated organisms. Standard intravenous immunoglobulins (IVIG) contain opsonic antibodies toward many such pathogens, including *Escherichia coli, Hemophilus influenzae, Klebsiella pneumoniae, Pseudomonas aeruginosa, Serratia marcenscens, Staph. aureus, Staph. epidermidis*, GBS and *Streptococcus pneumoniae.*[58–60] IVIG may also contain antibodies that neutralize toxins, immunomodulate T cells and macrophages, effect cytokine synthesis, B-cell function and complement activation. Patients with hypogammaglobulinemia can derive significant benefit from IVIG treatment.

Whether preterm neonates are aided by IVIG administration is less clear. Many prospective, randomized, controlled studies have evaluated the effectiveness of IVIG for prophylaxis against neonatal infections, but the results are somewhat conflicting. The largest was a multicenter, controlled trial conducted through the National Institute of Child Health and Human Development Neonatal Research Network.[61] It involved 2416 neonates with birth weights between 501 and 1500 g, who were randomized to receive either placebo or IVIG (Sandoglobulin) beginning in the first 72 hours of life with re-dosing every 14 days until the infant weighed 1800 g or was discharged from the hospital. The IVIG treatment failed significantly to reduce nosocomial infections (septicemia, meningitis or urinary tract infections), which occurred in 17.3% of the IVIG group and 19.5% of the control group. Although the total number of nosocomial infections was not reduced, a *post hoc* analysis of the organism-specific results indicated that IVIG was associated with fewer infections due to GBS.

Two recent meta-analyses have examined the effectiveness of IVIG in the prevention and treatment of neonatal infections.[62] Lacy and Ohlsson identified 19 randomized controlled trials involving premature and/or low birth weight infants and concluded that IVIG resulted in only a very minor reduction in infections. Specifically, the relative risk (and confidence intervals) among IVIG recipients were: for proven infection 0.81 (0.67–0.97); for sepsis 0.87 (0.66–1.13); and for death from all causes 0.85 (0.64–1.14). A subsequent meta-analysis by Jenson and Pollock indicated a statistically significant, although minimal, benefit of IVIG for the prevention of neonatal sepsis.[63] It is noteworthy that in this study the analysis of benefit was limited to the neonatal period, based on the assumption that benefit from IVIG would be more demonstrable during this period than during the entire hospitalization, when the development of nosocomial infections might reflect the contribution of numerous confounding factors. In view of the minimal benefit found in this study, the authors concluded that a cost-effectiveness analysis would be necessary to justify the routine administration of IVIG to preterm infants for prophylaxis against nosocomial infections.

Several explanations have been proposed for the lack of efficacy of IVIG in significantly reducing nosocomial infections among VLBW infants. First, preparations generally have low or undetectable titers of specific antibodies directed against relevant pathogens, such as CONS. In this regard, Fanaroff *et al* found no functional activity against CONS in any of the 4 batches of IVIG used in their trial.[61] Also, immaturity of other essential immune components in VLBW infants (complement, fibronectin and the quality and quantity of neutrophils) still exists despite an elevation in serum IgG concentrations. Thus, perhaps what is needed is a combined approach, involving IVIG containing high concentrations of relevant antibodies, along with administration of factors such as graulocyte colony-stimulating factor (G-CSF) that are aimed at improving multiple aspects of fetal host defense.

Finally, there are a few trials which have examined the ability of IVIG in conjunction with conventional therapy to treat (rather than to prevent) sepsis. Despite multiple variables and small sample sizes, meta-analyses of these studies indicate a benefit from using IVIG in neonates with sepsis.[64]

The administration of IVIG to preterm infants has not been associated with serious adverse effects. The potential exists, however, for transmission of viruses. The preparation process itself should be sufficient to inactivate viruses, including HIV and hepatitis B virus, while hepatitis C appears to be more resistant.[65] The possibility of suppression of immunity on the basis of decreased bacterial clearance, or decreased monocyte and neutrophil phagocytosis, has been postulated but is not a confirmed adverse consequence of IVIG administration to neonates.

Respiratory syncytial virus immune globulin intravenous (RSV-IGIV) has been recently approved by the Food and Drug Administration for use in the prevention of severe RSV lower respiratory tract disease in infants and children younger than 24 months with bronchopulmonary dysplasia (BPD) or a history of premature birth. RSV-IGIV is prepared from donors selected for high titers of RSV-neutralizing antibody and has been shown to be protective in several animal models.[66, 67] In a multicenter, randomized, controlled clinical trial, monthly RSV-IGIV infusions during the period of peak RSV activity in infants with underlying BPD, congenital heart disease or prematurity, resulted in a 65–85% reduction in RSV-associated disease severity and hospitalization.[68] Patients benefiting most were young children with BPD who had received oxygen therapy within the last 6 months and infants without BPD who were <32 weeks' gestation at birth and younger than 6 months at the start of the 'respiratory virus' season. These results have been recently confirmed by a multicenter, randomized, albumin placebo-controlled trial in 510 infants younger than 24 months with BPD and/or prematurity, in whom monthly RSV-IGIV infusions reduced RSV-associated illness frequency and severity by 40–60%.[69] Although clinical trials have demonstrated the efficacy of prophylactic RSV-IGIV, a recent cost-effectiveness analysis indicated that RSV-IGIV prophylaxis of all high-risk infants (FDA-approved indications) is unlikely to produce savings in medical resources but it does result in a favorable cost per year of life saved.[70] Adverse effects with RSV-IGIV are rare and usually consist of mild respiratory distress, fever and rash, and tend to be more severe in patients with cyanotic congenital heart disease. Current recommendations concerning the use of RSV-IGIV are shown in Table 10.1.[71]

In contrast, cytomegalovirus (CMV) immunoglobulin has not proven to be an effective prophylactic strategy. In a randomized, controlled study in multiple transfused premature neonates, administration of CMV immunoglobulin within 24 hours of the first transfusion

Table 10.1 Recommendations for RSV-IGIV prophylaxis.

1. RSV-IGIV should be considered for infants and children < 2 years with BPD who are currently receiving or have received oxygen therapy within the 6 months before the anticipated RSV season.
2. Infants ≤ 32 weeks of gestation without BPD or who do not meet the criteria in recommendation 1.
3. Infants in 1 and 2 who also have asymptomatic acyanotic congenital heart disease.
4. RSV-IGIV prophylaxis should be initiated before the onset of the RSV season and terminated at the end of the RSV season.
5. In infants and children receiving RSV-IGIV prophylaxis (750 mg/kg/dose), immunization with measles-mumps-rubella and varicella vaccines should be deferred for 9 months after the last dose.

Reproduced with permission from American Association of Pediatrics. Respiratory syncytial virus immune globulin intravenous: indications for use. *Pediatrics* 1997;**99**: 645.

and then at 10-day intervals, was associated with an incidence of CMV infection of 9.8% as compared with 11.2% in the placebo group.[72]

Granulocyte Colony-Stimulating Factor

Biology

Clonal maturation of hematopoietic progenitors proceeds under the regulatory influence of certain hematopoietic growth factors and interleukins. *In vitro*, when granulocyte progenitors are cultured in the presence of sufficient quantities of recombinant G-CSF (rG-CSF), colonies containing only neutrophils result.[73] Murine G-CSF was identified and purified by Nicola *et al*[74] and its actions on murine hematopoietic progenitors were first reported by Metcalf and Nicola.[75] In 1985, Nicola *et al* reported using receptor-binding competition and biological studies to demonstrate the presence of a human analog of murine G-CSF.[76] That same year, Welte *et al* purified human G-CSF from the human bladder carcinoma cell line 5637.[77] Two years later, Simmers *et al* reported that the gene encoding human G-CSF was located on the long arm of chromosome 17, band 11.2–21.[78]

G-CSF is a single polypeptide consisting of 207 amino acids, of which 30 constitute the leader sequence. Although the predicted molecular weight is 18 987 Da, the apparent molecular weight is 19 600 Da[79] due to glycosylation. Recombinant G-CSF produced by the bacterium *Escherichia coli* carrying a cDNA encoding the human gene, although not glycosylated, has the same activity as the native factor, with a specific activity of about 1×10^8 U/mg of protein.[79]

G-CSF is produced primarily by monocytes and macrophages, but it can also be generated by fibroblasts and endothelial cells.[80] Its actions include supporting the maturation of committed neutrophil progenitors, granulocyte colony-forming units (CFU-G), into clones of neutrophils; release of neutrophils from the bone marrow neutrophil storage pool into the blood; and up-regulation of neutrophil functions.[81] Specific neutrophil functions that increase after G-CSF exposure are chemotaxis, superoxide generation, phagocytosis and microbial killing.[80]

Administration of rG-CSF over a range of 1–500 μg/kg to normal adult animals or humans results in a dose-dependent increase in blood neutrophil concentrations.[82] With administration of high doses (>50 μg/kg), a transient neutropenia, due to margination, is observed for 10–40 min.[83] Following recovery from the neutropenia, a dose-dependent neutrophilia is observed, which is the kinetic result of release of neutrophils from the marrow neutrophil reserve. In healthy adult volunteers, single doses of 40 μg/kg resulted in a 4–5-fold increase in blood neutrophil concentration, with a return to the baseline values after about 48 hours.[84] In neutropenic patients, rG-CSF administration generally also results in a dose-proportional increase in blood neutrophils. In phase I/II trials in patients with cancer, myelodysplasia and congenital agranulocytosis, rG-CSF has resulted in elevations in blood neutrophils and diminutions in bacterial infections.[85, 86]

A number of observations suggest that G-CSF is not absolutely specific for neutrophil production. For instance, Lord *et al* observed that administration of very high doses of rG-CSF to mice produced an increase in circulating concentrations of monocytes as well as neutrophils.[87] Ikebucci *et al* reported that rG-CSF acts synergistically with interleukin (IL)-3 to shorten the G_0 period of multipotent progenitors, resulting in a faster emergence of these colonies in culture.[88] Duhrsen *et al* noted that following administration of rG-CSF, progenitors of all lineages were released into the circulation.[89]

The role of G-CSF in normal physiology was further defined by Lieschke *et al*, who produced a strain of mice that lacked G-CSF.[90] This was accomplished by targeted disruption of the G-CSF gene in embryonal stem cells. The G-CSF-deficient mice were viable, fertile and generally healthy, but had blood neutrophil concentrations of only about 20% that of normal mice. G-CSF-deficient mice also had significantly reduced macrophage progenitors, reduced numbers of circulating monocytes, and a reduced number of multipotent progenitors. Most strikingly, G-CSF-deficient mice failed to increase neutrophil production following infectious challenge or to show neutrophilia following infectious challenge, and had a very high susceptibility to death from infection. These defects could be experimentally remedied by the administration of rG-CSF.[90]

In otherwise normal mice made neutropenic by irradiation or administration of cytotoxic drugs, the administration of rG-CSF increases resistance to microbes such as *Pseudomonas* and *Candida*.[91] Similarly, primates show an increase in resistance to infection following administration of rG-CSF.[92] Humans who have received rG-CSF after anti-cancer treatment have higher blood neutrophil concentrations and fewer days of infection.[93, 94] rG-CSF has little dose-limiting toxicity, with reported adverse effects being mild and including rash, fever and discomfort from bones containing hematopoietic tissue.[95]

From the collective human and animal experiments, it appears that G-CSF is indeed the primary physiologic regulator of neutrophil production, although it is clearly not the only factor capable of this. It appears to be indispensable, however, for maintaining the normal steady-state production of neutrophils, and is important in rapid generation of neutrophils and their release from the neutrophil storage pool during infection.

Production by fetal/neonatal tissues

Using a specific ELISA, Cairo *et al* quantified G-CSF protein in the supernatants of unstimulated and stimulated mononuclear cells obtained from the blood of adults *vs* umbilical cord blood of term infants.[96] Supernatants of unstimulated cells contained undetectable quantities of G-CSF (< 50 pg/ml). Following stimulation, however, supernatants of adult cells contained significantly more G-CSF protein than did those of cord blood cells. Densitometry of Northern blots also revealed more G-CSF mRNA transcripts in adult than cord-blood mononuclear cells. The calculated number of G-CSF-binding sites per mature neutrophil, and their affinity for rG-CSF, were equal between cells obtained from adults and cord blood.

Schibler *et al*[97] observed that monocytes isolated from the blood of preterm infants generated less G-CSF protein *in vitro*, following stimulation with either lipopolysaccharide (LPS) or IL-1α. Other studies by Schibler *et al*[97] suggested that this relatively poor production of G-CSF by monocytes of preterm neonates was not counterbalanced by a heightened sensitivity of their G-CSF-responsive progenitors. In fact, the dose–response relationship was the same using progenitors from adults, term and preterm neonates. On the basis of the combined studies, they speculated that generation of comparatively low quantities of G-CSF by infected premature infants might partly explain their defective up-regulation of neutrophil production and function during infection.

English *et al*[98] stimulated leukocytes from neonates and adults with a variety of agonists, and assessed quantities of granulocyte/macrophage (GM)-CSF, G-CSF and M-CSF transcripts. Mononuclear cells from neonates accumulated only about 30% as much GM-CSF mRNA as did adult cells. Diminished GM-CSF production by mononuclear cells appeared to reflect decreased production by neonatal T lymphocytes. In fact, the accumulation of GM-CSF mRNA in monocytes of neonates and adults were similar, whereas neonatal T cells produced only ~25–50% as much GM-CSF mRNA and protein as did adult cells. The stimulated mononuclear cells, and purified monocytes, from neonates accumulated about the same concentrations of G-CSF mRNA as did those from adults. Using nuclear run-on assays, Lee *et al*[99] inferred that the decreased G-CSF protein production by fetal mononuclear cells was due to post-transcriptional instability as opposed to diminished G-CSF transcription.

Li *et al* have shown the placenta to be a significant potential source of G-CSF. Although the normal placenta, *in utero*, does not appear to produce large quantities of G-CSF, it has a tremendous capacity to do so.[100] Stimulation with bacterial endotoxin, IL-1 or other agonists, results in the production of marked quantitites of G-CSF. Similarly, chorioamnionitis is associated with placental G-CSF production and increased G-CSF concentrations in maternal and fetal serum.[101]

Blood concentrations in the perinatal period

The first report of umbilical cord blood concentrations of G-CSF was by Laver *et al.*[102] Precise quantification of the concentrations were not possible at that time, and a biological assay was employed. Nevertheless, it appeared that G-CSF concentrations in umbilical cord blood were significantly higher than in the blood of healthy adults. The first report of blood G-CSF concentrations in neonates using a specific ELISA was by Shimoda *et al,*[103] who quantified G-CSF in the umbilical cord blood of 59 term neonates; G-CSF was detected in only 10 (lower limit of detectability was 20 pg/ml). The detectable concentrations ranged between 20 and 57 pg/ml. No relationship was observed between the G-CSF concentration and the blood neutrophil concentration.

The first report of umbilical cord blood G-CSF concentrations from preterm infants was by Schibler *et al,*[97] who showed that in non-neutropenic neonates, serum G-CSF concentration were relatively low (92±34 pg/ml in 10 preterm neonates, 114±21 pg/ml in 16 term neonates, and 45 ± 12 pg/ml in 11 healthy adults). Serum G-CSF concentrations were markedly elevated in 8 neutropenic adults (2101±942 pg/ml) but were not in 7 neutropenic neonates (39±17 pg/ml). Cairo *et al* found that G-CSF concentration were somewhat higher in the umbilical cord blood of preterm than in term infants or adults, but found no differences in blood concentrations between umbilical cord blood and the blood from pregnant women in the third trimester.[81]

Gessler *et al* reported consecutively obtained serum G-CSF concentrations in term and preterm infants.[104] G-CSF in healthy infants peaked 7 hours after birth, followed by an increase in blood neutrophil concentrations. Neonates with signs of infection had higher G-CSF serum concentrations (mean 1300 pg/ml) than healthy neonates (170 pg/ml), although their concentrations were lower than reported in infected adults. Similar findings were reported in 613 neonates by Ikeno.[105] In 322 healthy neonates, G-CSF serum concentrations correlated with gestational age and blood neutrophil concentration; 95% of healthy term neonates had G-CSF concentrations of <100 pg/ml. Higher concentrations were observed in those with infections, fetal distress, premature rupture of membranes and asphyxia. Neonates with high G-CSF concentrations had high blood neutrophil counts. Russell *et al*[106] did not observe a correlation between serum G-CSF and gestational age, nor a correlation between serum G-CSF and blood neutrophil count. However, they agreed with Gessler *et al* and Ikeno that babies with suspected infection had higher serum G-CSF concentrations (mean 3100 pg/ml) than did healthy neonates (mean 32 pg/ml).

Paired samples of umbilical cord blood and maternal blood were reported by Bailie *et al*, who observed no association between the two.[107] Also, as with the report of Russell *et al*, no association was observed between blood neutrophil count and G-CSF concentration. Concordant with most other reports, Wilimas *et al* found that G-CSF concentrations were higher in neonates than in healthy adults, and that levels in preterm infants were somewhat higher than in term infants.[108]

In summary, term and preterm infants clearly are capable of generating G-CSF, and at the time of delivery they generally have serum G-CSF concentrations somewhat higher than healthy adults. During bacterial infections in newborn infants, serum G-CSF concentration certainly increases, but probably not to the concentrations achieved during infection in adults.

Addition to the treatment regimen of subjects with bacterial sepsis

Certain groups of patients who develop bacterial sepsis are at very high risk for death. These groups include those with underlying defects in antibacterial host defense, such as quantitative or qualitative defects in phagocytic immunity. Studies in experimental animals and clinical trials in humans have tested the hypothesis that inclusion of rG-CSF in the treatment regimen for bacterial sepsis will have a favorable risk/benefit ratio.

Animal studies. Cairo *et al* conducted several experiments in which rG-CSF was administered to newborn rat pups to determine whether it improved their capacity to withstand inoculation with group B streptococci.[109–112] A single dose of rG-CSF given to 1-day-old pups resulted in neutrophilia and a reduction in mortality following bacterial inoculation. The combination of rG-CSF and stem cell factor, or rG-CSF and IL-11, resulted in higher blood and bone marrow neutrophil concentrations, and better antibacterial resistance, than did G-CSF alone.

Smith *et al* inoculated 160 adult rabbits intratracheally with *Pasturella multocida.*[113] Twenty-four hours later treatment was begun with penicillin G and either rG-CSF (5–8 μg/kg/day for 5 days) or placebo injections (on the same schedule). Twenty-four parameters of organ function were serially followed, and all animals underwent histologic examination at the time of septic death, or when sacrificed on study day 6. Treatment with rG-CSF was associated with higher leukocyte concentrations by day 4, improved survival, and significantly increased inflammation in the liver, spleen and non-inoculated lung. No clinically-evident toxic effects occurred. The authors concluded that clinical trials of rG-CSF treatment in patients with septic shock and leukopenia were warranted.

Eichacher *et al* infected 54 2-year-old beagles with *Escherichia coli.*[114] Beginning 9 days before the inoculation, animals received 12 daily doses of G-CSF (5 μg/kg or 0.1 μg/kg) or a control. Survival was greater in the high-dose G-CSF group (14/17) than in the low-dose group (10/17) and controls (12/20). The high-dose G-CSF group also had better left ventricular ejection fractions, higher blood pressures and blood neutrophil concentrations, and lower serum endotoxin, tumor necrosis factor concentrations and blood bacterial counts.

Another potential method for diminishing the severity and sequelae of early-onset infection was investigated by Medlock *et al*[115] and Novales *et al*[116] using a pregnant rat model. They observed that a single dose (50 μg/kg) of recombinant G-CSF given to pregnant rats 1 day before delivery resulted in maternal and fetal peak G-CSF serum concentrations of 1200 ng/ml and 1.5 ng/ml, respectively. Despite the relatively low apparent transplacental passage, this concentration of G-CSF in the fetal rats was significantly elevated above the normal (undetectable) concentrations. Moreover, the increase in G-CSF concentrations was sufficient to stimulate neutrophil production, elevate blood neutrophil concentrations, and improve the outcome of the pups who were subsequently inoculated with group B β-hemolytic streptococci.

Human trials. Human trials of rG-CSF treatment of human neonates, to date, have sought answers to 3 experimental questions:

The first question is: *Will administration of rG-CSF to human neonates result in an elevated blood neutrophil concentration?* The first report of rG-CSF administration to a human neonate was by Roberts *et al.*[117] They described a 654 g small for gestational age infant delivered at 30 weeks' gestation by emergency cesarean section due to severe maternal hypertension. The infant was persistently neutropenic, and during the stay in the NICU developed 5 separate episodes of sepsis. Daily administration of rG-CSF, 10 μg/kg/day, resulted in neutrophilia. The dose was reduced, and then discontinued, and no further episodes of neutropenia or infection were observed over the next 7 months.

Gillan *et al*[118] randomized 42 newborn infants with suspected sepsis to three days of treatment, consisting of either placebo, 1, 5, or 10 μg rG-CSF/kg/day, or 5 vs 10 μg rG-CSF/kg every 12 hours (10 μg or 20 μg/kg/day). Twenty-four hours following a dose of ≥5 μg/kg/day circulating neutrophil concentrations were higher than the placebo recipients. A dose-dependent increase in blood neutrophils, bone marrow neutrophils, neutrophil C3bi expression, and marrow neutrophil progenitors were observed. The rG-CSF appeared to be well tolerated in all subjects.

Gilmore *et al* reported 2 neonates with alloimmune neutropenia who received 3–6 daily doses of G-CSF.[119] Their blood neutrophil concentration increased from 350 and 477/mm^3, respectively, to 3584 and 4320/mm^3 within 4 days. The counts remained elevated and the authors recommended rG-CSF treatment of neonates with alloimmune neutropenia.

La Gamma *et al* administered rG-CSF for 3 consecutive days to 9 preterm neonates who had neutropenia for >72 hours in association with severe maternal pregnancy-induced hypertension.[120] Absolute neutrophil counts increased nearly 4-fold within 48 hours with no obvious adverse effects. Makhlouf *et al*[121] treated 9 preterm infants, born to pre-eclamptic mothers, with 3 daily doses of rG-CSF (10 μg/kg) beginning within 24 hours of birth. Absolute neutrophil counts increased significantly in 8 within 6 hours of administration with no obvious adverse effect. Russell *et al* administered rG-CSF to 12 neutropenic preterm infants and all had a subsequent increase in blood neutrophil concentration.[122] Thus, administration of rG-CSF to newborn infants has similar effects on neutrophil production, function, pool sizes and blood concentrations to those in adults. Moreover, it appears that neonates with a variety of neutropenias experience an elevation in blood neutrophil concentration following administration of doses of as low as 5 μg/kg/day for 2–3 days.

The second question is: *Will administration of rG-CSF to women about to deliver an extremely preterm neonate cross from the maternal to the fetal circulation and induce granulocytopoiesis and elevated blood neutrophil concentrations in the fetus?* Calhoun *et al* performed a Phase I study to answer this question.[123] Twenty-two women about to deliver at <30 weeks' gestation were either given a 1 dose of G-CSF (25 μg/kg) or no such treatment. Twelve neonates were delivered to the 11 women given rG-CSF, of whom 10 were delivered within 30 hours (mean ± SD 10.8±8.9) of the G-CSF administration ('early delivery'), and 2 delivered after 54 and 108 hours, respectively. In the 'early delivery' group, maternal G-CSF concentrations and blood neutrophils were higher than in controls. However, no difference was seen in the cord blood neutrophil concentrations. In the 'late delivery group', although maternal serum and cord blood G-CSF concentrations were no different from controls, cord blood neutrophils were higher (25 900 and 17 700/μl) than in controls (3500±2000/μl; $p < 0.05$) and remained elevated for 1 week. Thus, administration of recombinant G-CSF to pregnant women with an imminent preterm delivery may result in transplacental passage of a measurable quantity of G-CSF, and this amount can have a biological effect on the fetus if the G-CSF is given at least 30 hours prior to the delivery. The hypothesis that maternal treatment with rG-CSF before preterm delivery will improve the neonatal outcome is now being tested.

The third question is: *What are the risks and benefits of treating neutropenic neonates with rG-CSF?* Initial clinical trials simply tested the hypothesis that rG-CSF increases blood neutrophil concentrations in neonates. Neonates with neutropenia and those with presumed bacterial infection were the subjects of these reports. Murray *et al*[124] used rG-CSF, with apparent success, to treat neonates with bacterial sepsis. However, to date, no placebo-controlled, randomized, controlled trials have tested the hypothesis that rG-CSF improves the outcome of human neonates with early-onset bacterial sepsis and no trials have been published that test the hypothesis that it improves the outcome of neonates with neutropenia secondary to maternal hypertension, necrotizing enterocolitis or late-onset bacterial sepsis. Thus, it is on the basis of animal studies, case reports and phase I clinical trials that rG-CSF is beginning to be used in many NICUs as an adjunct to the treatment of bacterial infections. Indeed, the promptness with which rG-CSF administration effects an increase in blood neutrophil concentration in many varieties of neonatal neutropenia is encouraging. Although adverse effects of rG-CSF treatment have not yet been described in neonates, it is prudent to await the results of phase III trials before rG-

CSF treatment becomes routine clinical practice in the treatment of infections in newborn infants.

Other Potential Adjuncts to Treatment

The pathogenesis of sepsis involves activation of several endogenous mediators. Lipopolysaccharide (LPS) in the outer cell wall of Gram-negative micro-organisms may be sufficient for several of the systemic manifestations of sepsis. Because of this, monoclonal IgM antibodies have been developed that bind the lipid A portion of LPS, and subsequently increase its phagocytosis and intravascular clearance. Results of 2 large clinical trials in adults, employing monoclonal antibodies directed against lipid A, showed a significant reduction in mortality. However, any benefit of this treatment would be limited to the subset of patients who have Gram-negative sepsis with organisms that possess a lipid A portion of LPS.[125, 126]

Other potential therapies for sepsis involve inhibitors of nitric oxide (NO), such as N^G-L-amino-arginine (L-NAME). Like other endogenous mediators of septic shock, NO has the potential both to protect and to harm the host. NO is a mediator with an important role in normal vascular homeostasis. Excess synthesis of NO has been proposed to mediate some of the vascular abnormalities noted during sepsis, therefore inhibition of its synthesis might be beneficial in this condition. In an *in vivo* adult rat model, Thiermann and Vane reported that L-NAME attenuated the hypotension induced by LPS administration.[127] In adult dogs, the hypotension induced by tumor necrosis factor administration was reversed by L-NAME administration.[128] In contrast, in animal models of GBS neonatal sepsis, infusion of L-NAME has been associated with detrimental hemodynamic effects.[129, 130] These conflicting results of the benefit of NO inhibitors in adult but not newborn animals may be due to differences between neonates and adults in the pathophysiology of septic shock. In neonates septic shock is more frequently accompanied by increased systemic and pulmonary vascular resistances, increased oxygen extraction and reduced systemic blood flow. Thus, the administration of a vasoconstrictor such as L-NAME can have serious hemodynamic consequences. Methylene blue, a soluble guanylate cyclase inhibitor, could provide an alternative to L-NAME for newborn infants. This approach has recently been used by Driscoll *et al* in 5 neonates with presumed septic shock. Methylene blue was given at a dose of 1 mg/kg during a 1-hour period.[131] After methylene blue infusion, blood pressure increased significantly in all patients and 3 were weaned from inotropic support within 72 hours. Although encouraging, these results need to be confirmed.

REFERENCES

1. Stoll BJ, Gordon T, Korones SB *et al.* Late-onset sepsis in very low birth weight neonates: A report from the National Institute of Child Health and Human Development Neonatal Research Network. *J Pediatr* 1996;**129**: 63.
2. Stoll BJ, Gordon T, Korones SB *et al.* Early-onset sepsis in very low birth weight neonates: A report from the National Institute of Child Health and Human Development Neonatal Research Network. *J Pediatr* 1996;**129**: 72.
3. Linder N, Ohel G, Gazit G, Keidar D, Tamir I and Reichman B. Neonatal sepsis after prolonged premature rupture of membranes. *J Perinatol* 1995;**15**: 6.
4. Svensson L, Ingemarsson I and Mardh PA. Chorioamnionitis and the isolation of microorganism from the placenta. *Obstet Gynecol* 1986;**67**: 403.
5. Raghavan M, Mondal GP, Bath BV and Srinivasav S. Perinatal risk factors in neonatal infections. *Ind J Pediatr* 1992;**59**: 35.
6. Hillier SL, Martius J, Krohn M, Kiviat N, Holmes KK and Eschenbach DA. A case-control study of chorioamnionic infection and histologic chorioamnionitis in prematurity. *N Engl J Med* 1978;**319**: 972.
7. Cassell GH, Waites KB, Gibbs RS and Davis JK. Role of *Ureaplasma urealyticum* in amnionitis. *Pediatr Infect Dis* 1986; **5(Suppl 6)**: S247.
8. Romero R and Mazor M. Infection and preterm labor. *Clin Obstet Gynecol* 1988;**31**: 553–584.
9. Galask RP, Varner MW, Petztold CR and Wilbur SL. Bacterial attachment to the chorioamniotic membranes. *Am J Obstet Gynecol* 1984;**148**: 915.
10. Romero R, Sibai B, Caritis S *et al.* Antibiotic treatment of preterm labor with intact membranes: a multicenter, randomized, double-blinded, placebo-controlled trial. *Am J Obstet Gynecol* 1993;**169**: 764.
11. Mercer BM and Arheart KL. Antimicrobial therapy in expectant management of preterm premature rupture of the membranes. *Lancet* 1995;**346**: 1271.
12. Egarter C, Leitich H, Karashwiesrf H, Husslein P, Kaider A and Schemper M. Antibiotic treatment in preterm premature rupture of membranes and neonatal morbidity: a meta-analysis. *Am J Obstet Gynecol* 1996;**174**: 589.
13. Steigman AJ, Bottone EJ and Hanna BA. Does intramuscular penicillin at delivery prevent group B beta hemolytic streptococcal disease of the newborn infant? (letter). *J Pediatr* 1975;**87**: 496.
14. American Academy of Pediatrics Committee on Infectious Diseases and Committee on Fetus and Newborn. Guidelines for prevention of group B streptococcal infection by chemoprophylaxis. *Pediatrics* 1992;**90**: 775.
15. American Academy of Pediatrics Committee on Infectious Diseases and Committee on Fetus and Newborn. Revised guidelines for prevention of early-onset group B streptococcal (GBS) infection. *Pediatrics* 1997;**99**: 489.
16. Tafari N, Ross S, Naeye RL, Judge DM and Marboe C. Mycoplasma 'T' strains and perinatal death. *Lancet* 1976;**i**: 108.
17. Cassell GH, Crouse DT, Waites KB, Rudd PT and Davis JK. Does *Ureaplasma urealyticum* cause respiratory disease in newborns? *Pediatr Infect Dis J* 1988;**7**: 535.

18. Waites KB, Crouse DT, Philips JB, Canupp KC and Cassell GH. Ureaplasma pneumonia and sepsis associated with persistent pulmonary hypertension of the newborn. *Pediatrics* 1989;**83**: 84.
19. Cassell GH, Waites KB, Crouse DT *et al.* Association of *Ureaplasma urealyticum* infection of the lower respiratory tract with chronic lung disease and death in very low birthweight infants. *Lancet* 1988;**ii**: 240.
20. Waites KB, Rudd PT, Crouse DT *et al.* Chronic *Ureaplasma urealyticum* and *Mycoplasma hominis* infection of central nervous system in preterm infants. *Lancet* 1988;**i**: 17.
21. Gardland S and Murton LJ. Neonatal meningitis caused by *Ureaplasma urealyticum. Pediatr Infect Dis* 1987;**6**: 868.
22. Sanchez PJ and Regan JA. Vertical transmission of *Ureaplasma urealyticum* in full term infants. *Pediatr Infect Dis J* 1987;**6**: 825.
23. Sanchez PJ. Perinatal transmission of *Ureaplasma urealyticum*: current concepts based on review of the literature. *Clin Infect Dis* 1993; **17 (Suppl 1)**: S107.
24. Sanchez PJ and Regan JA. Vertical transmission of *Ureaplasma urealyticum* from mothers to preterm infants. *Pediatr Infect Dis J* 1990;**9**: 398.
25. McCormack WM, Rosner B, Lee YH, Munoz A, Charles D and Kass EH. Effect on birth weight of erythromycin treatment of pregnant women. *Obstet Gynecol* 1987;**69**: 202.
26. Mercer BM, Moretti ML, Prevost RR and Sibai BM. Erythromycin therapy in preterm premature rupture of the membranes: a prospective, randomized trial of 220 patients. *Am J Obstet Gynecol* 1992;**166**: 794.
27. Walsh WF, Stanley S, Lally KP *et al. Ureaplasma urealyticum* demonstrated by open lung biopsy in newborns with chronic lung disease. *Pediatr Infect Dis J* 1991;**10**: 823.
28. Waites KB, Sims PJ, Crouse DT *et al.* Serum concentrations of erythromycin after intravenous infusion in preterm neonates treated for *Ureaplasma urealyticum* infection. *Pediatr Infect Dis J* 1994;**13**: 287.
29. Hentschel J, Abele HM and Peters J. *Ureaplasma urealyticum* in the cerebrospinal fluid of a premature infant. *Acta Paediatr* 1993;**82**: 690.
30. Senterfit LB. Antibiotic susceptibility testing of mycoplasmas. In: Tully JG and Razin S (eds) *Methods in Mycoplasmology*, vol 2. New York: Academic Press, 1983, pp 397–401.
31. Cummings MC and McCormack WM. Increased resistance of *Mycoplasma hominis* to tetracyclines. *Antimicrob Agents Chemother* 1990;**34**: 2297.
32. Taylor-Robinson D and Furr PM. Clinical antibiotic resistance of *Ureaplasma urealyticum. Pediatr Infect Dis J* 1986;5: S335.
33. Centers for Disease Control and Prevention. Nosocomial infections surveillance, 1984. *MMWR CDC Surveill Summ* 1986;**35(1SS)**: 17.
34. Gaynes RP, Edwards JR, Jarvis WR, Culver DH, Tolson JS, Martone WJ. Nosocomial infections among neonates in high-risk nurseries in the United States. *Pediatrics* 1996;**98**: 357.
35. Leyden JJ. Bacteriology of the newborn skin. In: Maibach H and Boisits EK (eds) *Neonatal Skin: Structure and Function*. New York, Marcel Dekker, 1982, p 167.

36. D'Angio CT, McGowan KL, Baumgart S, St Geme J and Harris MC. Surface colonization with coagulase negative staphylococci in premature neonates. *J Pediatr* 1989;**114**: 1029.
37. Davies AJ, Ward-Platt M, Kirk R, Marshall R, Speidel BD and Reeves DS . Is coagulase negative staphylococcal bacteremia in neonates a consequence of mechanical ventilation? *J Hosp Infect* 1984; 260.
38. Low DE, Schmidt BK, Kirpalani HM *et al.* An endemic strain of *Staphylococcus haemolyticus* colonizing and causing bacteremia in neonatal intensive care unit patients. *Pediatrics* 1992;**89**: 696.
39. Neumeister B, Kastner S, Conrad S, Klotz G and Bartmann P. Characterization of coagulase-negative staphylococci causing nosocomial infections in preterm infants. *Eur J Clin Microbiol Infect Dis* 1995;**14**: 856.
40. Charbonneau P, Harding I, Garaud JJ, Aubertin J, Brinet F and Dormat Y. Teicoplanin: a well-tolerated and easily administered alternative to vancomycin for gram-positive infections in intensive care patients. *Intensive Care Med* 1994;**20 (Suppl 4)**: S35.
41. De Lalla F and Tramarin A. A risk benefit assessment of teicoplanin in the treatment of infections. *Drug Safety* 1995;**13**: 17.
42. Parenti F. Structure and mechanism of action of teicoplanin. *J Hosp Infect* 1986; **7 (Suppl A)**: 79.
43. Cormican MG and Jones RN. Emerging resistance to antimicrobial agents in gram-positive bacteria. *Drugs* 1996;**51 (Suppl 1)**: 6.
44. O'Hare MD and Reynolds PE. Novel membrane proteins present in teicoplanin-resistant, vancomycin-sensitive, coagulase-negative *Staphylococcus* spp. *J Antimicrob Agents Chemother* 1992;**30**: 753.
45. Kacica MA, Horgan MJ, Ochoa L, Sandler R, Lepow ML and Venezia RA. Prevention of gram-positive sepsis in neonates weighing less than 1500 grams. *J Pediatr* 1994;**125**: 253.
46. Spafford PS, Sinkin RA, Cox C, Reubens L and Powell KR. Prevention of central venous catheter-related coagulase-negative staphylococcal sepsis in neonates. *J Pediatr* 1994;**125**: 259.
47. Moller JC, Nelskamp I, Jensen R, Gatermann S, Iven H and Gortner L. Teicoplanin pharmacology in prophylaxis for coagulase-negative staphylococcal sepsis of very low birthweight infants (letter). *Acta Paediatr* 1996;**85**: 638.
48. Butler KM and Baker CJ. Candida: An increasingly important pathogen in the nursery. *Pediatr Clin North Am* 1988;**35**: 543.
49. Baley JE, Kliegman RM, Annable WL, Dahms BB and Fanaroff AA. *Torupolopsis glabrata* sepsis appearing as necrotizing enterocolitis and endophthalmitis. *Am J Dis Child* 1984;**138**: 965.
50. Sanchez PJ and Cooper BH. *Candida lusitaniae*: Sepsis and meningitis in a neonate. *Pediatr Infect Dis J* 1987;**6**: 758.
51. Long JC and Keyserling HL. Catheter-related infection in infants due to an unusual lipophilic yeast – *Malassezia furfur*. *Pediatrics* 1985;**76**: 896.
52. Powell DA, Aungst J, Snedden S, Hanzen N and Brady M. Broviac catheter-related *Malassezia furfur* sepsis in five infants receiving intravenous fat emulsions. *J Pediatr* 1984;**105**: 987.

53. Ekenna O and Sheretz RJ. Factors affecting colonization and dissemination of *Candida albicans* from the gastrointestinal tract of mice. *Infect Immun* 1987;**55**: 1558.
54. Moise A, Landers S and Fraley K. Colonization and infection of umbilical catheters in newborn infants. *Pediatr Res* 1986;**20**: 1436 A.
55. Freeman JB, Lemire A and Maclean LD. Intravenous alimentation and septicemia. *Surg Gynecol Obstet* 1972;**135**: 708.
56. Curry CR and Quie PG. Fungal septicemia in patients receiving parenteral hyperalimentation. *N Engl J Med* 1971;**285**: 1221.
57. Sims ME, Yoo Y, You H, Salminen C and Walther FJ. Prophylactic oral nystatin and fungal infections in very-low-birthweight infants. *Am J Perinatol* 1988;**5**: 33.
58. Fischer GW, Wilson SR and Hunter KW. Functional characteristics of a modified immunoglobulin preparation for intravenous administration: summary of studies of opsonic and protective activity against group B streptococci. *J Clin Immunol* 1982;**2 (Suppl)**: 31S.
59. Hill HR, Augustine NH, Shigeoka AO. Comparative opsonic activity of intravenous gamma globulin preparations for common bacterial pathogens. *Am J Med* 1984;**76 (Suppl)**: 61.
60. Cryz SJ, Cross AS, Furer E, Chariatte N, Sadoff JC, Germanier R. Activity of intravenous immune globulins against Klebsiella. *J Lab Clin Med* 1986;**108**: 182.
61. Fanaroff AA, Korones SB, Wright LL *et al.* A controlled trial of intravenous immune globulin to reduce nosocomial infections in very-low-birth-weight infants. *N Engl J Med* 1994;**330**: 1107.
62. Lacy JB and Ohlsson A. Administration of intravenous immunoglobulins for prophylaxis or treatment of infection in preterm infants: meta-analyses. *Arch Dis Child* 1995;**72**: F151.
63. Jenson HB and Pollock BH. Meta-analyses of the effectiveness of intravenous immune globulin for prevention and treatment of neonatal sepsis. *Pediatrics* 1997;**99**: E2.
64. Baley JE and Fanaroff AA. Neonatal infections, Part 2: Specific infectious diseases and therapies. In: Sincler J and Bracken MB (eds) *Effective Care of the Newborn Infant*. Oxford: Oxford University Press, 1992, p 496.
65. Kliegman R, Clapp DW and Berger M. Targeted immunoglobulin therapy for the prevention of neonatal infections. *Rev Infect Dis* 1990;**12**: S443.
66. Siber GR, Leombruno D, Leszczynski *et al.* Comparison of antibody concentrations and protective activity of respiratory syncytial virus immune globulin and conventional immune globulin. *J Infect Dis* 1994;**169**: 1368.
67. Siber GR, Leszczynski J, Pena-Cruz V *et al.* Protective activity of human respiratory syncytial virus immune globulin prepared from donors screened by microneutralization assay. *J Infect Dis* 1992;**165**: 456.
68. Groothuis JR, Simoes EAF, Levin MJ, RSVIG Study Group. Prophylactic administration of respiratory syncitial virus immune globulin to high-risk infants and young children. *N Engl J Med* 1993;**329**: 1524.

69. Connor E, PREVENT Study Group. Reduction of RSV hospitalization among premature infants and infants with bronchopulmonary dysplasia using respiratory syncytial virus immune globulin prophylaxis. *Pediatrics* 1997;**99**: 93.
70. Hay JW, Hernest RL and Meissner HC. Respiratory syncytial virus immune globulin: a cost-effectiveness analysis. *Am J Managed Care* 1996: **2**: 851.
71. American Association of Pediatrics. Respiratory syncitial virus immune globulin intravenous: indications for use. *Pediatrics* 1997;**99**: 645.
72. Snydman DR, Werner BG, Meissner HC *et al.* Use of cytomegalovirus immunoglobulin in multiply transfused premature neonates. *Pediatr Infect Dis J* 1995;**14**: 34.
73. Demetri GD and Griffin JD. Granulocyte colony-stimulating factor and its receptor. *Blood* 1991;**78**: 2791.
74. Nicola NA, Metcalf D, Matsumoto M and Johnson GR. Purification of a factor inducing differentiation in murine myelomonocytic leukemia cells: identification as granulocyte colony-stimulating factor (G-CSF). *J Biol Chem* 1983;**258**: 9017.
75. Metcalf D and Nicola NA. Proliferation effects of purified granulocyte colony-stimulating factor (G-CSF) on normal mouse haematopoietic cells. *J Cell Physiol* 1983;**116**: 198.
76. Nicola NA, Begley CG and Metcalf D. Identification of the human analogue of a regulator that induces differentiation in murine leukaemic cells. *Nature* 1985;**314**: 125.
77. Welte K, Platzer E, Lu L *et al.* Purification and biochemical characterization for human pluripotent hematopoietic colony-stimulating factor. *Proc Natl Acad Sci USA* 1985;**82**: 1526.
78. Simmers RN, Webber LM, Shannon MF *et al.* Location of the G-CSF gene on chromosome 17 proximal to the breakpoint in the t(15;17) in acute promyelocytic leukemia. *Blood* 1987;**70**: 330.
79. Souza LM, Boone TC, Gabrilove J *et al.* Recombinant human granulocyte colony-stimulating factor: effects on normal and leukemic myeloid cells. *Science* 1986;**232**: 61.
80. Weisbart RH. Colony-stimulating factors and host defense. *Ann Intern Med* 1989;**110**: 297.
81. Cairo MS. Review of G-CSF and GM-CSF effects on neonatal neutrophil kinetics. *Am J Pediatr Hematol Oncol* 1989;**11**: 238.
82. Pojda Z, Molineux G and Dexter TM. Hemopoietic effects of short-term *in vivo* treatment of mice with various doses of rhG-CSF. *Exp Hematol* 1990;**18**: 27.
83. Okada Y, Kawagishi M and Kusaka M. Neutrophil kinetics of recombinant human granulocyte colony-stimulating factor-induced neutropenia in rats. *Life Sci* 1990;**47**: 65.
84. Welte K, Bonilla MA, Gillo AP *et al.* Recombinant human granulocyte colony-stimulating factor. *J Exp Med* 1987;**165**: 941.
85. Morstyn G, Souza LM, Keech J *et al.* Effect of granulocyte colony-stimulating factor on neutropenia induced by cytotoxic chemotherapy. *Lancet* 1988;**i**: 667.

86. Gabrilove JL, Jakubowski A, Scher H *et al.* Effect of granulocyte colony-stimulating factor on neutropenia and associated morbidity due to chemotherapy for transitional-cell carcinoma of the urothelium. *N Engl J Med* 1988;**318**: 1414.
87. Lord BI, Molineux G, Pojda Z, Souza LM, Merjod J-J, Dexter TM. Myeloid cell kinetics in mice treated with recombinant interleukin-3, granulocyte-colony-stimulating factor (CSF) or granulocyte-macrophage CSF *in vivo*. *Blood* 1991;**77**: 2154.
88. Ikebuchi K, Clark SC, Ihle JN *et al.* Granulocyte colony-stimulating factor enhances interleukin-3-dependent proliferation of multipotential hematopoietic progenitors. *Proc Natl Acad Sci USA* 1988;**85**: 3445.
89. Duhrsen U, Villeval J-L, Boyd J, Kannourakis G, Morstyn G and Metcalf D. Effects of recombinant human granulocyte colony-stimulating factor on hematopoietic progenitor cells in cancer patients. *Blood* 1994;**72**: 2074.
90. Lieschke GJ, Grail D, Hodgson G *et al.* Mice lacking granulocyte colony-stimulating factor have chronic neutropenia, granulocyte and macrophage progenitor cell deficiency, and impaired neutrophil mobilization. *Blood* 1994;**84**: 1737.
91. Matsumoto M, Matsubara S, Matsuno T *et al.* Protective effect of human colony-stimulating factor on microbial infection in neutropenic mice. *Infect Immun* 1987;**55**: 2715.
92. Welte K, Bonilla MA, Gillio AP *et al.* Recombinant human granulocyte-colony-stimulating factor: Effects on hematopoiesis in normal and cyclophosphamide-treated primates. *J Exp Med* 1987;**165**: 941.
93. Gabrilove JL, Jakubowski A, Scher H *et al.* Effect of granulocyte colony-stimulating factor on neutropenia and associated morbidity due to chemotherapy for transitional-cell carcinoma of the urothelium. *N Engl J Med* 1988;**318**: 1414.
94. Bronchud MH, Scarffe JH, Thatcher N *et al.* Phase I/II study of recombinant human granulocyte-colony-stimulating factor in patients receiving intensive chemotherapy for small cell cancer. *Br J Cancer* 1987;**56**: 809.
95. Morstyn G, Souza LM, Keech J *et al.* Effect of granulocyte colony-stimulating factor on neutropenia induced by cytotoxic chemotherapy. *Lancet* 1988;**i**: 667.
96. Cairo M, Suen Y, Knoppel E *et al.* Decreased G-CSF and IL-3 production and gene expression from mononuclear cells of newborn infants. *Pediatr Res* 1992;**31**: 574.
97. Schibler K, Liechty K, White W and Christensen R. Production of granulocyte-colony-stimulating factor *in vitro* by monocytes from preterm and term neonates. *Blood* 1993;**82**: 2478.
98. English BK, Hammond WP, Lewis DB, Brown CB and Wilson CB. Decreased granulocyte macrophage colony-stimulating factor production by human neonatal blood mononuclear cells and T cells. *Pediatr Res* 1992;**31**: 211.
99. Lee SM, Knoppel E, van de Ven C and Cairo MS. Transcriptional rates of granulocyte-macrophage colony-stimulating factor, granulocyte colony-stimulating factor, interleukin-3, and macrophage colony-stimulating factor genes in activated cord versus adult mononuclear cells: alteration in cytokine expression may be secondary to posttranscriptional instability. *Pediatr Res* 1993;**34**: 560.

100. Li Y, Calhoun DA, Polliotti BM, Sola MC, al-Mulla Z and Christensen RD. Production of granulocyte colony-stimulating factor by the human placenta at various stages of development. *Placenta* 1996;**17**: 611.
101. Li Y, Ohls R, Rosa C, Shah M, Richards DS and Christensen RD. Maternal and umbilical serum concentrations of granulocyte colony-stimulating factor and its messenger RNA during clinical chorioamnionitis. *Obstet Gynecol* 1995;**86**: 428.
102. Laver J, Duncan E, Abboud M *et al.* High levels of granulocyte and granulocyte-macrophage colony-stimulating factor in cord blood of normal full-term neonates. *J Pediatr* 1990;**116**: 627.
103. Shimoda K, Okamura S, Harada N, Omori F and Niho Y. Serum granulocyte colony-stimulating factor levels in umbilical cord blood of normal full-term infants. *Biomed Pharmacother* 1992;**46**: 337.
104. Gessler P, Kirchmann N, Kientsch-Engel R *et al.* Serum concentrations of granulocyte colony-stimulating factor in healthy term and preterm neonates and in those with various diseases including bacterial infections. *Blood* 1993;**82**: 3177.
105. Ikeno K. Increased granulocyte-colony stimulating factor levels in neonates with perinatal complications. *Acta Paediatr Jpn* 1994;**36**: 366.
106. Russell AR, Daview EG, McGuigan S *et al.* Plasma granulocyte-colony stimulating factor concentration in the early neonatal period. *Br J Haematol* 1994;**86**: 642.
107. Bailie KE, Irvine AE, Bridges JM and McClure BG. Granulocyte and granulocyte-macrophage colony-stimulating factors in cord and maternal serum at delivery. *Pediatr Res* 1994;**35**: 164.
108. Wilimas JA, Wall JE, Fairclough DL *et al.* A longitudinal study of granulocyte colony-stimulating factor levels and neutrophil counts in newborn infants. *J Pediatr Hematol Oncol* 1995;**17**: 176.
109. Cairo MS, Mauss D, Kammareddy S *et al.* Prophylactic or simultaneous administration of recombinant human granulocyte colony-stimulating factor in the treatment of group B streptococcal sepsis in neonatal rats. *Pediatr Res* 1990;**27**: 612.
110. Cairo MS, Plunkett J, Mauss D and van de Ven C. Seven-day administration of recombinant human granulocyte colony-stimulating factor to newborn rats: Modulation of neonatal neutrophilia, myelopoiesis, and group B streptococcus sepsis. *Blood* 1990;**76**: 1788.
111. Cairo MS, Plunkett J, Nguyen A and van de Ven C. Effect of stem cell factor with and without granulocyte colony-stimulating factor on neonatal hematopoiesis: *In vivo* induction of newborn myelopoiesis and reduction of mortality during experimental group B streptococcal sepsis. *Blood* 1992;**80**: 96.
112. Cairo MS, Plunkett J, Nguyen A *et al.* Effect of interleukin-11 with and without granulocyte colony-stimulating factor *in vivo* neonatal rat hematopoiesis: Induction of neonatal thrombocytosis by interleukin-11 and synergistic enhancement of neutrophilia by interleukin-11 plus granulocyte colony-stimulating factor. *Pediatr Res* 1993;**34**: 56.

113. Smith WS, Sumnicht GE, Sharpe RW, Samuelson D and Millard FE. Granulocyte colony-stimulating factor versus placebo in addition to penicillin G in a randomized blinded study of Gram-negative pneumonia sepsis: analysis of survival and multisystem organ failure. *Blood* 1995;**86**: 1301.
114. Eichacher PQ, Waisman Y, Natanson C *et al.* Cardiopulmonary effects of granulocyte colony-stimulating factor in a canine model of bacterial sepsis. *J Appl Physiol* 1994;**77**: 2366.
115. Medlock ES, Kaplan DL, Cecchini M, Ulich TR, del Castillo J and Andresen J. Granulocyte colony-stimulating factor crosses the placenta and stimulates fetal rat granulopoiesis. *Blood* 1993;**81**: 916.
116. Novales JS, Salva AM, Modanlou HD *et al.* Maternal administration of granulocyte colony-stimulating factor improves neonatal rat survival after a lethal group B streptococcal infection. *Blood* 1993;**81**: 923.
117. Roberts RL, Szelc CM, Scates SM *et al.* Neutropenia in an extremely premature infant treated with recombinant human granulocyte colony-stimulating factor. *Am J Dis Child* 1991;**145**: 808.
118. Gillian ER, Christensen RD, Suen Y *et al.* A randomized, placebo-controlled trial of recombinant granulocyte colony-stimulating factor administration in newborn infants with presumed sepsis: significant induction of peripheral and bone marrow neutrophilia. *Blood* 1994;**84**: 1427.
119. Gilmore MM, Stroneck DF and Korones DN. Treatment of alloimmune neonatal neutropenia with granulocyte colony-stimulating factor. *J Pediatr* 1994;**25**: 948.
120. La-Gamma EF, Alpha O and Kocherlakota P. Effect of granulocyte colony-stimulating factor on preeclampsia-associated neonatal neutropenia. *J Pediatr* 1995;**126**: 457.
121. Makhlouf RA, Doron MW, Bose CL, Price WA and Stiles AD. Administration of granulocyte colony-stimulating factor to neutropenic low birth weight infants of mothers with preeclampsia. *J Pediatr* 1995;**126**: 454.
122. Russell AR, Davies EG, Ball SE and Gordon-Smith E. Granulocyte colony stimulating factor treatment for neonatal neutropenia. *Arch Dis Child* 1995; **72**: F53.
123. Calhoun DA, Rosa C and Christensen RD. Administration of recombinant granulocyte colony-stimulating factor to women with an imminent preterm delivery. *Am J Obstet Gynecol* 1996;**174**: 1306.
124. Murray JC, McClain KL and Wearden ME. Using granulocyte colony-stimulating factor for neutropenia during neonatal sepsis. *Arch Pediatr Adolesc Med* 1994;**148**: 764.
125. Baumgartner JD and Glauser MP. Immunotherapy of endotoxemia and septicemia. *Immunobiology* 1993;**187**: 464.
126. Mehra IV, Gottlieb JE and Nash DB. Monoclonal antibody therapy for gram-negative sepsis: principles, applications, and controversies. *Pharmacotherapy* 1993;**13**: 128.
127. Thiermann C, Ruetten H, Wu CC and Vane JR. The multiple organ dysfunction syndrome caused by endotoxin in the rat: attenuation of liver dysfunction by inhibitors of nitric oxide synthetase. *Br J Pharmacol* 1995;**116**;2845.

128. Kilbourn RG, Gross SS, Jubran A *et al.* NG-methyl-L-arginine inhibits tumor necrosis factor-induced hypotension: implications for the involvement of nitric oxide. *Proc Natl Acad Sci USA* 1990;**87**: 3629.
129. Gibson RL, Berger JI, Redding GJ, Standaert TA, Mayock DE and Truog WE. Effect of nitric oxide synthase inhibition during group B streptococcal sepsis in neonatal piglets. *Pediatr Res* 1994;**36**: 776.
130. Meadow W, Rudinsky B, Bell A and Hipps R. Effects of inhibition of endothelium-derived relaxation factor on hemodynamics and oxygen utilization during group B streptococcal sepsis in piglets. *Crit Care Med* 1995;**23**: 705.
131. Driscoll W, Thurin S, Carrion V, Steinhorn RH and Morin III FC. Effect of methylene blue on refractory neonatal hypotension. *J Pediatr* 1996;**129**: 904.

11

Prenatal Diagnosis

Theresa L. Stewart and Diana W. Bianchi

As a result of the rapidly increasing number of prenatal diagnostic tests performed on pregnant women, neonatologists are frequently confronted with a wealth of clinical information about their patients long before they even touch them. The purpose of this chapter is to review the current indications and methods of prenatal genetic diagnosis and the information these tests convey, and to discuss what the results of these tests imply for the future care of the newborn infant. Neonatologists should strive to educate themselves about prenatal diagnosis to:

- understand physiologic and anatomic clues provided antenatally by their future patients;
- increase their awareness of potential late side effects of prenatal testing; and
- be able to answer questions from parents.

INDICATIONS FOR PRENATAL DIAGNOSIS

The process of prenatal diagnosis involves many steps. The most basic of these is the identification of those individuals who are appropriate candidates for the various prenatal diagnostic techniques. Genetic risk assessment must precede testing, because different procedures are associated with different medical risks to the mother and fetus. In general, the initial assessment takes into account the pregnant woman's prior reproductive and family histories and determines recurrence risk and the need for specific tests. Prenatal diagnosis is currently available for hundreds of different genetic conditions. No single fetus is tested for all of them. The indications for individual-specific prenatal diagnosis are given in Table 11.1.

Because the majority of newborns with chromosome abnormalities or major malformations are born to women with unremarkable reproductive and family histories, the development of population-based screening tests has generated much interest. Current population-based screening tests include maternal age, measurement of pregnancy-specific plasma proteins and first trimester sonographic assessment of the fetal nuchal membrane.

Maternal Age

A well known association exists between fetal chromosome aneuploidy and advanced maternal age, primarily due to errors in maternal meiosis I. Maternal age is used as an initial screen to determine who should be offered invasive prenatal cytogenetic diagnosis. A maternal age of 35 years at the time of delivery is used as a cut-off value, because the risk of a live-born infant with trisomy 21 (1/270) is approximately equal to the risk of a miscarriage following the amniocentesis procedure. Unfortunately, maternal age is a relatively inefficient screening tool, as only 20% of the infants with trisomy 21 are born to mothers over the age of 35 years.[1]

Screening on the basis of age alone misses 80% of affected liveborn infants. For this reason, much effort has been expended into developing other non-invasive tests that can accurately identify fetuses likely to be at high risk for Down syndrome. These are discussed below.

Table 11.1 Indication for prenatal diagnosis.

Prior family history	Type of test
Child with chromosome abnormality	Cytogenetic studies
Either parent balanced translocation carrier	Cytogenetic studies
Child with major malformation	Ultrasound examination
Affected individual with inborn error of metabolism	Biochemical or DNA studies
Affected individual with single gene disorder	DNA analysis (if mutation known)
Abnormal screening test	
Maternal serum screen	Ultrasound examination, cytogenetic studies
Ultrasound examination	Cytogenetic, DNA studies if indicated

Maternal Serum Screening

Screening pregnancies for congenital anomalies using prenatal serum biochemistry started with maternal serum alpha-fetoprotein (MSAFP) measurement in the 1970s. Alpha-fetoprotein is a glycoprotein produced by the fetus, and is the functional equivalent of adult albumin.[2] This protein is found in highest concentration in fetal blood. It is filtered by the fetal kidneys, distributed to the amniotic fluid, crosses the placenta, and can be measured in the maternal circulation. When a congenital defect exists that involves an opening of the fetal skin, such as an open neural tube defect, omphalocele or gastroschisis, the alpha-fetoprotein diffuses into the amniotic fluid in larger amounts than expected normally. As a result, the value in maternal serum is also elevated. When the association between fetal abnormalities and increased maternal serum AFP was realized, MSAFP screening for open neural tube defects became the standard of care in the early 1980s.[3, 4]

To facilitate collaboration between laboratories, MSAFP results are expressed relative to population-specific normal values, as multiples of the median (MoM). Traditionally, results of >2.5 MoM are considered abnormally high and <0.6 MoM are abnormally low. Both require further investigation.

In 1984, Merkatz *et al* reported an association between low MSAFP levels and fetal aneuploidy.[5] The MSAFP level and risk of Down syndrome were found to be independent of the age-related risk.[6] Therefore, age and MSAFP levels could be combined to establish a better estimate of Down syndrome risk. The discovery of altered MSAFP values in Down syndrome pregnancies encouraged researchers to begin evaluating other pregnancy-specific biochemical markers for their potential associations with fetal pathology.[7] In 1987, Bogart *et al* reported both high and low extremes of human chorionic gonadotropin (hCG) levels in pregnancies with chromosomally abnormal fetuses.[8] The next analyte that became part of serum screening protocols was unconjugated estriol (uE3), which is a protein product of the fetoplacental unit. Canick *et al* compared 22 pregnancies carrying fetuses with Down syndrome and 110 unaffected pregnancies, and found that maternal uE3 levels were significantly lower in the affected pregnancies.[9] Others have confirmed this finding and found it also to be independent of maternal age, hCG and MSAFP.[10] 'Triple screening', as it is now commonly called, can detect 60–65% of all Down syndrome pregnancies at a calculated false positive rate of 5%. The clinical application of serum screening during pregnancy has increased the Down syndrome detection rate by >2-fold compared to the previous rate using maternal age alone.

Both the American College of Obstetrics and Gynecology and the American College of Medical Genetics support the use of maternal serum markers for risk assessment of fetal chromosome abnormalities, but one specific combination is not recommended over another.

By analyzing the results of the triple screen, specific patterns associated with fetal defects can now be recognized (Table 11.2). Down syndrome pregnancies characteristically have low MSAFP and low uE3 levels with an elevated level of hCG. Fetuses with trisomy 18 typically have low levels for all 3 markers. It is important, however, to remember that the biochemical patterns typical for aneuploidy can be 'masked' in the presence of a co-existing open neural defect or an abdominal wall defect that increases the MSAFP.

In maternal serum screening, each separate protein is measured and compared to population standards. Using the result from each of the separate analytes, a likelihood ratio for Down syndrome is calculated. This ratio is then applied to the appropriate age-related risk to establish an overall risk estimation. Generally, if the risk of aneuploidy following serum screening is greater than the risk of miscarriage following amniocentesis (1/270), the woman is offered an amniocentesis. Prior to offering the patient amniocentesis, an assessment of the pregnancy and information regarding the triple screen is checked for accuracy. An ultrasound examination is performed to evaluate fetal anatomy, gestational age and number of fetuses present. The most common reason for an abnormal serum screening test is incorrect dating for the pregnancy (Table 11.3).

The application of maternal serum analytes has significantly increased the ability to identify fetal abnormalities in the second trimester of pregnancy; however, it would be more beneficial if the screening could be performed earlier in the pregnancy. Many other investigators are currently evaluating analytes that may be useful in the first trimester. Pregnancy-associated plasma protein A (PAPP-A) and the free β subunit of hCG appear to be good candidates to detect trisomy 21 pregnancies.[11]

Table 11.2 Specific patterns associated with abnormal serum screen.

	AFP	hCG	uE3
Trisomy 21	↓	↑	↔↓
Trisomy 18	↓	↓	↓
Anencephaly	↑↑	↔	↔↓

AFP = alpha-fetoprotein; hCG = human chorionic gonadotrophin; uE3 = unconjugated estriol.

Table 11.3 Differential diagnosis of abnormal maternal serum alpha-fetoprotein level.

High (>2.5 MoM)
Incorrect gestational dating
Multiple pregnancy
Threatened pregnancy loss or fetal demise
Fetomaternal hemorrhage
Anencephaly
Open spina bifida
Anterior abdominal wall defects
Congenital nephrosis
Acardia
Lesions of the placenta and umbilical cord
Turner syndrome
Cystic hygroma
Renal agenesis
Polycystic kidney disease
Epidermolysis bullosa
Hereditary persistence (autosomal dominant trait)
Low (<0.6 MoM)
Incorrect gestational dating
Trisomy 21
Trisomy 18
Intrauterine growth retardation

Nuchal Translucency Measurement

One of the most promising techniques currently being evaluated as a possible screen for the detection of Down syndrome in the general obstetric population is nuchal translucency (NT). NT is a measurement of the soft tissue in the posterior aspect of the fetal neck between the cervical spine and skin. It is usually performed in the first trimester and can be measured successfully by transabdominal ultrasound examination in approximately 95% of cases. The measurement is then compared with normal population values based upon gestational age. A risk assessment for trisomy 21 is then determined.[12] Using NT and maternal age together, 80% of Down syndrome pregnancies can be detected. Since this is measured during the first trimester, a comprehensive fetal anatomy scan cannot be adequately performed at the same time. Patients with a normal NT, but who are at risk for other anomalies, may require another ultrasound examination later in the pregnancy completely to assess fetal anatomy. In the United States, there has been controversy regarding the benefit of routine ultrasound examination to evaluate fetal anatomy. Therefore, incorporation of this limited first-trimester ultrasound examination into routine prenatal care may prove difficult. With this issue aside, NT appears to be an excellent screening tool. In addition to Down syndrome pregnancies, other anomalies have also been found to be associated with an increased NT, including other trisomies (18 and 13), Turner syndrome, sex chromosome aneuploidy, triploidy, cardiac anomalies and genetic syndromes such as Noonan, Jarcho-Levin and Smith-Lemli-Opitz.[13, 14]

INVASIVE PRENATAL DIAGNOSIS

All techniques of invasive prenatal diagnosis share the same goal of obtaining fetal nucleated cells for genetic analysis. The most clinical experience has been accrued with amniocentesis.

Amniocentesis

Amniocentesis had its beginnings in the 1880s when it was described for the treatment of polyhydramnios. In 1956, Fuchs and Riis demonstrated its safety and utility.[15] However, it was not until Steele and Breg in 1966 demonstrated the feasibility of amniotic fluid cell culture and karyotyping that its prenatal use blossomed.[16] As the availability of sonography increased in the late 1970s and early 1980s, the addition of ultrasound guidance for amniocentesis made it safer and easier to visualize the fetus during the procedure.[17] In a review of studies published from 1977 to 1985, Ager and Oliver demonstrated a miscarriage rate of 2.4–5.2% in patients who underwent amniocentesis.[18] The baseline miscarriage rate in the general population was 1.8–3.7%. Based on these findings, it was estimated that the procedure-related risk of amniocentesis was 0.2–2.1%. At the same time, Tabor *et al* performed a randomized trial of amniocentesis at 14–20 weeks' gestation versus ultrasound examination alone in 4606 low-risk women. They reported the fetal loss rate to be 1% higher in the group that underwent amniocentesis.[19]

'Traditional' or midtrimester amniocentesis is a procedure that is usually performed between 15 0/7 weeks' and 19 6/7 weeks' gestation, using a 22 gauge spinal needle that is inserted through the abdominal wall under direct ultrasound guidance. Approximately 20 cm^3 of amniotic fluid is removed. This fluid is then sent for fetal chromosome analysis, alpha-fetoprotein measurement and any other clinically indicated biochemical or DNA testing.

Complications from amniocentesis are well described. The rate of fetal loss following the procedure is usually quoted as 1/200 based on the studies cited above. Other complications include rupture of membranes and infection. Culture failure occurs in <1% of cases and requires that the procedure be repeated. Mosaicism occurs in approximately 0.05% of cases. True mosaicism refers to the presence of 2 different karyotypes in the same individual. The implications of this finding depend directly on the specific karyotypes observed and can raise very difficult counseling situations. A similiar phenomenon is that of pseudomosaicism. This is a laboratory artifact that arises in cell culture or sample preparation. Pseudomosaicism occurs when there is only one or a small number of abnormal cells in a single culture or clone. Since this is a reflection of laboratory culture, these results are generally not reported to the patient and are of no significance to the pregnancy.

Early amniocentesis

One of the main disadvantages of midtrimester amniocentesis is its timing. Many women desire information much sooner in the pregnancy than in the second trimester. The psychological benefits of early prenatal diagnosis are obvious. Although chorionic villus sampling (CVS) (see below) provides the benefits of early diagnosis, the number of obstetricians trained in this technique is limited in the United States. Many more obstetricians are well trained and qualified to perform amniocentesis. In addition, the specimen handling and processing for CVS is much more labor intensive compared with amniotic fluid. The question has therefore arisen as to the feasibility, safety and accuracy of performing amniocentesis at an earlier gestation. 'Early' amniocentesis is the term generally applied when the procedure is performed between 11 0/7 weeks and 14 6/7 weeks' gestation.

The technique is similiar to that described for midtrimester amniocentesis except that less fluid is removed (approximately 1 cm^3 per week of gestation). Early amniocentesis is technically more difficult to perform than the later procedure, which relates to differences in fetal and maternal anatomy early in gestation, such as the size of the uterus. Since the uterus is smaller, it is more likely that maternal bowel will be lying between the uterus and the abdominal wall, thereby obstructing the path that the needle needs to transverse. The other major anatomical difficulty is the relationship between amnion and chorion. At approximately 14–15 weeks' gestation, these 2 membranes fuse together and then fuse with the uterine wall. When amniocentesis is performed prior to this fusion, the membranes often create a tent around the needle, making it more difficult to enter the amniotic cavity. Either of these 2 anatomical problems can lead to an unsuccessful procedure or rupture of the membranes and pregnancy loss.

The safety of early amniocentesis is currently being evaluated, and a slightly increased risk to the pregnancy, when compared to the midtrimester procedure, has already been noted. The risk is directly related to the gestational age, with the earliest procedure having the greatest risk.[20] Two randomized trials comparing early amniocentesis with other prenatal diagnosis procedures have been published. In 1994, Nicolaides *et al* compared early amniocentesis with CVS and found a 4.7% increase in spontaneous losses in the early amniocentesis group.[21] These results contrasted with those of Johnson *et al*, who found no increase in loss rate between 349 women who underwent early amniocentesis versus 346 women who underwent midtrimester amniocentesis.[22] Multiple non-randomized studies looking at the safety of early amniocentesis have been published,[23] and their results support early amniocentesis as a safe procedure with loss rates similiar to the other invasive prenatal diagnostic procedures (approximately 1–2%). Preliminary results of a randomized trial of early amniocentesis versus transabdominal CVS indicate an increased incidence of clubfoot in the early aminocentesis group.

Molecular cytogenetic studies

Significant advances have occurred in the ability to use DNA probes in the prenatal setting. Normally, a karyotype is performed on amniocytes that have undergone cell culture and are halted in metaphase. In certain settings, it may be useful to have rapid (within 48 hours) information on the fetus' chromosome status. A technique known as fluorescence *in situ* hybridization (FISH) can be performed using DNA probes unique to chromosomes 13, 18, 21, X and Y on non-dividing (interphase cells). Each probe hybridizes to a single copy of its corresponding chromosome. The probes are conjugated to fluorescent dyes. The laboratory technician can count areas of hybridization (colored dots) and rapidly determine if an abnormal number of chromosomes is present.

Another exciting development is the use of DNA probes that hybridize to areas of the genome that would not normally be detected by conventional metaphase chromosome analysis. Such probes detect microdeletions. The most commonly used prenatally is the one that detects a chromosome 22q11 microdeletion seen in DiGeorge syndrome. Many centers are routinely ruling out DiGeorge syndrome in all fetuses diagnosed antenally as having a conotruncal cardiac defect.

Chorionic Villus Sampling

The desire to make prenatal diagnosis available in the first trimester inspired the development of CVS. It was introduced experimentally in

1968 by Mohr.[24] It was first described for clinical use by a Chinese group in 1975 to determine fetal gender.

CVS is usually performed at 10 weeks' gestation and a transcervical or transabdominal approach is used. Both techniques are performed under direct ultrasound guidance and both have proven to be safe. In transcervical sampling, a thin catheter is placed under aseptic conditions through the cervix and passed parallel to the placenta almost to its distal margin. A syringe is attached to the catheter and the villi are aspirated and collected. With transabdominally performed procedures, a needle is placed through the abdominal and uterine walls to lie within the chorion frondosum; it is passed along the placenta and villi are aspirated. The approach used for an individual patient is determined by her specific anatomy and the experience and preference of the person performing the procedure.

Due to the close juxtaposition of the fetal villi and maternal decidual tissue in the chorionic villus sample, it is usually necessary to have a technician nearby immediately to dissect away the contaminating maternal cells. The resulting fetal sample is then divided into 2 preparations: direct and cultured. The direct preparation consists mainly of cytotrophoblast and syncytiotrophoblast; cells are dividing rapidly and a metaphase analysis is possible within hours. The cultured preparation consists of fetal mesenchymal cells, capillaries and fetal blood. Maternal contamination is more likely to be detected in the cultured preparation. In the case of a chromosomally abnormal result, fetal blood in the CVS supernatant can provide additional information.[25]

The safety of CVS has been evaluated in a number of studies. The Canadian Collaborative CVS/Amniocentesis Trial group (1989) was a prospective randomized trial involving 2391 women and 11 centers, comparing CVS performed at 9–12 weeks' gestation, versus amniocentesis performed at 15–17 weeks. The total fetal loss rates were 7.6% and 7.0% for the CVS and amniocentesis groups, respectively.[26] In the CVS group, 9.9% of the women required a subsequent amniocentesis due to difficulty with the CVS or problems with the laboratory analysis. In the US Collaborative CVS study, also published in 1989, the pregnancy outcomes of patients undergoing CVS were compared with patients undergoing amniocentesis at 16 weeks' gestation. This non-randomized study involved 2278 CVS patients and 671 amniocentesis patients. The total loss in the CVS group exceeded that of the amniocentesis group by 0.8%.[27] Results of a consensus conference held by the Centers for Disease Control (CDC) and the National Institutes of Health indicate that the risk of miscarriage after CVS is of the order of 0.5–1.0%.[28]

Complications other than fetal loss have also been described for CVS. In 1991, Firth *et al* were the first to report an increased incidence of limb defects in infants born following CVS: 5 cases of limb defects among 289 patients who underwent CVS.[29] Since that time there has been much debate regarding the role of CVS in the etiology of limb defects. Mahoney reported no increase in limb defects over the baseline population incidence.[30] Although there may be some association between very early (before 8 weeks) CVS and limb malformations, this association appears to be complicated by type of catheter, sample size, number of passes and operator experience. The World Health Organization performed a follow-up study and did not find any evidence of limb reduction defects in CVS procedures performed after 8 weeks' gestation.[31] The CDC recommends quoting a CVS-procedure-related risk of limb malformation of 1:3000 cases.[28]

Both mosaicism and pseudomosaicism, as described with amniocentesis, have been documented in CVS samples. An additional finding that has been recognized with the increased clinical utilization of CVS is that of confined placental mosaicism (CPM). CPM is a true biologic dichotomy that exists between the chromosomal constitution of placental and fetal tissue. It results from mutations in the trophoblast or extraembryonic mesodermal progenitor cells and has an incidence of 1% in CVS cases.[32] The exact significance of this finding needs further evaluation. A number of studies have reported a higher incidence of adverse perinatal outcome in pregnancies complicated by CPM. Kalousek *et al* reported an increase of intrauterine growth restriction (IUGR) in pregnancies complicated by CPM.[33] Wapner *et al* subsequently found a higher fetal loss rate (8.6%) in patients with CPM compared to patients with normal karyotypes (3.4%), but did not find any difference in rates of IUGR.[34] Until the significance of CPM can be defined more precisely, patients need to be counseled concerning these uncertanties and understand that additional testing, including amniocentesis, may be required after CVS.

The presence of mosaic trisomy in a CVS result may alert the clinician to the possibility that *disomic rescue* has occurred in the fetus. This implies that the fetus originated as a trisomic conceptus, but subsequently lost the extra copy of the chromosome. In one-third of cases, the fetus will be left with both chromosome homologs from one parent, i.e. the parent who had the non-disjunctional event. In some situations, particularly for chromosomes that contain imprinted genes, pathology can result from having *uniparental disomy*.[35] This is being increasingly recognized as an important cause of Prader-Willi syndrome, in which many cases originate in trisomy 15 conceptuses that lose the paternal contribution of chromosome 15.

Cordocentesis

Percutaneous umbilical blood sampling or cordocentesis is the process of obtaining fetal blood by accessing the umbilical cord under ultrasound guidance. A 20-gauge needle is placed into the umbilical vein at the site where the cord inserts into the placenta. Cordocentesis is most commonly performed to evaluate fetal anemia in cases of isoimmunization.

For prenatal diagnostic purposes, this same technique can be used to obtain fetal leukocytes as a source of cells for rapid karyotyping. Clinical indications for cordocentesis include: advanced gestations in which the karyotype from amniocentesis may be delayed due to poor cell growth, or confirmation of a fetal karyotype when mosaicism is found on a prior CVS or amniocentesis sample.[36] The risk of pregnancy loss from a cordocentesis procedure is related to gestational age, but in general is of the order of 1–2%.[37]

Fetal Biopsy and Fetoscopy

Fetal tissue sampling can be performed to evaluate fetal skin, liver and muscle disorders. This invasive procedure is reserved for genetic disorders in which biochemical or DNA analysis is unavailable or uninformative. Although initially these procedures were performed by fetoscopy,[38] they are currently performed by percutaneous biopsy under direct ultrasound guidance.

This technique has been most widely used in the area of genodermatosis (Table 11.4). Genodermatoses are genetic skin disorders that are often fatal. Currently, many of these disorders cannot be diagnosed by any other method except skin biopsy. Fetal skin biopsies are optimally performed between 17 and 20 weeks' gestation; the risk of pregnancy loss when performed by fetoscopy is 5%.[38] Risks to the pregnancy for liver and muscle biopsies are currently unknown because of limited clinical experience. Over time the ability to diagnose these disorders by biochemical or DNA analysis has increased and therefore the indications for fetal biopsy have decreased. Fetal liver biopsy has been successful in diagnosing certain inborn errors of metabolism that cannot currently be diagnosed by DNA analysis, e.g. carbamoyl-phosphate synthetase deficiency,[39] non-ketotic hyperglycemia, glucose-6-phosphate deficiency[40] and, in certain families, ornithine transcarbamylase deficiency.[41] As with the skin disorders, the molecular basis of many of

Table 11.4 Genodermatoses prenatally detectable by fetal skin sampling. Modified from Ref. 53.

Anhidrotic ectodermal dysplasia
Bulbous congenital ichthyosiform erythroderma
Epidermolysis bulbous dystrophia
Epidermolysis bullosa dystrophia
Epidermolysis bullosa lethalis
Harlequin ichthyosis
Hypohidrotic ectodermal dysplasia
Non-bullous ichthyosiform erythroderma
Oculocutaneous albinism
Sjogren-Larsson syndrome

these disorders is becoming known, facilitating the safer procedures of CVS or amniocentesis for DNA diagnosis.[42]

Fetoscopy is the placement of an endoscope within the amniotic cavity to obtain direct visualization of the fetus. The risk of pregnancy loss associated with the procedure is approximately 5%.[38] Fetoscopy may be indicated to evaluate for subtle genetic malformations not readily identifiable by ultrasound examination. However, as ultrasound technology has improved, the situations where this might significantly improve diagnostic abilities are extremely rare.

Preimplantation Genetic Diagnosis

Preimplantation genetic diagnosis is the application of DNA or chromosomal analysis to the earliest components of pregnancy – oocyte, blastomere or blastocyst. Within a few specialized laboratories worldwide, single-cell genetic analysis is performed in conjunction with *in vitro* fertilization with the aim of establishing only genetically normal pregnancies in couples that are at high risk for genetic disorders. By performing the testing prior to implantation, the couple can avoid issues of termination later in pregnancy. However, only approximately 15% of couples with normal fertility who undergo this type of procedure have a 'take home' baby.[43] Furthermore, in 3 of 34 babies born following this technique, a diagnostic error had been made.[43]

Because of the experimental nature of these procedures, couples who undergo preimplantation diagnosis are also offered traditional prenatal diagnostic methods (CVS or amniocentesis) later in the pregnancy for confirmation of the diagnosis.

NON-INVASIVE PRENATAL DIAGNOSIS

Concern regarding procedure-related complications has shifted emphasis to prenatal diagnostic techniques that carry no risk of miscarriage. Ultrasound examination is particularly significant for the neonatologist because antenatal identification of fetal anatomic abnormalities may change the site of delivery to a tertiary medical center.

Ultrasound Examination

Ultrasound examination is an extremely powerful diagnostic tool in the field of obstetrics. The prenatal indications for its use are numerous and continue to increase.[44] Although obstetricians rely on ultrasound examination almost daily in their clinical practice, the efficacy of routine ultrasound examination during pregnancy continues to be debated.[45] Much of the debate has centered around the RADIUS (Routine Antenal Diagnostic Imaging by Ultrasound) study.[45, 46] In brief, this was a prospective randomized study comparing routine ultrasound examination versus selective (clinically indicated only) use in a 'low risk' pregnant population. The primary outcome evaluated was perinatal morbidity and mortality. The study's authors reported no difference in pregnancy outcome between the 2 groups.[45] There has been criticism and controversy concerning the conclusions of this study.[47] However, many lessons were learned as a result of the study. During the RADIUS trial, the anomaly detection rate was only 35%. The study was carried out in multiple centers and the detection rate varied significantly between them. In non-tertiary centers, where a majority of the scans were performed, the detection rate of fetal anomalies was only 13%. Many studies have been published since the RADIUS trial evaluating the sensitivity of ultrasound examination for prenatal diagnosis. Using current technology in tertiary centers, the detection rate of fetal anomalies is of the order of 50–60%.[48]

Fortunately, many of the severest anomalies tend to have the highest detection rates. Gonsalves *et al* looked at the sensitivity of prenatal ultrasound examination and their overall detection rate was 53%.[48] However, they reported an overall 89% detection rate for lethal anomalies, including 79% for CNS anomalies, 32% for cardiac anomalies, 76% for respiratory system anomalies, 37% for gastrointestinal anomalies and 91% for urinary tract abnormalities. The sensitivity was higher in patients who were considered to be at 'high risk' (i.e. previous history of abnormality, abnormal serum screen, advanced maternal age).

Because ultrasound examination can successfully detect many fetal anomalies, patients and physicians sometimes misunderstand that a normal study does not guarantee the complete absence of anomalies. Pregnant patients need to be counseled regarding the limitations of ultrasound examination.

Fetal Cells in Maternal Circulation

Because all nucleated fetal cells from the same individual contain identical genetic information, research efforts are focusing on the non-invasive isolation of fetal cells from maternal blood. Advances in molecular genetic analytic techniques, such as FISH and the polymerase chain reaction (PCR), combined with innovation in cell separation methods and a better understanding of the immunobiology of feto-maternal cell transfer, bode well for the incorporation of this approach into routine prenatal care.[49]

Target fetal cell types that cross the placenta and circulate in maternal blood include the trophoblast and granulocyte; most efforts, however, are concentrated on the nucleated erythrocyte. Cytogenetic diagnoses already made from isolated fetal cells include trisomies 18 and 21, 47 XXY, 69 XXX and 69 XXY. An increasing number of single gene mutations have been diagnosed as well, including β globin mutations. Finally, this technique has been used to exclude Duchenne muscular dystrophy and determine fetal Rhesus D genotype and inheritance of HLA-DR and DQ α alleles.

Based upon encouraging reports of successful cytogenetic diagnoses using FISH on interphase fetal nucleated erythrocytes, the US National Institute of Child Health and Human Development has instituted a multicenter clinical trial designed to assess the accuracy, sensitivity, specificity and positive predictive value of this technique for the non-invasive detection of fetal chromosome aneuploidy.

OUTCOME OF PRENATAL DIAGNOSIS

Genetic Counseling

Many prenatal diagnostic centers work with genetic counselors, masters-trained health care providers, who take a 3-generational family history and ask specific questions designed to elicit the need for specialized tests.[50] Genetic counselors also advise the patient regarding the risk–benefit ratios for certain procedures. Most importantly, they serve as a patient advocate and continuity link for prospective parents facing the birth of a child with an abnormality. Whereas it is usually the physician who interprets the results of the diagnostic tests, it is the genetic counselor who fully discusses the options for the couple following the diagnosis of an abnormality. Genetic counseling is non-directive, and adequate emotional and psychological support must be available for the parents.

Multidisciplinary Fetal Treatment Team

Formation of a multidisciplinary fetal treatment team allows pediatric subspecialists (including neonatologists) the opportunity to participate in the care of the fetal patient. Many opportunities for fetal treatment following prenatal diagnosis exist. These may include:

- maternal administration of corticosteroids to a female fetus diagnosed by DNA analysis to have congenital adrenal hyperplasia;
- insertion of a catheter into the fetal bladder to permit drainage of fetal urine in the setting of posterior urethral valves; and
- *in utero* transfusion of paternal bone marrow in a male fetus diagnosed with X-linked severe combined immunodeficiency disease.[51]

It is increasingly important that neonatologists become active participants in discussions that involve treatment of the fetus, as it is pediatricians who have background knowledge in the long-term aspects of the abnormal childhood condition.

Identification of Clinically Silent Newborn Findings by Prenatal Diagnosis

One of the rarely discussed aspects of prenatal diagnosis is its ability to identify abnormalities that would not be apparent on the typical newborn physical examination. Examples of this include choroid plexus cyst (CPC), echogenic bowel, borderline ventriculomegaly and minimal hydronephrosis. Many pediatricians face a dilemma in deciding how to follow-up on mildly abnormal prenatal sonographic findings. A comprehensive clinical research agenda is needed to study this phenomenon.[52]

SUMMARY

Despite the concerns aired above, tremendous scientific and technical advances over the past 20 years have enabled improved and more precise prenatal diagnosis of fetal conditions. Currently, emphasis is being placed on more accurate and cost-effective methods of identifying fetuses at risk by using population-based screening techniqes. Furthermore, testing is moving earlier into the first trimester, using the less invasive methods of sonography and maternal blood analysis. As the Human Genome Project moves towards completion, and the sequence of all human genes becomes known, it is conceivable that one day all fetuses will have prenatal DNA diagnosis via the DNA chip technology that is currently available.

REFERENCES

1. Verloes A, Schoos R, Herens C, Vintens A and Koulischer L. A prenatal trisomy 21 screening program using 2-fetoprotein, human chorionic gonadotropin, and free estriol assays on maternal dried blood. *Am J Obstet Gynecol* 1995;**172**: 167–174.
2. Bergstrand CG. Alphafetoprotein in paediatrics. *Acta Paediatr Scand* 1986;**75**: 1.
3. Brock DJH and Sutcliffe RG. Alpha-fetoprotein in the antenatal diagnosis of anencephaly and spina bifida. *Lancet* 1972;**ii**: 197.
4. Ferguson-Smith MA. The reduction of anencephalic and spina bifida births by maternal serum alpha-fetoprotein screening. *Br Med Bull* 1983;**39**: 365.
5. Merkatz IR, Nitowsky HM, Macri JN and Johnson WE. An association between low maternal serum alpha-fetoprotein and fetal chromosomal abnormalities. *Am J Obstet Gynecol* 1984;**148**: 886–894.
6. Cuckle HS, Wald NJ and Lindenbaum RH. Maternal serum alpha-fetoprotein measurement: A screening test for Down syndrome. *Lancet* 1984;**ii**: 413.
7. Chard T, Lowings C and Kitau MJ. Alpha-fetoprotein and chorionic gonadotrophin levels in relation to Down's syndrome [letter]. *Lancet* 1984;**ii**: 750.
8. Bogart MH, Pandian MR and Jones OW. Abnormal maternal serum chorionic gonadotrophin levels in pregnancies with fetal chromosome abnormalities. *Prenat Diagn* 1987;**7**: 623–630.
9. Canick JA, Knight GJ, Palomaki GE, Haddow JE, Cuckle HS and Wald NJ. Low second trimester maternal serum unconjugated oestriol in pregnancies with Down syndrome. *Br J Obstet Gynaecol* 1988;**95**: 330–333.
10. Wald NJ, Cuckle HS, Demsem JW, Nanchahal K, Canick JA and Haddow JE. Maternal serum unconjugated estriol as an antenatal screening for Down's syndrome. *Br J Obstet Gynaecol* 1988;**95**: 334–341.
11. Brambati B, Tului L, Shrimanker K *et al.* Serum PAPP-A and free B-hCG are first trimester screening markers for Down syndrome. *Prenat Diagn* 1994;**14**: 1043–1047.
12. Pandya PP, Snijders RJ, Johnson SJ, Brizot M and Nicolaides KH. Screening for fetal trisomies by maternal age and nuchal translucency thickness at 10 to 14 weeks of gestation. *Br J Obstet Gynaecol* 1995;**102**: 957–962.

13. Hyett JA, Clayton PT, Moscoso G and Nicolaides KH. Increased first trimester nuchal translucency as a prenatal manifestation of Smith-Lemli-Opitz syndrome. *Am J Med Genet* 1995;**58**: 374–376.
14. Hyett JA, Perdu M, Sharland GK, Snijders RS and Nicolaides KH. Increased nuchal translucency at 10–14 weeks of gestation as a marker for major cardiac defects. *Ultrasound Obstet Gynecol* 1997;**10**: 272–276.
15. Fuchs F and Riis P. Antenatal sex determination. *Nature* 1956;**177**: 330.
16. Steele MW and Breg WR. Chromosome analysis of human amniotic fluid cells. *Lancet* 1966;**i**: 383–385.
17. Benacerraf BR and Frigoletto FD. Amniocentesis under continuous ultrasound guidance: a series of 232 cases. *Obstet Gynecol* 1983;**62**: 760–763
18. Ager RP and Oliver RW. *The Risks of Mid-Trimester Amniocentesis*. Lancashire: Biological Materials Analysis Research Unit, Dept. Biological Sciences, University of Salford, 1986, p 179.
19. Tabor A, Madsen M, Obel EB, Philip J, Bang J and Noergard-Peterson B. Randomised controlled trial of genetic amniocentesis in 4606 low-risk women. Lancet 1986;**i**: 1287–1293.
20. Stripparo L, Buscaglia M, Longatti L *et al*. Genetic amniocentesis: 505 cases performed before the sixteenth week of gestation. *Prenat Diagn* 1990;**10**: 359–364.
21. Nicolaides K, de Lourdes Brizot M, Patel F and Snijders R. Comparison of chorionic villus sampling and amniocentesis for fetal karyotyping at 10–13 weeks' gestation. *Lancet* 1994;**344**: 435–439.
22. Johnson J, Wilson RD, Winsor EJ, Singer J, Dansereau J and Kalousek DK. The early amniocentesis study: a randomized clinical trial of early amniocentesis versus mid-trimester amniocentesis. *Fetal Diagn Ther* 1996;**11**: 85–93.
23. Wilson RD. Early amniocentesis: A clinical review. *Prenat Diagn* 1995;**15**: 1259–1273.
24. Mohr J. Foetal genetic diagnosis: development of techniques for early sampling of foetal cells. *Acta Path Microbiol Scand* 1968;**73**: 73–77.
25. Mavrou A, Zheng Y-L, Kolialexi A, Metaxotou C and Bianchi DW. Fetal nucleated erythrocytes (NRBCs) in chorionic villus sample supernatant fluids: and additional source of fetal material for karyotype confirmation. *Prenat Diagn* 1997;**17**: 643–650.
26. Canadian Collaborative CVS–Amniocentesis Clinical Trial Group. Multicenter randomized clinical trial of chorionic villus sampling and amniocentesis. First report. *Lancet* 1989;**i**: 1–7.
27. Rhoads GG, Jackson LG, Schlessman SE *et al*. The safety and efficacy of chorionic villus sampling for early diagnosis of cytogenetic abnormalities. *N Engl J Med* 1989;**320**: 609–663.
28. Centers for Disease Control & Prevention. Chorionic villus sampling and amniocentesis: recommendations and prenatal counseling. *MMWR* 1995;**44**: 1–12.
29. Firth HV, Boyd PA, Chamberlain P, MacKenzie IZ, Lindenbaum RH and Huson SM. Limb abnormalities and chorionic villus sampling. *Lancet* 1991;**338**: 51.

30. Mahoney MJ. Limb abnormalities and chorionic villus sampling. *Lancet* 1991;**337**: 1422–1423.
31. Kuliev AM, Modell B, Jackson L *et al.* Risk evaluation of CVS. *Prenat Diagn* 1993;**13**: 197–209.
32. Bianchi DW, Wilkins-Haug LE, Enders AC and Hay ED. Origin of extra-embryonic mesoderm: Relevance to chorionic villus sampling. *Am J Med Genet* 1993;**46**: 542–550.
33. Kalousek DK, Howard-Peebles PN, Olson SB *et al.* Confirmation of CVS mosaicism in term placentae and high frequency of intrauterine growth retardation association with confined placental mosaicism. *Prenat Diagn* 1991;**12**: 626–627.
34. Wapner RJ, Simpson JL, Golbus MS *et al.* Chorionic villus mosaicism: association with fetal loss but not with adverse perinatal outcome. *Prenat Diagn* 1992;**12**: 347–355.
35. Ledbetter DH and Engel E. Uniparental disomy in humans: development of an imprinting map and its implications for prenatal diagnosis. *Hum Mol Genet* 1995;**4**: 1757–1764.
36. Gosden C, Nicolaides KH and Rodeck CH. Fetal blood sampling in investigation of chromosomal mosaicism in amniotic fluid cell culture. *Lancet* 1988;**i**: 613.
37. Ghidini A, Sepulveda W, Lockwood CJ and Romero R. Complications of fetal blood sampling. *Am J Obstet Gynecol* 1993;**168**: 1339–1344.
38. Rodeck CH and Nicolaides KH. Fetoscopy and fetal tissue sampling. *Br Med Bull* 1983;**39**: 332–337.
39. Piceni-Sereni L, Bachman C, Pfister U *et al.* Prenatal diagnosis of carbamoyl-phosphate synthetase deficiency by fetal liver biopsy. *Prenat Diagn* 1988;**8**: 307.
40. Golbus MS, Simpson TJ, Koresawa M *et al.* The prenatal determination of glucose-6-phosphatase activity by fetal liver biopsy. *Prenat Diagn* 1988;**8**: 401.
41. Holzgreve W and Golbus MS. Prenatal diagnosis of ornithine transcarbamylase deficiency utilizing fetal liver biopsy. *Am J Hum Genet* 1984;**36**: 320–328. 1995;**58**: 374–376.
42. Nussbaum RL, Boggs BA, Beaudet AL *et al.* New mutation and prenatal diagnosis in ornithine transcarbamylase deficiency. *Am J Hum Genet* 1986;**38**: 149.
43. Harper J. Preimplantation diagnosis of inherited disease by embryo biopsy. An update of the world figures. *J Assist Reprod Genet* 1996;**13**: 90–95.
44. *Ultrasound in Pregnancy*. ACOG Technical Bulletin #187. ACOG, 1993.
45. Ewigman BG, Crane JP, Frigoletto FD, Lefevre ML, Bain RP, McNeills D and the RADIUS Study Group. A randomized trial of prenatal ultrasound screening in a low risk population. Impact on perinatal outcome. *N Engl J Med* 1993;**329**: 821–827.
46. Lefevre ML, Bain RP, Ewigman BG, Frigoletto FD, Crane JP, McNeills D and the RADIUS Study Group. A randomized trial of prenatal ultrasound screening. Impact on maternal management and outcome. *Am J Obstet Gynecol* 1993;**169**: 483–489.
47. Gonsalves LF and Romero R. A critical appraisal of the RADIUS Study. *Fetus* 1993;**3**: 7–18.

48. Gonsalves LF, Jeanty P and Piper JM. The accuracy of prenatal ultrasonography in detecting congenital anomalies. *Am J Obstet Gynecol* 1994;**171**: 1606–1612.
49. Bianchi DW. Progress in the genetic analysis of fetal cells circulating in maternal blood. *Curr Opin Obstet Gynecol* 1997;**9**: 121–125.
50. Inati MN, Lazar EC and Haskin-Leahy L. The role of the genetic counselor in a perinatal unit. *Semin Perinatol* 1994;**18**: 133–139.
51. Flake AW, Roncarlo M-G, Puck JM *et al.* Treatment of X-linked severe combined immunodeficiency by *in utero* transplantation of paternal bone marrow. *N Engl J Med* 1996;**335**: 1806–1810.
52. Nichols VG and Bianchi DW. Prenatal pediatrics: Traditional specialty definitions no longer apply. *Pediatrics* 1996;**97**: 729–732.
53. Golbus MS and Cadrin CR. Fetal tissue sampling. In: Kuller JA, Chescheir NC, Cefalo RC (eds) Prenatal Diagnosis and Reproductive Genetics. St Louis, Mosby. 1996, pp. 159–169.

12

What is New in the Management of Preterm Labor?

David S. McKenna and Jay D. Iams

INDICATED VERSUS SPONTANEOUS PRETERM BIRTH

Preterm birth occurs at a rate of 7.2% of liveborn infants and is the leading cause of perinatal mortality and morbidity. It is important to differentiate between *indicated* and *spontaneous* preterm births. Indicated preterm births occur secondary to maternal medical or obstetric disorders that place the fetus or mother at risk. Examples are severe pre-eclampsia, diabetes, placenta previa, fetal red cell iso-immunization and intrauterine growth restriction. Indicated preterm births account for 20–30% of premature births. The etiologies for indicated preterm births may be recurrent and their prevention focuses on prevention and treatment of the underlying disorder.

Spontaneous preterm births (SPTBs) occur after preterm labor (PTL), preterm premature rupture of membranes (PPROM) or related diagnoses. They account for approximately 75% of premature births. This category includes deliveries that occur after amnionitis, with or without PPROM, and in patients with an 'incompetent' cervix.

PATHOGENESIS OF SPONTANEOUS PREMATURITY

Maternal Risk Factors

Characteristics associated with an increased risk of preterm birth are shown in Table 12.1. Despite these associations, more than one-half of SPTBs occur in women who have no apparent risk factors. An individual risk factor rarely operates independently to cause SPTB; instead, factors function together as pieces in a larger puzzle which ultimately leads to a common clinical presentation: PPROM or PTL. Risk factors can be targeted for potential interventional therapies, but to date no interventional trial that has attempted to eliminate a single mutable recurrent risk factor has succeeded in reducing the rate of SPTB. The risk factor of history of previous SPTB provides a helpful estimation of risk of recurrent SPTB. The recurrence risk rises as the number of prior SPTBs increases and increases further as the gestational of the prior preterm birth decreases.[1]

Ischemia, Infection, the Fetus and the Uterus

Injuries to the uteroplacental interface or chorioamniotic infection may lead to a maternal and/or fetal inflammatory response that results in uterine contractions and cervical ripening. Abnormalities of the placenta and an increased prevalence of poor intrauterine growth,[2–6] positive amniotic fluid cultures in 20–30% of women delivering early,[7] and elevated fetal proinflammatory cytokine levels[8] have all been reported in premature births.

Two current theories integrate infectious causes and uterine factors as causes of SPTB. The first proposes that uterine contractions open the cervix which then allows the ascent of organisms and the resultant infection and inflammation.[9] The uterine contractions are postulated to occur due to the loss of the natural hormonal inhibition. The second theory places the uterine contractions at the end of a process that begins with microbes ascending through a short or dilated cervix to produce inflammation with a maternal and fetal response. This leads to the production of prostinoids which cause cervical ripening and contractions.[10]

Model for the Pathogenesis of Preterm Birth

Preterm birth is best understood in the context of a model which integrates multiple risk factors. A basis for explaining the pathogenesis of disease produced by multiple risk factors already exists in the understanding of atherosclerotic cardiovascular disease (ASCVD). The model

Table 12.1 Characteristics associated with preterm birth.

Demographic factors
Black race
Low socioeconomic status
Age <18 or >40 years
Strenuous work
High personal stress
Past obstetrical or gynecological factors
History of previous spontaneous preterm birth
Cervical injury or abnormality
Uterine anomaly or fibroids
Current pregnancy factors
Poor nutrition
Low pre-pregnancy weight
Absent or poor prenatal care
Anemia (hemoglobin <10 g/dl)
Cigarette smoking
Bacteruria
Genital colonization or infection
Premature cervical dilation >1 cm

for the pathogenesis of ASCVD integrates multiple potentially mutable variables (e.g. serum cholesterol, blood pressure, cigarette smoking and blood glucose), along with multiple immutable variables (e.g. family history, age and gender). The integrated variables may result in a common outcome (coronary vessel occlusion) which may present in a number of clinical scenarios (e.g. myocardial infarction, angina or rhythm disturbances).

Recurrent SPTB can also be understood by a model that is analogous to the model for ASCVD.[11] The SPTB model integrates variables such as uterine volume and contraction frequency, microbial colonization of the genital tract, injury to the fetal-maternal interface, fetal paracrine signals for labor, and host resistance to labor such as cervical competence and resistance to infection. The common outcome in the model is SPTB which may initially present as PTL, PPROM or chorioamnionitis.

PREVENTION OF SPONTANEOUS PRETERM BIRTH

Primary Care

Primary care is the elimination or reduction of a risk for a specific disease in an entire population. This requires a good understanding of the pathophysiology of the disease. Effective primary interventions have not been demonstrated for the prevention of SPTB. In order to validate a primary care intervention program, the program would have to be shown to be easy and inexpensive to apply to all women of child-bearing age and to result in a reduced incidence of preterm birth.

Secondary Care

Secondary care selects individuals with increased risk for surveillance and prophylactic treatment. The key to success of secondary health care strategies is identification of the at-risk population and the availability of risk-reduction measures. For SPTB, secondary care strategies include screening programs based on clinical or laboratory tests, and therapeutic interventions such as bedrest, antibiotic therapy and cervical cerclage.

Screening programs

Many screening tests for the identification of women at risk for SPTB have been suggested, including clinical, biochemical, biophysical and microbial screens. A simple detailed obstetrical history can identify many major risk factors for SPTB:

- history of prior preterm delivery between 18 and 36 weeks;[12]
- multiple gestation;
- vaginal bleeding after the first trimester;[13]
- low pre-pregnancy weight (<19.8 kg/m).[14]

These risk factors should be screened for during routine prenatal care visits for every woman. If a risk factor is identified, then further investigation is warranted.

Fetal fibronectin (fFN) is an extracellular matrix protein that is normally found in the fetal membranes and decidua. The presence of fFN in the cervix or vagina after the 20th week is abnormal and may indicate disruption of the attachment of the membranes to the decidua. Data from 2929 women enrolled in the National Institute of Child Health and Human Development (NICHD) Preterm Prediction Study indicated that a single positive fFN performed at 24–26 weeks' gestation may identify up to 60% of women destined to deliver before 28 weeks.[15] The sensitivity of this test at 24 weeks for SPTB before 35 weeks was 20%. Other biochemical screening tests have been proposed recently, such as maternal salivary estriol and maternal serum relaxin, but have not been evaluated in large trials.

The biophysical tests that have been studied as screens for increased risk of SPTB include home uterine activity monitoring (HUAM), digital cervical examination and cervical sonography. The use of HUAM as a screening tool has not been fully evaluated; however, its large expense may be prohibitive. Digital examination of the cervix showing premature dilatation and effacement has been associated with an increased risk of subsequent SPTB.[16] However, in a randomized trial there were no differences in rates of preterm birth between 2803 women followed with serial digital cervical examination when compared with 2799 women in whom this examination was not routinely performed.[17] Transvaginal cervical sonographic measurement of cervical length has been reported to identify women at risk for SPTB on the basis of cervical length <10th percentile, below 25 mm at 24–28 weeks' gestation.[18] However, this data has not been tested in an interventional trial and cervical sonography can be expensive and requires the operator to go through an extensive learning curve.

Microbial screens (e.g. for bacterial vaginosis or group B streptococcus) have been tested as screening tools but cannot be recommended because of the high prevalence of positive results, the large variance in declaring a positive test result, and the paucity of successful interventional trials.

A combination of screening tests may improve the efficacy of screening for women at risk for SPTB. The NICHD Preterm Prediction Study found that a positive maternal history of previous SPTB, the presence of cervicovaginal fFN at 24–26 weeks' gestation and cervical length <10th percentile at 24–28 weeks were associated with a 6–8 fold increased risk of SPTB in the current pregnancy.[12]

Therapeutic Interventions

The association of various risk factors with SPTB has led to interventional trials aimed at reducing preterm birth, but this approach has not been successful. The existing interventional trials include those aimed at early identification of PTL through patient education, pharmacologic suppression of uterine contractions, antimicrobial therapy of vaginal micro-organisms, cerclage sutures to bolster the cervix, reduction of maternal stress, improved access to prenatal care, and reduced physical activity. The lack of success of these trials is not surprising when the ASCVD multifactorial model of SPTB is considered. SPTBs occur when the sum of the 'triggers' or stimuli for labor exceed the ability of the maternal host to resist labor. The stimulus or trigger contributed by each individual risk factor is rarely sufficient to reach the threshold necessary to initiate SPTB. Elimination of a single risk factor is unlikely in this model to produce a substantial decrease in SPTB.

EVALUATION OF SUSPECTED PRETERM LABOR AND PRETERM PREMATURE RUPTURE OF MEMBRANES

A major shortfall in studies of PTL has been accurate diagnosis. The diagnosis has traditionally been made by the combination of persistent uterine contractions and change in the dilatation or effacement of the cervix by digital exam. Approximately 40% of subjects in clinical randomized trials of tocolytics, diagnosed with PTL and treated with placebo, delivered at term,[19] indicating the poor positive predictive value of traditional methods of diagnosis of PTL.

The symptoms and signs of early PTL are non-specific and are not necessarily the same as those of labor at term. The symptoms are prevalent among normal healthy women and include menstrual like cramps, low back pain, increased vaginal discharge, and a balling-up sensation in the abdomen. Screening for symptomatology relies on the clinician's awareness to question patients at every obstetrical visit and investigate positive responses.

The use of HUAM for the early diagnosis of PTL has been ineffective. Meta-analyses of the published reports have concluded that HUAM as currently employed as an early diagnosis technique is ineffective in reducing preterm birth in at-risk women.[20]

Digital examination of the cervix is imprecise when the cervical dilation is <3 cm. Effacement and consistency are highly subjective. Digital examination is a poor predictor of early PTL, but the use of more components of the Bishop score may improve the predictive value.

Cervical sonography

A cervical length of 30 mm or more by transvaginal sonography is good evidence that appreciable effacement has not occurred. Seventy patients with threatened PTL were evaluated with cervical sonography and it was found that wedging of the cervix and short cervical length were significantly associated with preterm delivery (sensitivity 100%, specificity 74.5%).[21] Several other studies have confirmed these findings.

Fetal fibronectin

fFN was approved by the United States Food and Drug Administration (FDA) in 1995 as an aid in the diagnosis of PTL. Three studies have compared fFN to traditional methods of diagnosing PTL.[22–24] The greatest clinical utility of fFN lies in the negative predictive value (>96%) as a test to avoid overdiagnosis and treatment. The combination of fFN and transvaginal sonography have been shown to improve the diagnostic accuracy compared to either test alone.[25] Recently, the use of cervical interleukin-6 has been shown to be a promising biochemical marker for the early diagnosis of PTL,[26] but larger scale trials will need to be conducted to validate the routine use of IL-6.

Maternal evaluation

During the initial evaluation for PTL, all patients should undergo a sterile speculum exam and assessment of fetal well-being. The sterile speculum examination should include visualization of the cervix, cervical cultures for gonorrhea, chlamydia and group B streptococcus, swab for fFN, and evaluation for rupture of membranes. Ruptured membranes is usually suspected when the patient gives a history of a gush of fluid and subsequent leaking, but the symptoms may be more subtle, e.g. an increase in vaginal discharge. For this reason, a digital exam should not be performed until the diagnosis of PPROM is excluded. Membrane rupture is usually diagnosed by the presence of amniotic fluid pooling in the vagina, a positive nitrazine test and positive ferning. If the diagnosis of PPROM has been excluded, then a digital examination of the cervix should be performed and transvaginal sonography of the cervix should be considered whenever the cervix is not completely effaced. Digital examinations or transvaginal sonography should not be performed in patients with confirmed or suspected cases of PPROM. Even a single digital exam of the cervix in patients with PPROM increases the risk of amnionitis and neonatal infection and decreases the latency period until delivery.[27, 28] Usually, adequate visualization of the cervix can be accomplished with the sterile speculum examination and this will identify those patients with advanced dilatation of the cervix. Digital examination of the cervix in patients with PPROM should not be performed until delivery is anticipated within 24 hours.

Fetal evaluation

Fetal well-being should be assessed by a non-stress test and fetal ultrasonography for presentation, estimated fetal weight, estimated gestational age, amniotic fluid volume, placental location, and an examination of fetal anatomy for the presence of anomalies. Many fetal anomalies and aneuploidies will be found by sonography, but a normal examination does not rule out all anomalies or aneuploidies. For example, ultrasound of trisomy 21 infants detects major structural defects in only about 30% of the cases.[29, 30] If the diagnosis of PPROM is equivocal, the presence of oligohydramnios can help with confirmation, and occasionally amniocentesis is performed with instillation of indigo carmine dye as a test for PPROM.

Putting it all together and counseling the family

At this point, the information obtained from the history and maternal and fetal evaluations can be assimilated to formulate a plan. Indications for immediate delivery such as maternal chorioamnionitis or prolapsed umbilical cord need to be ruled out. Available records should be reviewed and an accurate estimation of the fetal gestational age determined and used to estimate the fetal risks of delivery versus the maternal and fetal risks of prolonging the gestation.

Most families are not familiar with the complexities of care required for an extremely premature infant in the intensive care unit and after discharge. Information needs to be provided in small segments with frequent repetition to assure understanding. An explanation of supportive measures necessary in the intensive care unit, potential complications, and long-term support should be provided.

Goals of treatment and a delivery plan should be discussed with the family. The family should be provided with the most accurate estimate of survival and morbidity, preferably based on the current literature and the institution's own data. Maternal and fetal risks and benefits of different modes of delivery should be discussed with the family in a non-directive fashion and a decision made based on the expectations for survival and morbidity. The goals of treatment, degree of perinatal intervention, and planned route of delivery must be documented in the patient's chart.

MANAGEMENT OF PRETERM LABOR AND PRETERM PREMATURE RUPTURE OF MEMBRANES

Tertiary Care

Tertiary care, i.e. treatment after the diagnosis has been made, has no effect on the incidence of disease; the goals are a reduction in mortality and morbidity. For SPTB, tertiary care includes prompt diagnosis and referral, treatment of the primary diagnosis and ancillary care. The initial goal of treatment of women with preterm labor or PPROM is to delay delivery long enough to allow 3 interventions that have been shown to reduce neonatal morbidity and mortality:

- maternal transfer
- glucocorticoids
- antibiotic prophylaxis to prevent neonatal group B streptococcus infection.

Maternal and neonatal transfer

Transfer of low birth weight (LBW) infants after birth began in the 1970s and led to dramatic improvements in neonatal outcomes. Transfer of the mother with the fetus *in utero*, whenever possible, became preferable after reports of improved neonatal survival and reduced morbidity for inborn versus outborn infants. Maternal transfer is a priority for preterm delivery ≤32 weeks' gestation and the obstetrician's assessment and evaluation of PTL or PPROM should be aimed at this goal.

Antenatal glucocorticoids

Liggins and Howe in 1972 reported a reduction in respiratory distress syndrome (RDS) in premature infants born to women treated with antenatal glucocorticoids.[31] Subsequent studies have confirmed this work and demonstrated additional benefits including reduced incidence and severity of intraventricular hemorrhage (IV_H), necrotizing enterocolitis (NEC), and decreased perinatal mortality.[32–40] Two glucocorticoid regimens have been studied: betamethasone 12 mg IM Q24h for 2 doses and dexamethasone 6 mg IM Q6h for 4 doses. The two regimens have been found to be equivalent in prevention of neonatal morbidity and mortality.

Glucocorticoids were underutilized in the 1980s and early 1990s despite overwhelming evidence of their benefit from experimental models and randomized controlled trials. The NICHD Neonatal Research Network in a study of 9949 premature infants born at a mean gestational age of 28.1 weeks found that only 19% were exposed to antenatal glucocorticoids, with 65% of these receiving a complete course.[41] In 1994 the National Institutes of Health Consensus Conference Development Panel recommended that antenatal treatment with glucocorticoids be considered for all fetuses at risk for preterm delivery between 24 and 34 weeks, and in circumstances of PPROM at <30–32 weeks' gestation, in the absence of clinical chorioamnionitis, due to the high risk of IV_H at these gestational ages.[42] The use of antenatal glucocorticoids has significantly increased since the Consensus Conference's recommendations.

Several questions about the antenatal glucocorticoid use that remain to be answered:

- Is repeat dosing efficacious and safe in patients who are undelivered after 1 week of initial dosing?
- What are the fetal and maternal impacts of the diabetogenic effect of administration of glucocorticoids to women with insulin-dependent diabetes, gestational diabetes and impaired glucose tolerance?

- Does the long-term use (e.g. repeat dosing) have an effect on membrane strength and predispose to PROM?
- Are glucocorticoids efficacious in multifetal gestations and what is the appropriate dosing?

These questions are the subjects of several current multicenter trials and recommendations for the use of glucocorticoids in the above circumstances will have to await the published results.

The use of antenatal glucocorticoids in the setting of PPROM is controversial. One of the major deterrents to steroid use in mothers with PPROM has been fear of fetal and maternal immunosuppression resulting in increased infectious morbidity, but two large studies noted neither increased neonatal nor maternal infections.[43, 44] The risk of infection in the setting of PPROM needs to be weighted against the potential benefits; this is where the controversy lies. Two meta-analyses of steroid trials in patients with PPROM returned different conclusions depending upon the use or exclusion of data from 2 controversial studies by Morales *et al*[46–47] The impact of the Morales studies on the 2 meta-analyses is significant: the studies contain the largest sample sizes in the meta-analyses, have the largest reported reduction in RDS with steroid use, and higher rates of RDS in the control groups than those in other studies.[48] Exclusion of the studies by Morales *et al* from either meta-analysis results in failure to show a beneficial effect of glucocorticoids for reducing RDS in the setting of PPROM. Reduced IV_H was associated with steroid use in both meta-analyses and lead to the NICHD and ACOG recommendation that glucocorticoids be used in the setting of PPROM at gestational ages <32 weeks.

Administration of antenatal glucocorticoids should be a priority due to their unequivocal benefits in the setting of intact membranes at 24–34 weeks' gestation, and in the setting of PPROM at 24–32 weeks. Glucocorticoids should be administered once a diagnosis is made and prior to maternal transport. The use of glucocorticoids in the setting of PPROM does have a clear benefit in reducing IVH up to 32 weeks' gestation, but their use for RDS prophylaxis remains unsubstantiated.

Antibiotics

There are 2 reasons for administering prophylactic antibiotics to women with PTL or PPROM. The first is to reduce the risk of neonatal group B streptococcal (GBS) infection. PTL and PPROM are major risk factors for early-onset GBS infection. Women presenting with PTL or PPROM should be cultured for GBS and prophylactic antibiotics administered. Antibiotic therapy should continue until a negative culture result is obtained, or for at least 7 days if the culture is positive. The second reason is to prolong gestation by targeting a broad range of micro-organisms that have been implicated in the pathogenesis of SPTB. Randomized placebo-controlled trials of prophylactic broad-spectrum antibiotics in patients with intact membranes have failed to demonstrate improvements in the interval to delivery, mean birth weight, or the incidence of PPROM and amnionitis.[49] A NICHD trial of 614 women with PPROM randomized to either expectant management or treatment with ampicillin and erythromycin found the antibiotic group to have significantly less morbidity and a prolonged latency period.[50] In addition to giving antibiotics for GBS prophylaxis to all women with PPROM and PTL, broader-spectrum coverage should be considered for women with PPROM.

Tocolysis

Studies of tocolytic drugs have failed to show a reduction in SPTB in treated subjects. However, there is good evidence that tocolytics can prolong gestation by at least 48 hours. All currently used tocolytic agents cross the placenta and the incidence of neonatal side effects is greatest when the fetus is born close to a period of high-dose parenteral therapy. In cases of PPROM, tocolysis may be considered to allow time for maternal transport, antenatal glucocorticoids and antibiotics, but has not been shown to be beneficial for longer than that.

β-Sympathomimetic agents. The efficacy of β-mimetic agents has been examined in numerous clinical trials. A meta-analysis of the randomized trials found β-mimetic agents to be most successful in prolonging pregnancy for at least 24 hours.[19] There was no advantage for the treated groups compared to placebo controls in the frequency of LBW <2500 g, severe RDS or perinatal death. The main advantage of β-mimetic agents are their ability to delay delivery long enough to allow for maternal transport and the administration of glucocorticoids and antibiotics.

A number of maternal side effects are common. Most are mild and only result in maternal discomfort, such as tachycardia, apprehension, nausea and vomiting and jitteriness. Other maternal side effects can be life-threatening such as pulmonary edema, myometrial ischemia, cardiac dysrhythmias, hypotension, and hyperglycemia and hypokalemia. Neonatal side effects include an increased risk of IV_H,[51] hypoglycemia, hypocalcemia and ileus.[52]

Magnesium sulfate. Intravenous magnesium sulfate has been safely used in obstetrics for seizure prophylaxis in pre-eclampsia for almost 60 years.

The efficacy of magnesium sulfate as a tocolytic is even less proven than that of β-sympathomimetic agents. Randomized studies of magnesium sulfate compared to β-sympathomimetics found no differences in tocolytic effect; however, the power of these studies was insufficient.[53, 54]

Cox *et al* compared magnesium sulfate to no tocolysis and found no differences in duration of pregnancy, birth weight, neonatal morbidity or perinatal mortality.[55] Overall, the studies suggest some delay in delivery associated with magnesium sulfate, but the agent does not appear to be a highly effective tocolytic agent. Magnesium sulfate, similar to the β-sympathomimetic agents, can be considered as a temporizing agent that allows for maternal transfer and treatment with ancillary agents.

Maternal side effects are relatively rare compared to those from the β-sympathomimetics. The commonest include flushing, nausea, vomiting, headache, generalized muscle weakness, diplopia and shortness of breath. More severe complications include pulmonary edema and cardiorespiratory arrest from toxicity at higher dosages, usually secondary to administration error. Neonatal side effects are minimal and include lethargy, hypotonia and respiratory depression. Recently, there has been interest in the beneficial neonatal effects of magnesium sulfate. Preliminary reports have suggested that antenatal magnesium sulfate treatment is associated with lower frequencies of cerebral palsy and IV_H.[56–58] Several multicenter randomized placebo controlled trials to investigate the effects of antenatal magnesium sulfate are underway.

Prostaglandin synthetase inhibitors. The commonest agent studied in this class has been indomethacin, but sulindac, naproxen, aspirin and fenoprofen have also been clinically used. The efficacy of indomethacin in placebo-controlled trials has been very promising. Two small studies have shown that indomethacin is superior to placebo in delaying delivery for 48 hours and for up to 7 days.[59, 60] Unfortunately, the clinical use of indomethacin is limited by its unfavorable fetal and neonatal side-effect profile.

Maternal side effects are usually mild and consist of nausea, heartburn and vomiting. More serious are reports of gastrointestinal bleeding, alterations in coagulation, thrombocytopenia and bronchospasm in women with drug-induced asthma. Usually, the serious maternal side effects occur only in women with predisposing disorders such as peptic ulcer disease.

Fetal and neonatal side effects are potentially much more serious than maternal side effects. Three principal side effects: constriction of the ductus arteriosis, oligohydramnios and neonatal pulmonary hypertension. The ductal constriction is due to the inhibition of prostaglandin E_2 formation. The incidence of ductal constriction is relatively low (5–10%) prior to 32 weeks' gestation, but increases significantly thereafter.[61] It is usually transient and responds to discontinuation of the drug. Oligohydramnios is common, dose related and reversible. It is due to reduced fetal urine production secondary to a reduction in the normal prostaglandin inhibition of antidiuretic hormone and by direct effects on renal blood flow. Primary pulmonary hypertension in the neonate has been associated with the use of indomethacin for >48 hours.[62] Other complications that have been reported to be associated with indomethacin use include necrotizing enterocolitis, small bowel perforation, patent ductus arteriosus, jaundice IV_H. Due to the broad and potentially serious fetal and neonatal side effect profiles, indomethacin usage for tocolysis is usually limited to periods of 48 hours or less at gestations <32 weeks.

Calcium channel blockers. These are rapidly absorbed after oral and sublingual administration and have potential use as tocolytics. Nifedipine and nicardipine have received the most attention as tocolytic agents due to their ability selectively to inhibit uterine contractions. Nifedipine has been compared to ritodrine in several studies and has been shown to be either equal or superior in delaying delivery with fewer side effects.[63, 64]

Maternal side effects are mild and most commonly include headache, flushing, dizziness and nausea. Their use in conjunction with magnesium sulfate should be avoided due to the risk of skeletal muscle blockade.[65, 66] Fetal side effects were initially a concern due to animal studies reporting reduction in uteroplacental blood flow, fetal bradycardia and hypoxic myocardial depression with calcium channel blockers other than nifedipine.[67, 68] Subsequent animal studies of nifedipine have not shown such effects unless used in supertherapeutic doses. Human studies have not shown an effect on Doppler flow studies of the fetal and uteroplacental circulations, Apgar scores or umbilical blood gas values.[69–71] Based on these data, nifedipine is considered to be a safe agent for tocolytic use and some centers have begun to use it as the tocolytic of first choice. The other calcium channel blockers cannot be considered safe for use at this time.

Other tocolytic agents. Agents that are currently under study include the oxytocin antagonist atosiban, the nitric oxide donor glycerol trinitrate and nitroglycerin. Preliminary reports are promising for these new agents in their ability to arrest maternal contractions with a favorable maternal and neonatal side-effect profile. Their efficacy compared to current tocolytics will need to be demonstrated prior to their recommendation for use.

LABOR AND DELIVERY OF THE PRETERM INFANT

When tocolysis has failed to prolong the gestation and delivery is imminent, specialized care of the LBW fetus is needed. Survival and morbidity issues should be discussed again with the family to develop a clear understanding of expectations. In particular, a plan for the mode of delivery needs to be made, and special attention paid to fetal monitoring, maternal anesthesia and delivery procedures.

It is always difficult to determine appropriate intervention for a fetus at the margin of viability (i.e. <800 g or <26 weeks). Questions that need to be addressed include:

- Is the fetal heart rate going to be monitored?
- Will a cesarean section be performed for non-reassuring fetal heart rate patterns?
- Should elective cesarean section be performed for breech presentation?
- Will the neonatal resuscitation team attend the delivery?
- How far will the resuscitation go?

The answers to these questions are known to influence the outcome in extremely LBW infants as demonstrated in several studies. Paul *et al* demonstrated that infants judged to be previable have significantly higher mortality rates than do infants of the same weight and gestational age who have received intensive intrapartum care.[72] An analysis of 713 infants <1000 g at 11 universities found that aggressive management is associated with increased overall survival, increased intact survival and, unfortunately, increased severe neurologic morbidity.[73]

Vaginal delivery is the preferred route when the preterm infant is in the cephalic presentation. Prophylactic cesarean section has been advocated in the past but is not justified by available data. Several large studies have failed to note improvement in perinatal morbidity or mortality with routine cesarean birth for LBW infants.[74–76] Furthermore, these studies did not show an advantage to cesarean delivery for breech presentation in infants weighing <750 g. The decision to proceed with cesarean whether for prophylactic or obstetrical reasons is difficult at the extremes of viability and requires the consideration that improvements in survival may result in a child with severe physical and mental impairment.

CONCLUSIONS

Three main objectives have been discussed in this chapter. The first is that in order to improve the morbidity and mortality of preterm birth, a comprehensive approach, similar to that used to combat ASCAD, needs to be developed and adopted. Primary and secondary care plans for the prevention of SPTB should be evaluated. Secondly, there are 3 tertiary interventions that have been proven to have a positive influence on neonatal morbidity and mortality: maternal transfer, antenatal glucocorticoids and antibiotics. Tocolysis is justified to 'buy time' in order to accomplish these interventions as long as there are no maternal or fetal contraindications to prolonging pregnancy for 24–48 hours. Finally, more accurate methods of diagnosis of PTL will improve the identification of those patients who need treatment and help insure that only patients with PTL are enrolled in future interventional trials.

REFERENCES

1. Mercer BM, Goldenberg RL, Moawad A *et al.* Prediction of spontaneous prematurity based on prior obstetric outcome (abstract). *Am J Obstet Gynecol* 1995;**172**: 404.
2. Tamura RK, Sabbagha RE, Depp OR *et al.* Diminished growth in fetuses born preterm after spontaneous labor or rupture of membranes. *Am J Obstet Gynecol* 1984;**148**: 1105.
3. MacGregor SN, Sabbagha RE, Tamura RK *et al.* Differing fetal growth patterns in pregnancies complicated by preterm labor. *Obstet Gynecol* 1988;**72**: 834
4. Ott WJ. Intrauterine growth retardation and preterm delivery. *Am J Obstet Gynecol* 1993;**168**: 1710.
5. Hediger ML, Scholl TO, Schall JI *et al.* Fetal growth and the etiology of preterm delivery. *Obstet Gynecol* 1995;**85**: 175.
6. Salafia CM, Vogel CA, Vintzeleos AM *et al.* Placental pathologic findings in preterm birth. *Am J Obstet Gynecol* 1991;**165**: 934.
7. Romero R, Sirtori M, Oyarzun E *et al.* Infection and labor V: prevalence, microbiology, and clinical significance of intraamniotic infection in women with preterm labor and intact membranes. *Am J Obstet Gynecol* 1989;**161**: 817.
8. Romero R, Gomez R, Ghezzi F *et al.* The onset of spontaneous preterm parturition is preceded by an intense pro-inflammatory cytokine response in the human fetus. *Am J Obstet Gynecol* 1997;**176**: S3 (abstract).
9. MacDonald PC and Casey ML. The accumulation of prostaglandins (PGs) in amniotic fluid is an after effect of labor and not indicative of a role for PGE_2 or PGF_2 alpha in the initiation of human parturition. *J Clin Endocrinol Metab* 1993;**76**: 1332.

10. Romero R, Masor M, Munoz H *et al.* The preterm labor syndrome. *Ann NY Acad Sci* 1994;**734**: 414.
11. Creasy RK. Preterm birth prevention: where are we? *Am J Obstet Gynecol* 1993;**168**: 1223.
12. Iams JD *et al* from the National Institute of Child Health and Human Development Maternal Fetal Medicine Unit Network. The preterm prediction study: A model for estimation of risk of spontaneous preterm birth in parous women. *Am J Obstet Gynecol* 1998; **178(5)**: 1035–1040.
13. Ekwo EE, Gosselink CA and Moawad A. Unfavorable outcome in penultimate pregnancy and premature rupture of membranes in successive pregnancy. *Obstet Gynecol* 1992;**80**: 166.
14. Kramer MS, Coates AL, Michoud MC *et al.* Maternal anthropometry and idiopathic preterm labor. *Obstet Gynecol* 1995;**86**: 744.
15. Goldenberg R, Mercer BM, Meis PJ *et al.* The preterm prediction study: Early fetal fibronectin testing predicts early spontaneous preterm birth. *Am J Obstet Gynecol* 1996;**87**: 643.
16. Papiernik E, Bouyer J, Collin D *et al.* Precocious cervical ripening and preterm labor. *Obstet Gynecol* 1986;**67**: 238.
17. Buekens P, Alexander S, Boutsen M *et al.* Randomized controlled trial of routine cervical examinations in pregnancy. *Lancet* 1994;**344**: 841.
18. Iams JD, Goldenberg RL, Meis PJ *et al.* The length of the cervix and the risk of spontaneous premature delivery. *N Engl J Med* 1996;**334**: 567.
19. King JF, Grand A, Keirse MJN *et al.* Betamimetics in preterm labour: an overview of randomized controlled trials. *Br J Obstet Gynaecol* 1988;**95**: 211.
20. Grimes DA and Schultz KF. Randomized controlled trials of home uterine activity monitoring: a review and critique. *Obstet Gynecol* 1992;**79**: 137.
21. Timor-Tritsch IE, Boozarjomehri F, Masakowski MA *et al.* Can a 'snapshot' sagittal view of the cervix by transvaginal ultrasonography predict active labor? *Am J Obstet Gynecol* 1996;**174**: 990.
22. Iams JD, Casal D, McGregor JA *et al.* Fetal fibronectin improves the accuracy of diagnosis of preterm labor. *Am J Obstet Gynecol* 1995;**173**: 141.
23. Peaceman AM, Andrews WW, Thorp JM *et al.* Fetal fibronectin as a predictor of preterm birth in symptomatic patients – A multicenter trial. *Am J Obstet Gynecol* 1996;**174**: 303(abstract).
24. Adeza Biomedical. Presentation to the United States Food and Drug Administration. April 6, 1995.
25. Rizzo G, Capponi A, Arduini D *et al.* The value of fetal fibronectin in cervical and vaginal secretions and of ultrasonographic examination of the uterine cervix in predicting premature delivery for patients with preterm labor and intact membranes. *Am J Obstet Gynecol* 1996;**175**: 1146.
26. Rizzo G, Capponi A, Rinaldo D *et al.* Interleukin-6 concentrations in cervical secretions identify microbial invasion of the amniotic cavity in patients with preterm labor and intact membranes. *Am J Obstet Gynecol* 1996;**175**: 812.
27. Schutte M, Treffers P, Kloosterman G *et al.* Management of premature rupture of membranes: the risk of vaginal examination to the infant. *Am J Obstet Gynecol* 1983;**146**: 395.

28. Lewis DF, Major CA, Towers CV *et al.* Effects of digital vaginal examinations on latency period in preterm premature rupture of membranes. *Obstet Gynecol* 1992;**80**: 630.
29. Benaceraff BR, Gelman R and Frigoletto FD. Sonographic identification of second-trimester fetuses with Down syndrome. *N Engl J Med* 1987;**317**: 1371.
30. Nyberg DA, Resta RG, Luthy DA *et al.* Prenatal sonographic findings of Down syndrome: review of 94 cases. *Obstet Gynecol* 1990;**76**: 370.
31. Liggens GC and Howie RN. A controlled trial of antepartum glucocorticoid treatment for prevention of the respiratory distress syndrome in premature infants. *Pediatrics* 1972;**50**: 515.
32. Crowley PA. Antenatal corticosteroid therapy. A meta-analysis of the randomized trials. *Am J Obstet Gynecol* 1995;**173**: 322.
33. Garite TJ, Rumney PJ, Briggs GG *et al.* A randomized, placebo-controlled trial of betamethasone for the prevention of respiratory distress syndrome. *Am J Obstet Gynecol* 1992;**166**: 646.
34. Eronen M, Kari A and Posonon E. The effect of antenatal dexamethasone administration on the fetal and neonatal ductus arteriosis. A randomized double-blind study. *Am J Dis Child* 1993;**147**: 187.
35. Kari MA, Hallman M, Eronen M *et al.* Prenatal dexamethasone treatment in conjunction with rescue therapy of human surfactant: randomized placebo-controlled multicenter study. *Pediatrics* 1994;**93**: 730.
36. Jobe AH, Mitchell BR and Gunkel JH. Beneficial effects of the combined use of prenatal corticosteroids and post-natal surfactant on preterm infants. *Am J Obstet Gynecol* 1993;**168**: 508.
37. Andrews EB, Marcucci G, White A *et al.* Associations between use of antenatal corticosteroids and neonatal outcomes within the Exosurf Neonatal Treatment Investigational New Drug Study Group. *Am J Obstet Gynecol* 1995;**173**: 290.
38. Farrell EE, Silver RK, Kimberlin LV *et al.* Impact of antenatal dexamethasone administration on respiratory distress syndrome in surfactant-treated infants. *Am J Obstet Gynecol* 1989;**161**: 628.
39. Ment LR, Oh W, Ehrenkrantz RA *et al.* Antenatal steroids, delivery mode, and intraventricular hemorrhage in preterm infants. *Am J Obstet Gynecol* 1995;**172**: 795.
40. Gardner MO, Goldenberg RL, Gaudier FL *et al.* Predicting low Apgar scores of infants weighing less than 1000 grams: the effect of corticosteroids. *Obstet Gynecol* 1995;**85**: 170.
41. Wright LL, Verter J, Younes N *et al.* Antenatal corticosteroid administration and neonatal outcome in very low birth weight infants: The NICHD Neonatal Research Network. *Am J Obstet Gynecol* 1995;**173**: 269.
42. National Institutes of Health Consensus Development Conference Statement. Effect of corticosteroids for fetal maturation on perinatal outcome, February 28–March 2, 1994. *Am J Obstet Gynecol* 1995;**173**: 246.
43. Collaborative Group on Antenatal Steroid Therapy. Effect of antenatal dexamethasone administration on the prevention of respiratory distress syndrome. *Am J Obstet Gynecol* 1981;**141**: 276.

44. Liggins GC. The prevention of RDS by maternal betamethasone administration. In: Moore TD (ed) *Lung Maturation and the Prevention of Hyaline Membrane Disease*. Report of the Seventieth Ross Conference on Pediatric Research. Columbus, OH: Ross Laboratories, 1976, p 97.
45. Ohlsson A. Treatments of preterm premature rupture of the membranes: a meta-analysis. *Am J Obstet Gynecol* 1989;**160**: 890.
46. Morales WJ, Diebel ND, Lazar AJ *et al.* The effect of antenatal dexamethasone on the prevention of respiratory distress syndrome in preterm gestation with premature rupture of the membranes. *Am J Obstet Gynecol* 1986;**154**: 591.
47. Morales WJ, Angel JL, O'Brien WF *et al.* Use of ampicillin and corticosteroids in premature rupture of membranes: A randomized study. *Obstet Gynecol* 1989;**73**: 721.
48. Imseis HM and Iams JD. Glucocorticoid use in patients with preterm premature rupture of the fetal membranes. *Semin Perinatol* 1996;**20**: 439.
49. Romero R, Sibai B, Caritis S *et al.* Antibiotic treatment of preterm labor with intact membranes: a multicenter, randomized, double-blinded, placebo-controlled trial. *Am J Obstet Gynecol* 1993;**169**: 764.
50. Mecer B, Miodovnik M, Thurnau R *et al.* A multicenter randomized masked trial of antibiotic vs. placebo therapy after preterm rupture of the membranes. *Am J Obstet Gynecol* 1996;**174**: 304(abstract).
51. Groome LJ, Goldenberg RL, Cliver SP *et al.* Neonatal periventricular-intraventricular hemorrhage after maternal beta-sympathomimetic tocolysis. The March of Dimes Multicenter Study Group. *Am J Obstet Gynecol* 1992;**167**: 873.
52. Epstein M, Nicholls E and Stubblefield P. Neonatal hypoglycemia after beta-sympathomimetic tocolytic therapy. *Pediatrics* 1979;**94**: 449.
53. Miller YM, Keane MWD and Horger EO. A comparison of magnesium sulfate and terbutaline for the arrest of preterm labor. *J Reprod Med* 1982;**27**: 348.
54. Hollander DI, Nagey DA and Pupkin MJ. Magnesium sulfate and ritodrine hydrochloride: a randomized comparison. *Am J Obstet Gynecol* 1987;**156**: 631.
55. Cox SM, Sherman LM and Leveno KJ. Randomized investigation of magnesium sulfate for prevention of preterm birth. *Am J Obstet Gynecol* 1990;**163**: 767.
56. Nelson KB and Grether J. Effect of $MgSO_4$ therapy on cerebral palsy rates in infants < 1500 grams. *J Pediatr* 1995;**95**: 263.
57. Bottoms S, Paul R, Iams JD *et al.* Obstetrical determinants of neonatal survival in extremely low birth weight infants. *Am J Obstet Gynecol* 1994;**170**: 383.
58. Hauth JL, Goldenberg RL, Nelson KG *et al.* Reduction of cerebral palsy rates with maternal $MgSO_4$ treatment in newborns weighing 500–1000 grams. *Am J Obstet Gynecol* 1995;**172**: 419(abstract).
59. Neibyl J, Blake D, White R *et al.* The inhibition of premature labor with indomethacin. *Am J Obstet Gynecol* 1980;**136**: 1014.
60. Zuckerman H, Shalev E, Gilad G *et al.* Further study of the inhibition of premature labor by indomethacin. Parts I&II. *J Perinat Med* 1984;**12**: 19 and 25.
61. Moise K. Effect of advancing gestational age on the frequency of fetal ductal constriction in association with maternal indomethacin use. *Am J Obstet Gynecol* 1994;**168**: 1350.

62. Manchester D, Margolis H and Sheldon R. Possible association between maternal indomethacin therapy and primary pulmonary hypertension of the newborn. *Am J Obstet Gynecol* 1976;**126**: 467.
63. Ulmsten U, Anderson KE and Wingerup L. Treatment of preterm labor with the calcium antagonist nifedipine. *Arch Gynecol* 1980;**229**: 1.
64. Read MD and Wellby DE. The use of a calcium antagonist (nifedipine) to suppress preterm labor. *Br J Obstet Gynaecol* 1986;**93**: 933.
65. Snyder SW and Cardwell MS. Neuromuscular blockade with magnesium sulfate and nifedipine. *Am J Obstet Gynecol* 1989;**161**: 35.
66. Ben-Ami M, Galadi Y and Shalev E. The combination of magnesium sulphate and nifedipine: a cause of neuromuscular blockade. *Br J Obstet Gynaecol* 1994;**101**: 262.
67. Parisi VM, Salinas J and Stockmar EJ. Fetal vascular responses to maternal nicardipine administration in the hypertensive ewe. *Am J Obstet Gynecol* 1989;**161**: 1035.
68. Parisi VM, Salinas J and Stockmar EJ. Placental vascular responses to maternal nicardipine administration in the hypertensive ewe. *Am J Obstet Gynecol* 1989;**161**: 1039.
69. Mari G, Kirshon B, Moise KJ *et al.* Doppler assessment of the fetal and uteroplacental circulation during nifedipine therapy for preterm labor. *Am J Obstet Gynecol* 1989;**161**: 1514.
70. Murray C, Haverkamp AD, Orleans M *et al.* Nifedipine for the treatment of preterm labor. *Am J Obstet Gynecol* 1992;**167**: 52.
71. Ray D, Dyson D and Crites Y. Nifedipine tocolysis and neonatal acid-base status at delivery. *Am J Obstet Gynecol* 1994;**170**: 387(abstract).
72. Paul R, Koh K and Monfared A. Obstetric factors influencing outcome in infants weighing from 1000 to 1500 grams. *Am J Obstet Gynecol* 1979;**133**: 503.
73. Bottoms SF, Paul RH, Iams JD *et al.* Obstetrical determinants of neonatal survival: influence of willingness to perform cesarean delivery on survival of extremely low birth weight infants. *Am J Obstet Gynecol* 1997; **176**(5): 960–966.
74. Malloy MH, Rhoads GG, Schramm W *et al.* Increasing cesarean section rates in very low-birth-weight infants, effect on outcome. *JAMA* 1989;**262**: 1475.
75. Kitchen W, Ford GW, Doyle LW *et al.* Cesarean section or vaginal delivery at 24 to 28 weeks gestation: comparison of survival and neonatal and two-year morbidity. *Obstet Gynecol* 1985;**66**: 149.
76. Malloy MH, Onstad L, Wright E *et al.* The effect of cesarean delivery on birth outcome in very low birth weight infants. *Obstet Gynecol* 1991;**77**: 498.

Index

Note: tables in **bold**; figures in *italic*

47 XXY 245
69 XXX 245
69 XXY 245

Acetylcholine 74, 122
Acidosis 15
Acinetobacter 36
Age, maternal 233
Agranulocytosis, congenital 215
Albuterol 160
Alcohol 96, 98
Alkaline phosphatase 52
α-fetoprotein 234, **236**
Amblyopia 184
Amicon minifilter 17, 19
Amino acids 8
Aminoglycosides 8, 32, 33
Ammonium 9
Amniocentesis 237–9
Amnionitis 251
Amphotericin B 210
Ampicillin 31, 204
Angiotensin II 6
Angiotensin converting enzyme inhibitors 6
Anisometropia 184, 191
Antibiotics
- changing policy on 33–4
- duration 34–8
- in early-onset sepsis 31–2
- in late-onset sepsis 32–3
- negative blood culture 34–5
- positive blood culture 35–7
- in PPROM 260–1
- prophylactic antepartum 203–4
- prophylaxis, neonatal 30–1
- toxicity 34

Antidiuretic hormone (ADH) 8
Antro-duodenal manometry 131
Anuria 11
Apert's disorder 94
Apnoea 120, 129
Apoptosis 95
Asphyxia, perinatal, severe 28
Aspiration syndromes 141
Aspirin 262
Astrocytes 97, 98
Atherosclerotic cardiovascular disease (ASCVD) 252–3, 255
ATN 10
Atosiban 263
Autoimmune disease 134
Autoregulation of renal blood flow 6, 7

β blockers 65
Betamethasone 259
Bicarbonate 8, 15
Biopsy, fetal 242–4
Bishop score 256
Blood pressure
- adequate 80
- observational studies 66–70
- in preterm infant 66–71
- raising 75–80
- rules of thumb 70–1, 80

Blood urea concentration 47
Blood urea nitrogen (BUN) 10, 11, 163
Bone mineral content 52

Borderline ventriculomegaly 246
Brain
fatty acids and 99–101
growth, fetal 94–5
neonatal, development 101–3
weight 101
Breastfeeding a preterm baby 53–4
see also milk, human
Bronchomalacia 158
Bronchopulmonary dysplasia (BPD) 157–70, 213
cardiopulmonary physiology 158
co-ordination of care 165–8
management strategies 159–61
pathogenesis and clinical course 161–5
Bronchospasm 129

Calcium 98
absorption 52
in milk 50–1, 52
Calcium channel blockers 263
Calcium polystyrene sulphate 15
Candida infection 36, 133, 134, 201, 208, 216
Candida albicans 201, 210
Candida arapsilosis 210
Candida glabrata 210
Candida lusitaniae 210
Carbamoyl-phosphate synthetase deficiency 242
Cardiovascular disease 126
Cardiovascular function, fetal and neonatal 63–5
Cataracts 185
Cdx1/Cdx2 119
Cdx_2 gene 113
Cdx_{26} gene 113
Cephalosporin, third-generation 32, 33
Cerebellar granular cells 97
Cerebral injury in very low birthweight infant 72–3
Cerebral neurones 97
Cerebrosides 100
Cervical sonography 255, 256
Chloramphenicol 207
Chloride reabsorption 8
Cholesterol, unesterified 100
Chorioamnionitis 25, 201, 203, 205, 217, 253, 258
Chorionic villus sampling (CVS) 238, 239–42
Choroid plexus cyst (CPC) 246
Citrobacter 34
Clindamycin 207
Clostridia 209
Cloxacillin 32, 33
Coagulase-negative staphylococci (CONS) 201, 208, 209, 210
Cobra venom factor 149
Colitis 134
pseudomembranous 134
Collagen 114
Colloid 72
Colon
endoscopy 134
motor activity 126–9
Colonoscopy 132–3
Confined placental mosaicism (CPM) 241
Continuous arteriovenous diahaemofiltration *18*, 19
Continuous arteriovenous haemofiltration 16–19, *18*
Continuous venovenous haemofiltration *18*, 19–20
Copper deficiency 95
Cor pulmonale 158, 160, 163
Cordocentesis 242
Coronary arteries in very low birthweight infant 73
Corpus callosum 94
Cortical plate 94
Corticosteroids 79–80, 123
inhaled 160
systemic 160–1
Countercurrent immunoelectrophoresis 28
C-reactive protein (CRP) 26
Creamatocrit test 47
Creatinine clearance 2–3, *3*, *4*
Crouzon's disorder 94

Cryotherapy ablation of retina 182, 186
Crypt stem cell 112, 113
Cyanotic congenital heart disease 213
Cyclomydril 188
Cytomegalovirus 213–14

Dexamethasone 160, 259
Diabetes, gestational 259
Diabetes mellitus 95, 251
  insulin-dependent 259
Dialysis in acute renal failure 15–20, **16**
Diaphragmatic hernia, congenital 141
Diencephalon 94
DiGeorge syndrome 239
Digital cervical examination 254–6
Disomic rescue 241
DNA probes 239
Dobutamine 76, 77–8
Docosahexaenoic acid (DHA) 100–1
Dopamine 76, 77, 79
Down syndrome 233, 234, 235, 236–7, 245
D-penicillamine 181
DQ α alleles 245
Drosophila 118
Duchenne muscular dystrophy 245
Ductus arteriosis, constriction 262
Duocal 47
Duodenitis 134
Duodenum, investigation 130–1
Dysfunctional programming 98
Dysmorphogenesis, brain 94

Echocardiography 164
Echogenic bowel 246
Electrical impedance tomography (EIT) 131
Electrogastrography 131
ELISA 216
Endocrine cells 112, 113
Endoscopy, neonatal 132–4
Endothelin signalling pathway 116–17
Enoximone 78
Enteric bacilli, Gram-negative 32
Enteric ganglioneuromatosis 117
Enteric nervous system 115–18
Enterobacter 34, 201, 208
Enterococci (faecal streptococci) 24, 32, 208
  vancomycin-resistant (VRE) 31
Enterocytes, absorptive 112, 113
Enx (*Hox 11L1*) 119
Erythromycin 206–7
Escherichia coli 31, 201, 208, 211, 214, 219
Extracorporeal membrane oxygenation (ECMO) 144, 152

Familial exudative vitreoretinopathy (FEVR) 180
Fatty acids
  n-3 deficiency 100
  and neonatal brain growth 99–101
FC-75 146
Fenoprofen 262
Fetal alcohol syndrome 98
Fetal fibronectin (fFN) 254, 256–7
Fetoscopy 242–3
Fibroblast growth factor receptor defects 94
Fibronectin 114
  fetal (fFN) 254, 256–7
Fluorescence *in situ* hybridization 239
5-Fluorocytosine 210
Folic acid deficiency 95–6
Food allergy 134
Fore gut, functional development 119–29
Fractional sodium excretion 3–4, *5*, 12–13
Frank Starling mechanism 75
Frontal occipital circumference (FOC) 163
Fungaemia 31
Fungal infections 210
Fusbacterium 201
FUSH 245

Gambro AK-10 19
Gastric acid secretion 121–2
Gastric emptying 126, 130
Gastric function 123–6

Gastric hydrophobicity 122–3
Gastric pH in newborns 122
Gastric surfactant 123
Gastric ulcers 121, 134
Gastrin 121, 122
Gastritis 123, 134
  haemorrhagic 123
Gastrointestinal tract
  development 111–19
  fore gut, functional development 119–29
  motor function, investigation 131
  neonatal, investigation 129–34
  in very low birthweight infant 74
Gastro-oesophageal reflux 126, 129, 130, 134
Gastroscopy 132, 133
Genetic counselling 245–6
Genodematoses 242, **243**
Gentamicin 204, 208
Glaucoma 185
Glial cells 97, 116
Glioblasts 116
Glomerular filtration rate (GFR)
  in fetus 2, 4
  neonatal 11
  in newborn 4–6
Glomerulonephritis 10
Glucocorticoids 74
  antenatal 259–60
Glucose 8
Glucose-6-phosphate deficiency 242
α-Glucosidase 113
β-Glucosidase 113
Glutamic acid 98
Glutamine 98
Glycerol trinitrate 263
Glycosaminoglycans, sulphated 114
Glycosphingolipids 100
Goblet cells 112, 113
Granulocyte colony-forming units (CFU-G) 215
Granulocyte colony-stimulating factor (G-CSF) 212, 214–22
Granulocyte/macrophage (GM)-CSF 217
Group B streptococcus (GBS) 24, 26, 31, 201, 203, 204, *205–6*, 211, 219, 255, 260–1
  pneumonia 35
Growth cones 97
Growth factors 94

Haemodialysis 16
Haemofiltration 16, 19
Haemophilus influenzae 211
Haemorrhage, intraventicular 67, 181, 269
Helical CT 149
Heparin infusion 19
Hepatitis 211
Hepatitis B 213
Hepatitis C 213
High-frequency ventilation 152
High-resolution computed tomography (HRCT) 149
Hirschsprung's disease 117
Histamine 122
Histidine 98
HIV 213
HIV-1 infection 55
HLA-DR 245
Holoprosencephaly 94
Home uterine activity monitoring (HUAM) 254, 255, 256
Homeobox genes 113, 118–19
Homocysteine 96
Hox genes 118–19
  Hox A4 119
  Hox C4 119
  Hox D13 119
Human chorionic gonadotropin (hCG) 234
Hyaline membrane disease (HMD) 25, 200
Hyaluronic acid 114
Hydrocortisone 79
Hydrogen ions 9
Hydronephrosis 246
Hydroxyapatite 51
Hypercalcaemia 51
Hypercalciuria 51

Hypergastrinaemia, neonatal 121
Hyperglycaemia, non-ketotic 242
Hyperkalaemia 14
Hyperphenylalaninaemia 98
Hyperphosphataemia 14
Hypertension
  neonatal pulmonary 262, 263
  pregnancy-induced 29, 220
  pulmonary 158, 164
  see also blood pressure
Hypocalcaemia 14, 17
Hypogammaglobulinaemia 211
Hypomagnesaemia 14
Hyponatraemia 7
Hypotension 65, 70
Hypovolaemia 13–14, 65, 75
Hypoxaemia 164

Immature:total neutrophil (IT) ratio 26
Immunoglobulin, intravenous 211–14
Immunoglobulin G (IgG) 211
Indigo carmine dye 257
Indomethacin 74, 75, 123, 181, 262, 263
Infections, neonatal, early-onset 201–7
Inositol supplementation 181–2
Inotropes 76–9
Integrins 114
Interleukins
  IL-1 217
  IL-1α 216
  IL-3 215
  IL-6 257
International Classification of ROP (ICROP) 176
Interstitial nephritis 10
Intestine
  cytodifferentiation in 113–14
  epithelial mesenchymal interactions 114–15
  see also gastrointestinal tract
Intrapartum antimicrobial prophylaxis (IAP) 26, *27*
Intrauterine growth restriction (IUGR) 241, 251
Intrauterine infections (IUI) 201
Intrauterine ischaemia 95
Intravenous immunoglobulin 211–14
Intraventricular haemorrhage 67, 181, 269
Intrinsic renal failure 10
Iodine deficiency 95
Ipatropium bromide 160
Iron deficiency 95

Jarcho-Levin syndrome 237
Jaundice 263
Juxtamedullary nephrons 2, 5

Kidney
  morphological development 1–2, *2*
  in very low birthweight infant 72
Kjeldahl technique 47
Klebsiella 34, 201
Klebsiella pneumoniae 211

β-Lactamase production 209
Lactase 114
Lactoferrin 44
Laminin-2 115
Laser photocoagulation of retina 182
Late metabolic acidosis (LMA) of prematurity 9
Latex particle agglutination (LPA) 28
Leigh's encephalopathy 95
Leukocoria 185
Lignoceric acid 101
Limb defects 241
Lincomycin 207
Lipopolysaccharide (LPS) 216, 222
Liquid-assisted ventilation (LAV) 141, 143
Listeria 29, 32
Listeria monocytogenes 31, 35, 38
Liver biopsy, fetal 242
Liver in very low birthweight infant 72
L-NAME 222
Long-chain polyunsaturated fatty acids (LCPUFA) 45, 100
Long-chain triglyceride 126]
Loop of Henle 8–9

Magnesium sulphate 261–2

Malassezia furfur 210
Malnutrition 96–8
Manganese deficiency 95
Manometry
antro-duodenal 131
oesophageal 130
Maternal salivary oestriol 254
Maternal serum α-fetoprotein (MSAFP) 234, **236**
Maternal serum relaxin 254
Maternal serum screening 234–5
M-CSF 217
Meconium aspiration 29, 147
Medium chain triglyceride 126
Medullary interstitial hypertonicity 8
Meningitis 32, 35, 38, 203, 207, 209, 212
Mesencephalon 94
Metabolic bone disease of prematurity 51–2
Metaclopramide 53–4
Metanephros 1
Metered dose inhaler (MDI) 160
Methicillin 32
Methicillin resistance 209
Methicillin-resistance *Staphyloccus aureus* (MRSA) 32, 33
5,10-Methylene tetrahydrofolate reductase (MTHFR) 96
Metoprolol 65
β-2 Microglobulin 8
Microvillous atrophy 134
Migrating motor complex (MMC) activity 127
Milk banks 55
Milk, formula 126
brain growth and 99, 101
feed tolerance 44–5
infection and 44
Milk, human 126
brain growth and 99, 101
calcium, phosphorus and vitamin D 50–3
diet, growth and neurological development 45
energy 46–7
feed tolerance 44–5
infection and 44
non-nutritional outcomes of feeding 43–5
protein 46, 47–50
storing and administering 54–5
term and preterm 46
Milk, mammalian 96–7
Milrinone 78
Mitochondria 63, 99
Modified Bernoulli equation 164
Monoclonal antibodies 222
Mosaicism 238, 241
Mucosa *124*, *125*
Mucosal defence 122–3
Multidisciplinary fetal treatment team 246
Multiple endocrine neoplasia, types 2A and 2B 117
Mycoplasma hominis 205, 207
Myelination 97, 101
Myelodysplasia 215
Myocardium
in extreme preterm infant 63
in very low birthweight infant 73
Myopia 184, 191

Na^+ K^+ ATPase 77, 113, 121
Naproxen 262
Near-drowning 141
Necrotizing enterocolitis 15, 44–5, 74, 134, 203, 221, 263, 269
Nephrogenesis 2
Nervonic acid 101
Neural crest 94, 115–16
Neural tube 94
Neural tube defects 234
Neuroblasts 116
Neurohypophysis 94
Neurones 116
Neurotrophic factor, glial-derived 116
Neurotrophins 98
Neutropenia 29
Niacin deficiency 96
Nidogen 114
Nifedipine 263

Nitric oxide 148, 222
Nitrogen
  fecal retention 49
  in milk 47–50
  urea 47
Nitroglycerin 263
Non-ketotic hyperglycaemia 242
Non-steroidal anti-inflammatory drugs 6
Non-volatile acid (NVA) 9
Noonan syndrome 237
Norepinephrine 78
Norrie's disease 180
Northern blotting 216
Nosocomial infections, neonatal 200, 207–10
Nuchal translucency measurement 236–7
Nystatin 31, 210

Oculo-cardiac reflex 188
Oesophagitis 120, 123, 130, 133
Oesophagus
  functional development 120–1
  investigation 129–30
Olfactory bulb 94
Oligodendrocyte 97, 98
Oligodendroglia 97
Oligohydramnios 257, 262, 263
Oliguria 10, 11
Ophthalmia neonatorum 204
Opsonic antibody 211
Ornithine transcarbamylase deficiency 242
Oxacillin 208

Pac-X machine 16
Pancuronium 72
Paneth cells 112, 113
Paralogous group 118, 119
Partial liquid ventilation (PLV) 144, 146–7
Pasteurella multocida 219
Patent ductus arteriosis (PDA) 74–5, 162, 181, 263
PAX 6 gene 94
Penicillin 31, 32, 208
Penicillin G 204
Peptidases 113
Perflubron 141, 146, 149, 150
Perflurochemical (PFC) liquids 140–52
  anti-inflammatory activity 149–50
  clinical experiences 150–1, **151**
  drug delivery 148
  lavage 147–8
  lung expansion 150
  non-respiratory support applications 147–50
  physical properties 141–3, **142**
  pulmonary imaging 148–9
  respiratory support applications 143–7
Perfusion, suboptimal, in very low birth weight infant 65–6
Peritoneal dialysis 15–16
Perlecan 114
Peroxisomes 99
Periventricular leukomalacia 67
Phenobarbitol 133
Phenobarbitone 72
Phenylalanine 98
Phenylephrine 188
Phenylketonuria 95
Phosphate, inorganic 9
Phosphatidylcholine 100
Phosphatidylethanolamine 100
Phosphatidylinositol 100
Phosphatidylserine 100
Phosphoglycerols 99, 100
Phospholipids 100
Phosphorus
  deficiency 51
  in milk 50, 51–2
Phosphosphingolipids 100
Placenta praevia 251
Plain film X-rays 149
Plasma expanders 75–6
Play therapy 165
Pneumococci 24
Pneumonia 25, 26, 120, 141, 203
Pneumonitis 205
Pneumothorax 181

Polyhydramnios 237
Polymerase chain reaction (PCR) 245
Post-renal failure 10
Potassium reabsorption 8
Potter sequence 4
Prader-Willi syndrome 241
Pre-eclampsia 29, 251, 261
Pregnancy-associated plasma protein A (PAPP-A) 235
Preimplantation genetic diagnosis 243
Premature lung disease 141
Prematurity, spontaneous
  evaluation 256–8
  indicated versus 251
  labour and delivery 264
  management 258–64
  pathogenesis 252–3
  prevention 253–5
  primary care 253–4
  secondary care 254–5
Prenatal diagnosis
  indications 232–7, **233**
  invasive 237–43
  non-invasive 243–5
  outcome 245–6
Pre-renal failure 6, 10
Preterm labor (PTL) 251, 252, 253
Programmed cell death 95
Prolonged preterm rupture of membranes (PPROM) 24, 26, 28, 203, 207, 218, 251, 252, 253
  evaluation 256–8
  management 258–64
Prostaglandin E 263
Prostaglandin synthetase inhibitors 262–3
Prostaglandins 6
Protein in milk 46, 47–50
Protein supplements 50
Proximal tubular function 6–8
Proximal tubular reabsorption 8
Pseudomonas 36, 201, 216
Pseudomonas aeruginosa 211
Pseudomosaicism 238, 241
Pulmonary hypertension 158, 164
Pulmonary hypoplasia 141, 150
Pulmonary venous resistance 163
Pulse oximetry 164
Purkinje cells 97
Pyridoxine (vitamin B6) deficiency 96
Pyruvate dehydrogenase complex (PDH) 96
Pyruvate dehydrogenase deficiency 95

Rabies 211
Red cell isoimmunization, fetal 251
Renal failure, acute (ARF), neonatal 6, 9–20
  aetiology 10
  causes **11**
  conservative management 13–15
  definition 9–10
  diagnosis 11–13
  dialysis 15–20
  incidence 10
Renal failure, chronic, congenital 10
Renal failure index (RFI) 12–13
Renal function
  in fetus 2–4
  in newborn 4–9
Renal plasma flow (RPF) in newborn 4–6
Renal vein thrombosis 12
Respiratory distress syndrome 25–6, 73, 126, 129, 141, 146, 203, 213, 259, 260
Respiratory syncytial virus 165
Respiratory syncytial virus immune globulin intravenous (RSV-IGIV) 213, **214**
Ret proto-oncogene 117
Ret tyrosine kinase receptor 117
Retina
  injury 178–9
  normal growth 178
  repair/healing 179–80
Retinal detachment 182, 183–4, 186
Retinopathy of prematurity 174–91
  changing picture and classification 174–7
  co-morbidities 175
  genetics 180

Retinopathy of prematurity *(Continued)*
  pathophysiology 178–80
  prevention 180–2
  screening/tracking programme 186–91
  treatment 182–6
Retrolental fibroplasia *see* retinopathy of prematurity
Rhesus D genotype 245
Riboflavin 54
Rifampicin 209
Rimar 101 146
Ritodrine 263

Salbutamol 14
Schizencephaly 94
Seldinger technique 15
Selenium deficiency 95
Sepsis 141
  early-onset (EOS) 24–9
  late-onset (LOS) 29–30
Septicaemia 37–8, 212
Septo-optic dysplasia 95
Serratia marcenscens 211
Sex chromosome aneuploidy 237
Skin biopsy, fetal 242
Small bowel perforation 263
Small intestine
  motor activity 126–9
  mucosa 112–13
Smith-Lemli-Opitz syndrome 237
Smoke inhalation 141
Sodium 9
  in milk 46
  reabsorption 8
  urinary loss 7
Sodium bicarbonate 15
Somatostatin 121
Sphingomyelins 100
Stable isotope breath test 131
Staphylcocci, coagulase-negative 32, 36
Staphylococcus aureus 32, 54, 208, 209, 211
  methicillin-resistance 32, 33
Staphylococcus epidermidis 208, 209, 211
Staphylococcus haemolyticus 208, 209
Steroids, prenatal 181
Stomach
  functional development 121
  investigation 130–1
Streptococcal antigen 28
Streptococcus, Group B *see* Group B streptococcus
Streptococcus agalactiae 203
Streptococcus pneumoniae 211
Streptococcus viridans 201
Stress ulceration 123
Subcapsular nephrons 2
Sulindac 262
Surfactant therapy 181
β-Sympathomimetics 261, 262
Synaptosomes 95, 99

Taurine 98
Teicoplanin 209, 210
Tenascin 114, 115
Tenckhoff catheter 15
Tetanus 211
Tetracyclines 207
Tidal liquid ventilation (TLV) 144–6
Tocolysis 261
Tolazoline 6, 123
Total neutrophil count 26
Tracheobronchomalacia 163
Transcription factors 94, 98
Transcutaneous oxygen tension 164
Transient tachypnoea of the newborn (TTN) 25
Tricuspid regurgitation 164
'Triple screening' 234
Triploidy 237
Trisomy 13 237
Trisomy 15 242
Trisomy 18 235, 18 237, 18 245
Trisomy 21 *see* Down syndrome
Tropicamide 188
Tryptophan 98
Turner syndrome 237
24 hour pH monitoring 129
Tyrosine 98

Ulcers
gastric 121, 134
stress 123
Ultrasonography
gastric 130
of kidneys and urinary tract 12
maternal screening 243, 244–5
Umbilical cord, prolapsed 258
Uniparental disomy 241
Ureaplasma urealyticum 201, 205–7
Urinary indices 12–13, **13**
Urinary tract infections 212
Urine
flow rate 3
osmolality 8
output
production 2
sodium loss 7
in very low birthweight infant 73

Vancomycin 30–1, 32, 33, 208–9, 210
Vancomycin-resistant enterococci (VRE) 31
Vascular development 64
Vascular endothelial growth factor 178
Vascular resistance 64
Ventricular size and function 64
Ventriculomegaly, borderline 246
Virtual bronchoscopy 149
Vitamin A 54
Vitamin A deficiency 96
Vitamin B_1(thiamine) deficiency 96
Vitamin B_6(pyridoxine) deficiency 96
Vitamin D 52
Vitamin E prophylaxis 181

Wet lung CXR 26

Zinc 98
Zinc deficiency 95